AF835702

GEORGE WASHINGTON UNIVERSITY
PAUL HIMMELFARB HEALTH SCIENCES LIBRARY
2300 EYE STREET, N. W.
WASHINGTON, D. C. 20037
DISCARDED

THALASSEMIA: RECENT ADVANCES IN DETECTION AND TREATMENT

RECENT TITLES PUBLISHED BY ALAN R. LISS, INC.
FOR MARCH OF DIMES BIRTH DEFECTS FOUNDATION

Birth Defects Compendium, Second Edition, Daniel Bergsma, *Editor*

BIRTH DEFECTS: ORIGINAL ARTICLE SERIES

1981 — Volume XVII

No. 1 **Annual Review of Birth Defects, 1980, The Fetus and the Newborn,** Proceedings of the 1980 New York City Birth Defects Conference, Arthur D. Bloom and L. Stanley James, *Editors*
No. 2 **Morphogenesis and Malformation of the Skin,** Richard J. Blandau, *Editor*
No. 3 **Pregnancy and Childbearing During Adolescence: Research Priorities for the 1980s,** Elizabeth R. McAnarney and Gabriel Stickle, *Editors*
No. 4 **Reproductive Pasts, Reproductive Futures: Genetic Counseling and Its Effectiveness,** James R. Sorenson, Judith P. Swazey, and Norman A. Scotch
No. 6 **Perinatal Parental Behavior: Nursing Research and Implications for Newborn Health,** Regina Placzek Lederman, *Conference Coordinator–Consulting Editor*, and Beverly S. Raff, *Editor*

1982 — Volume 18

No. 1 **Craniofacial Anomalies: New Perspectives,** Carlos F. Salinas, *Editor*
No. 3A **Annual Review of Birth Defects, 1981, Prenatal Diagnosis and Mechanisms of Teratogenesis,** William L. Nyhan and Kenneth Lyons Jones, *Editors*
No. 3B **Annual Review of Birth Defects, 1981, Dysmorphology,** William L. Nyhan and Kenneth Lyons Jones, *Editors*
No. 4 **Children With Sex Chromosome Aneuploidy: Follow-Up Studies,** Donald A. Stewart, *Editor*
No. 5 **Cumulative Index: Birth Defects: Original Article Series Volumes I (1965)–XVI (1980),** Natalie W. Paul, *Editor*
No. 6 **Genetic Eye Diseases: Retinitis Pigmentosa and Other Inherited Eye Disorders,** Edward Cotlier, Irene H. Maumenee, and Elaine R. Berman, *Editors*
No. 7 **Thalassemia: Recent Advances in Detection and Treatment,** Antonio Cao, Ugo Carcassi, and Peter T. Rowley, *Editors*

GEORGE WASHINGTON UNIVERSITY
PAUL HIMMELFARB HEALTH SCIENCES LIBRARY
2300 EYE STREET, N. W.
WASHINGTON, D. C. 20037
DISCARDED

March of Dimes Birth Defects Foundation
Birth Defects: Original Article Series, Volume 18, Number 7, 1982

THALASSEMIA: RECENT ADVANCES IN DETECTION AND TREATMENT

International Symposium Held June 7-11, 1981, in S. Margherita di Pula, Cagliari, Sardinia, Italy, Sponsored by March of Dimes Birth Defects Foundation

Editors:

Antonio Cao, MD
Ugo Carcassi, MD
Universita di Cagliari
Sardinia, Italy

Peter T. Rowley, MD
University of Rochester
Rochester, New York

Associate Editor:

Natalie W. Paul
March of Dimes Birth Defects Foundation

Assistant Editors:

Elizabeth O'Brien Eakin
Florence Dickman
March of Dimes Birth Defects Foundation

ALAN R. LISS, INC., NEW YORK

To enhance medical communication in the birth defects field, the March of Dimes Birth Defects Foundation publishes the *Birth Defects Compendium (Second Edition),* an *Original Article Series, Syndrome Identification,* a *Reprint Series,* and provides a series of films and related brochures.

Further information can be obtained from:

Professional Education Department
March of Dimes Birth Defects Foundation
1275 Mamaroneck Avenue
White Plains, New York 10605

Published by:
Alan R. Liss, Inc.
150 Fifth Avenue
New York, New York 10011

Copyright © 1982 by March of Dimes Birth Defects Foundation

All rights reserved. No part of this publication may be reproduced or transmitted in any form or by any means, electronic or mechanical, including photocopying and recording, or by any information storage and retrieval system, without permission in writing from the copyright holder.

Views expressed in articles published are the authors', and are not to be attributed to the March of Dimes Birth Defects Foundation or its editors unless expressly so stated.

Library of Congress Cataloging in Publication Data

Main entry under title:

Thalassemia : recent advances in detection and treatment.

(Birth defects original article series ; v. 18, no. 7)
Includes index.
1. Thalassemia--Congresses. I. Cao, Antonio. II. Carcassi, Ugo. III. Rowley, Peter T. IV. Paul, Natalie W. IV. March of Dimes Birth Defects Foundation. VI. Series. [DNLM: 1. Thalassemia--Congresses. W1 BI966 v.18 no. 7 / WH 170 R295 1981]
RG626.B63 vol. 18, no.7 [RC641.7.T5] 616.1'52 82-16179
ISBN 0-8451-1051-9

Printed in the United States of America.

RG
626
.B63
v.18
no.7
1981

The **March of Dimes Birth Defects Foundation** is dedicated to the goals of preventing birth defects and ameliorating their consequences for patients, families, and society.

As part of our efforts to achieve these goals, we sponsor, or participate in, a variety of scientific meetings where all questions relating to birth defects are freely discussed. Through our professional education program we speed the dissemination of information by publishing the proceedings of these and other meetings. From time to time, we also reprint pertinent journal articles to help achieve our goal. Now and then, in the course of these articles or discussions, individual viewpoints may be expressed which go beyond the purely scientific and into controversial matters. It should be noted, therefore, that personal viewpoints about such matters will not be censored but this does not constitute an endorsement of them by the **March of Dimes Birth Defects Foundation.**

Contents

Contributors

M. Addis, 2nd Pediatric Clinic, University of Cagliari, Sardinia, Italy **[303]**

Sarah Agosti-Vallerino, Microcytemia Center of Galliera Hospital, Via A. Volta, 8, Genova, Italy **[189]**

Vassiliki Aleporou-Marinou, National Unit for Prevention of Thalassemia, Section of Prenatal Diagnosis, "Vassilvevs Pavlos" Hospital, Athens 609, Greece **[293]**

Blanche P. Alter, Polly Annenberg Levee Hematology Center, Departments of Medicine and Pediatrics, Mount Sinai School of Medicine, New York, NY 10029 **[111,263]**

Ester Alvino, Centro Diagnosi Prenatale, II Clinica Ostetrica e Ginecologica, Università di Roma, Rome, Italy **[313]**

A. Angius, 2nd Pediatric Clinic, University of Cagliari, Via Porcell, I, 09100 Sardinia, Italy **[303]**

M. Antimi, Divisione di Ematologia, Ospedale S. Eugenio, Rome, Italy **[203]**

Aris Antsaklis, 1st Department of Obstetrics and Gynecology, University of Athens, "Alexandra" Maternity Hospital, Athens 611, Greece **[293]**

F. Argiolu, Clinica Pediatrica 2a, University of Cagliari, Via Porcell, I, 09100 Cagliari, Sardinia, Italy **[355]**

Michael Baird, Department of Medicine, Department of Human Genetics and Development, Department of Pediatrics, College of Physicians and Surgeons of Columbia University, New York, NY 10032 **[45]**

Arthur Bank, Department of Medicine, Department of Human Genetics and Development, Department of Pediatrics, College of Physicians and Surgeons of Columbia University, New York, NY 10032 **[45]**

Francesco Battista, Centro Microcitemia, Ospedale Civile, Taranto, Italy **[195]**

Edward J. Benz, Jr., Department of Medicine, Yale University School of Medicine, New Haven, CT 06510 **[51]**

Francesco Bernardi, Centro di Studi Biochimici sul Morbo di Cooley, Cassa di Risparmio di Ferrara, University of Ferrara, 44100 Ferrara, Italy **[61]**

Yves Beuzard, Unité de Recherches sur les Anémies, INSERM U. 91, Hôpital Henri Mondor, 94010 Creteil, France **[117]**

Ida Bianco, Centro delle Microcitemie, Via Treviso n. 29, Rome, Italy **[141]**

Pasquale Bilotta, Centro Diagnosi Prenatale, II Clinica Ostetrica e Ginecologica, Università di Roma, Rome, Italy **[313]**

Jacqueline Bouguet, Unité de Recherches sur les Anémies, INSERM U. 91, Hôpital Henri Mondor, 94010 Creteil, France **[117]**

The bold face numbers in brackets following an author's affiliation is the opening page number of that author's paper.

Bruno Brambati, Perinatal Unit, First Institute of Obstetrics and Gynaecology, University of Milan, Milan, Italy **[317]**

Carlo Brancati, Centro di Studi Della Microcitemia, Via F. lli Cervi, 1, 87100 Cosenza, Italy **[147]**

Maurizio Bresadola, Centro Diagnosi Prenatale, II Clinica Ostetrica e Ginecologica, Università di Roma, Rome, Italy **[313]**

Janine Breton-Gorius, Unité de Recherches sur les Anémies, INSERM U. 91, Hôpital Henri Mondor, 94010 Creteil, France **[117]**

C. Bunch, MRC Molecular Haematology Unit, Nuffield Department Clinical Medicine, University of Oxford, John Radcliffe Hospital, Oxford OX3 9DU, England **[103]**

Enrico Cacace, School of Medicine, University of Cagliari, Sardinia, Italy **[165]**

Angelo Cantù-Rajnoldi, Department of Haematology, Istituti Clinici de Perfezionamento, Milan, Italy **[317]**

Antonio Cao, Director of the Institute of Clinic and Biology of Developmental Age, University of Cagliari, c/o Ospedale Regionale delle Microcitemie, Via Jenner (Casella Postale 251), 09100 Cagliari, Sardinia, Italy **[157,303,355]**

Ugo Carcassi, Director of 1st Institute of Clinical Medicine, School of Medicine, University of Cagliari, Sardinia, Italy **[165]**

Concetta Carestia, International Institute of Genetics and Biophysics, CNR, Naples, Italy **[177]**

M. Cecconi, Divisione di Ematologia, Ospedale S. Eugenio, Rome, Italy **[203]**

Judy C. Chang, Howard Hughes Medical Institute Laboratory, Division of Molecular Hematology, Department of Medicine, University of California, San Francisco, CA 94143 **[275]**

Paolo Cianciulli, Divisione di Ematologia, Ospedale S. Eugenio, Rome, Italy **[203]**

J.B. Clegg, MRC Molecular Haematology Unit, Nuffield Department of Medicine, University of Oxford, John Radcliffe Hospital, Headington, Oxford OX3 9DU, England **[15]**

Paola Comi, Centro Studio Patologia Cellulare, CNR, Milan, Italy **[65,131]**

Francesco Conconi, Centro di Studi Biochimici sul Morbo di Cooley, Cassa de Risparmio di Ferrara, University of Ferrara, 44100 Ferrara, Italy **[61]**

Pietro Congedo, Centro delle Microcitemie, Via Treviso n. 29, Rome, Italy **[141]**

G. Cornacchia, Clinica Pediatrica 2a, University of Cagliari, Via Porcell, I, 09100 Cagliari, Sardinia, Italy **[355]**

P. Cossu, Clinica Pediatrica 2a, University of Cagliari, Via Porcell, I, 09100 Cagliari, Sardinia, Italy **[355]**

Bruno Dallapiccola, Istituto di Genetica Medica, Università di Roma, Rome, Italy **[313]**

Fabrizio De Gado, Centro Diagnosi Prenatale, II Clinica Ostetrica e Ginecologica, Università di Roma, Rome, Italy **[313]**

Laura Del Senno, Centro di Studi Biochimici sul Morbo di Cooley, Cassa di Risparmio di Ferrara, University of Ferrara, 44100 Ferrara, Italy **[61]**

Stefano De Virgiliis, Clinica Pediatrica 2a, University of Cagliari, Via Porcell, I, 09100 Cagliari, Sardinia, Italy **[355]**

Andrée M. Dozy, Howard Hughes Medical Institute Laboratory, Division of Molecular Hematology, Department of Medicine, University of California, San Francisco, CA 94143 **[275]**

M. Catherine Driscoll, Department of Medicine, Department of Human Genetics and Development, Department of Pediatrics, College of Physicians and Surgeons of Columbia University, New York, NY 10032 **[45]**

A.M. Falchi, 2nd Pediatric Clinic, University of Cagliari, Via Porcell, I, 09100 Sardinia, Italy **[303]**

Maurizio Ferrari, Department of Haematology, Istituti Clinici de Perfezionamento, Milan, Italy **[317]**

A. Ferreli, Clinica Pediatrica 2a, University of Cagliari, Via Porcell, I, 09100 Cagliari, Sardinia, Italy **[355]**

Phaedon Fessas, 1st Department of Medicine, University of Athens, "Vassilevs Parlos" Hospital, Athens 609, Greece **[293]**

Lawrence Fisher, Department of Psychiatry, The Veterans Administration Medical Center, Fresno, CA 93703 **[231]**

D.M. Flynn, Department of Paediatrics, Royal Free Hospital, London, NW3 2QG, England **[347]**

Bernard G. Forget, Departments of Medicine and Human Genetics, Yale University School of Medicine, New Haven, CT 06510 **[51]**

Suthat Fucharoen, The Thalassemia Center, Faculty of Graduate Studies, Mahidol University, Bangkok 10700, Thailand **[213]**

Mario Furbetta, Institute of Clinic and Biology of Developmental Age, University of Cagliari, c/o Ospedale Regionale delle Microcitemie, Via Jenner (Casella Postale 251), 09100 Cagliari, Sardinia, Italy **[157,303]**

Marco Gabbianelli, Istituto Superiore de Sanitá, Laboratorio di Patologia non Infettiva, Viale Regina Elena, 299, 00161, Rome, Italy **[203]**

Renzo Galanello, Institute of Clinic and Biology of Developmental Age, University of Cagliari, c/o Ospedale Regionale delle Microcitemie, Via Jenner (Casella Postale 251), 09100 Cagliari, Sardinia, Italy **[157,303]**

Adele Giampaolo, Istituto Superiore di Sanitá Laboratorio de Patologia non Infettiva, Viale Regina Elena, 299, 00161 Rome, Italy **[203]**

Alessandro Massimo Gianni, Clinica Medica (I), University of Milan, Milan, Italy **[65,131]**

Barbara Giglioni, Centro Studio Patologia Cellulare, CNR, Milan, Italy **[65,131]**

Bruno Graziani, Centro delle Microcitemie, Via Treviso n. 29, Rome, Italy **[141]**

Joseph Graziano, College of Physicians and Surgeons of Columbia University, Div. of Pediatric Pharmacology, New York, NY 10032 **[339]**

Raffaella Guerriero, Istituto Superiore di Sanitá, Laboratorio di Patologia non Infettiva, Viale Regina Elena, 299, 00161 Rome, Italy **[203]**

D.R. Higgs, MRC Molecular Haematology Unit, Nuffield Department of Medicine, University of Oxford, John Radcliffe Hospital, Headington, Oxford OX3 9DU, England **[15]**

A.V. Hoffbrand, Department of Paediatrics and Haematology, Royal Free Hospital, London, NW3 2QG, England **[347]**

Titus H.J. Huisman, Department of Cell and Molecular Biology, Director, Comprehensive Sickle Cell Center, Medical College of Georgia, Augusta, GA 30912 **[83]**

Giovanni Ivaldi, Microcytemia Center of Galliera Hospital, Via A. Volta, 8, Genova, Italy **[189]**

Michael M. Kaback, Departments of Pediatrics and Medicine, UCLA School of Medicine, Associate Chief, Division of Medical Genetics, Harbor-UCLA Medical Center, Torrance, CA 90502 **[243]**

Yuet Wai Kan, Howard Hughes Medical Institute Laboratory, Division of Molecular Hematology, Department of Medicine, University of California, San Francisco, CA 94143 **[35,275]**

Judith Kantor, Clinical Hematology Branch, National Heart, Lung, and Blood Institute, National Institutes of Health, Bethesda, MD 20205. Present address: Department of Biochemistry, Basic Science Building, Medical Dental Schools, Georgetown University, Washington D.C., 20007 **[69]**

Photini Karababa, National Unit for Prevention of Thalassemia, Section of Prenatal Diagnosis, "Vassilevs Parlos" Hospital, Athens 609, Greece **[293]**

Arturo Lania, International Institute of Genetics and Biophysics, CNR, Napoli, Italy **[177]**

Hermann Lehmann, Department of Biochemistry, University of Cambridge, Cambridge CB2 IQW, England **[1]**

Daniela Leone-Da Passano, Microcytemia Center of Galliera Hospital, Via A. Volta, 8, Genova, Italy **[189]**

Maria Lerone, Centro delle Microcitemie, Via Treviso n. 29, Rome, Italy **[141]**

Timothy Ley, Clinical Hematology Branch, National Heart, Lung, and Blood Institute, National Institutes of Health, Bethesda, MD 20205 **[69]**

Stephen A. Liebhaber, Department of Human Genetics, University of Pennsylvania, Philadelphia, PA 19104 **[35]**

Mack Lipkin, Jr., Rockfeller Foundation, 1133 Avenue of the Americas, New York, NY 10036 **[231]**

Maurizio Longinotti, Interdisciplinary Laboratory for Thalassemia and Favism, Institute of Clinica Medica, University of Sassari, viale San Pietro 8, Sassari 07100, Italy **[169]**

Dimitris Loukopoulos, 1st Department of Medicine, University of Athens, "Vassilevs Pavlos" Hospital, Athens 609, Greece **[293]**

Leo Lupi, Divisione Pediatrica 29, Ospedale Cardarelli, Napoli, Italy **[177]**

Lucio Luzzatto, International Institute of Genetics and Biophysics, CNR, Napoli, Italy **[177]**

L. Maccioni, 2nd Pediatric Clinic, University of Cagliari, Via Porcell, I, 09100 Sardinia, Italy **[303]**

Guiseppe Malcangi, Clinica Medica II, Policlinico, 70124 Bari, Italy **[195]**

Giovanna Marchetti, Centro di Studi Biochimici sul Morbo di Cooley, Cassa di Risparmio di Ferrara, University of Ferrara, 44100 Ferrara, Italy **[61]**

Marino Marinucci, Istituto Superiore di Sanitá, Laboratorio di Patologia non Infettiva, Viale Regina Elena, 299, 00161 Rome, Italy **[203,313]**

Bruno Masala, Interdisciplinary Laboratory for Thalassemia and Favism, Institute of General Physiology and Biological Chemistry, University of Sassari, via Muroni 25, Sassari 07100, Italy **[169]**

Guiseppe Masera, Clinica Pediatrica "G.D. De Marchi," Via Commenda, 9, 20122 Milano, Italy **[325]**

M. Masi, Divisione di Ematologia, Ospedale S. Eugenio, Rome, Italy **[203]**

Adriana Massa, Istituto Superiore di Sanitá, Laboratorio di Patologia non Infettiva, Viale Regina Elena, 299, 00161 Rome, Italy **[203,313]**

Gianfranco Mastroberardino, Istituto Patologia Medica (VI), University of Rome, Rome, Italy **[131]**

Antonella Mastrobuono, Divisione Ematologia, Ospedale Cardarelli, Napoli, Italy **[177]**

Fulvio Mavilio, Istituto Superiore di Sanitá, Laboratorio di Patologia non Infettiva, Viale Regina Elena, 299, 00161 Rome, Italy **[203]**

Quirico Mela, School of Medicine, University of Cagliari, Sardinia, Italy **[165]**

M.A. Melis, 2nd Pediatric Clinic, University of Cagliari, Via Porcell, I, 09100 Sardinia, Italy **[303]**

Anna Rita Migliaccio, Istituto Patologia Medica, II Faculty, University of Naples, Naples, Italy **[131]**

Giovanni Migliaccio, Istituto Patologia Medica, II Faculty, University of Naples, Naples, Italy **[131]**

Bernadette Modell, Honorary Consultant in Perinatal Medicine, Department of Obstetrics and Gynaecology, University College Hospital, London, WCIE 6AU England **[285,329]**

Michele Monaco, Centro Microcitemie, Ospedale Civile, Foggia, Italy **[195]**

Mary Mouzouras, Department of Obstetrics and Gynaecology, University College Hospital, London, WCIE 6AU England **[285]**

Filippo Muratore, Centro Microcitemie, Ospedale "Fazzi," Lecce, Italy **[195]**

David G. Nathan, Division of Hematology/Ontology of Children's Hospital Medical Center, Sidney Farber Cancer Institute, Department of Pediatrics, Harvard Medical School, Boston, MA 02115 **[111]**

Umberto Nicolini, Perinatal Unit, First Institute of Obstetrics and Gynaecology, University of Milan, Milan, Italy **[317]**

Arthur W. Nienhuis, Clinical Hematology Branch, National Heart, Lung, and Blood Institute, National Institutes of Health, Bethesda, MD 20205 **[69]**

A. Nucaro, Clinica Pediatrica 2a, University of Cagliari, Via Porcell, I, 09100 Cagliari, Sardinia, Italy **[355]**

Sergio Ottolenghi, Centro Studio Patologia Cellulare, CNR, Istituto Patologia Generale, University of Milan, Milan, Italy **[65,131]**

Antonio Pachì, Centro Diagnosi Prenatale, II Clinica Ostetrica e Ginecologica, Università di Roma, Rome, Italy **[313]**

Rosalba Paesano, Centro Diagnosi Prenatale, II Clinica Ostetrica e Ginecologica, Università di Roma, Rome, Italy **[313]**

E. Paglietti, 2nd Pediatric Clinic, University of Cagliari, Via Porcell, I, 09100 Sardinia, Italy **[303]**

John Panourgias, National Unit for Prevention of Thalassemia, Section of Prenatal Diagnosis, "Vassilevs Pavlos" Hospital, Athens 609, Greece **[293]**

Maria Isola Parodi, Microcytemia Center of Galliera Hospital, Via A. Volta, 8, Genova, Italy **[189]**

Guiseppe Passiu, School of Medicine, University of Cagliari, Sardinia, Italy **[165]**

Guglielmina Pepe, Department of Biochemistry, Rutgers Medical School, Piscataway, NJ 08854 **[69,177]**

Robert G. Pergolizzi, Department of Medicine, Department of Human Genetics and Development, Department of Pediatrics, College of Physicians and Surgeons of Columbia University, New York, NY 10032 **[45]**

Guiseppe Perpignano, School of Medicine, University of Cagliari, Sardinia, Italy **[165]**

Carla Perrotta, Centro di Studi Biochimici sul Morbo di Cooley, Cassa di Risparmio di Ferrara, University of Ferrara, 44100 Ferrara, Italy **[61]**

Cesare Peschle, Laboratorio Patologia non Infettiva, Istituto Superiore di Sanitá, Viale Regina Elena, Roma, Italy **[131]**

Anna Pietrapertosa, Clinica Medica II, Policlinico, 70124 Bari, Italy **[195]**

Aldo Pintus, School of Medicine, University of Cagliari, Sardinia, Italy **[165]**

Sergio Piomelli, Department of Pediatric Hematology/Oncology, College of Physicians and Surgeons of Columbia University, New York, NY 10032 **[339]**

Dina Politis, Hellenic Red Cross, Athens, Greece **[347]**

Donatella Ponzini, Centro delle Microcitemie, Via Treviso n. 29 Rome, Italy **[141]**

G. Pratesi, Divisione di Ematologia, Ospedale S. Eugenio, Rome, Italy **[203]**

L. Pressley, MRC Molecular Haematology Unit, Nuffield Department of Medicine, University of Oxford, John Radcliffe Hospital, Headington, Oxford OX3 9DU, England **[15]**

Angelo Putignano, Clinica Medica II, Policlinico, 70124 Bari, Italy **[195]**

Eliezer A. Rachmilewitz, Department of Hematology, Hadassah University Hospital, Jerusalem, Israel **[219]**

M. Rais, Clinica Pediatrica 2a, University of Cagliari, Via Porcell, I, 09100 Cagliari, Sardinia, Italy **[355]**

Charles H. Rodeck, Department of Obstetrics and Gynaecology, King's College Hospital, London, S.E. 5, England **[255]**

Jean Rosa, Unité de Recherches sur les Anémies, INSERM U. 91, Hôpital Henri Mondor, 94010 Creteil, France **[117]**

C. Rosatelli, 2nd Pediatric Clinic, University of Cagliari, Via Porcell, I, 09100 Sardinia, Italy **[303]**

Philippe Rouyer-Fessard, Unité de Recherches sur les Anémies, INSERM U. 91, Hôpital Henri Mondor, 94010 Creteil, France **[117]**

Peter T. Rowley, University of Rochester School of Medicine, Rochester, NY 14642 **[231]**

R. Ruggeri, 2nd Pediatric Clinic, University of Cagliari, Via Porcell, I, 09100 Sardinia, Italy **[303]**

Guiseppe Russo, Clinica Pediatrica, Città Universitaria, Viale Andrea Doria, Catania, Italy **[185]**

G. Sanna, Clinica Pediatrica 2a, University of Cagliari, Via Porcell, I, 09100 Cagliari, Sardinia, Italy **[355]**

Gennaro Sansone, Chair of Human Genetics, Microcytemia Center of Galliera Hospital, Via A. Volta 8, Genova, Italy **[189]**

M.T. Scalas, 2nd Pediatric Clinic, University of Cagliari, Via Porcell, I, 09100 Sardinia, Italy **[303]**

Guiseppina Villy Sciarratta, Microcytemia Center of Galliera Hospital, Via A. Volta, 8, Genova, Italy **[189]**

Beryl E. Serjeant, Medical Research Council Laboratories, University of the West Indies, Mona, Kingston 7, Jamaica, W.I. **[223]**

Graham R. Serjeant, Director, Medical Research Council Laboratories, University of The West Indies, Mona, Kingston 7, Jamaica, W.I. **[223]**

Dhira Sonakul, Department of Pathology, Siriraj Hospital, Mahidol University, Bangkok, 10700, Thailand **[213]**

Sally E. Spence, Department of Medicine, Department of Human Genetics and Development, Department of Pediatrics, College of Physicians and Surgeons of Columbia University, New York, NY 10032 **[45]**

Nadia M. Sposi, Istituto Superiore di Sanitá, Laboratorio di Patologia non Infettiva, Viale Regina Elena, 299, 00161 Rome, Italy **[203,313]**

Richard A. Spritz, Department of Medical Genetics, Henry Mall, University of Wisconsin, Madison, WI 53706 **[51]**

Antonio Tagarelli, Centro di Studi Della Microcitemia, Via F. 11i Cervi, 1, 87100, Cosenza, Italy **[147]**

Joseph Tam, Clinical Hematology Branch, National Heart, Lung, and Blood Institute, National Institutes of Health, Bethesda, MD 20205. Present address: Dept. of Biochemistry, University of Hong Kong, Li Shu Fan Building, Sassoon Road, Hong Kong **[69]**

Nunzia Tannoia, Clinica Medica II, Policlinico, 70124, Bari, Italy **[195]**

Roberto Taramelli, Centro Studi per la Patologia Cellulare, Istituto di Patologia Generale, Università di Milano, via Mangiagalli 31, 20133 Milano, Italy **[65]**

Leonardo Tentori, Director, Laboratorio di Patologia Infettiva, Istituto Superiore di Sanitá, Viale Regina Elena, 299, 00161 Rome, Italy **[203,313]**

Ugo Testa, Unité de Recherches sur les Anémies, INSERM U. 91, Hôpital Henri Mondor, 94010 Creteil, France **[117]**

E. Donnall Thomas, Department of Medicine, University of Washington, School of Medicine, Fred Hutchinson Cancer Research Center, Seattle, WA 98104 **[361]**

Monique Titeux, Unité de Recherches sur les Anémies, INSERM U. 91, Hôpital Henri Mondor, 94010 Creteil, France **[117]**

C. Toccafondi, Clinica Pediatrica 2a, University of Cagliari, Via Porcell, I, 09100 Cagliari, Sardinia, Italy **[355]**

T. Tuveri, 2nd Pediatric Clinic, University of Cagliari, Via Porcell, I, 09100 Sardinia, Italy **[303]**

William Vainchenker, Unité de Recherches sur les Anémies, INSERM U. 91, Hôpital Henri Mondor, 94010 Creteil, France **[117]**

Maria Valente, Centro delle Microcitemie, Via Treviso n. 29, Rome, Italy **[141]**

Marco Vignetti, Laboratorio di Patologia non Infettiva, Istituto Superiore di Sanitá, Rome, Italy **[313]**

Calogero Vullo, Arcispedale S. Anna, Divisione Pediatria, 44100 Ferrara, Italy **[199]**

J. Wainscoat, MRC Molecular Haematology Unit, Nuffield Department of Medicine, University of Oxford, John Radcliffe Hospital, Headington, Oxford OX3 9DU, England **[15]**

Prawase Wasi, Division of Hematology, Department of Medicine, Siriraj Hospital, Mahidol University, Bangkok 10700, Thailand **[213]**

D. J. Weatherall, MRC Molecular Haematology Unit, Nuffield Department of Clinical Medicine, John Radcliffe Hospital, Headington, Oxford OX3 9DU, England **[15]**

Sherman M. Weissman, Departments of Medicine and Human Genetics, Yale University School of Medicine, New Haven, CT 06510 **[51]**

Robert Williamson, Department of Biochemistry, St. Mary's Hospital Medical School, University of London, London, W2 1PG, England **[29]**

W.G. Wood, MRC Molecular Haematology Unit, Nuffield Department of Medicine, University of Oxford, John Radcliffe Hospital, Headington, Oxford OX3 9DU, England **[15,103]**

Praparn Youngchaiyud, Division of Chest Medicine, Department of Medicine, Siriraj Hospital, Mahidol University, Bangkok 10700, Thailand **[213]**

Preface

In the last few years there have been tremendous advances in the study of thalassemia syndromes. The fascinating progress realized in molecular biology has resulted in the development of sophisticated techniques for the analysis of human genes. By the application of these techniques to the thalassemia field considerable progress in the elucidation of the molecular basis of many thalassemia syndromes has been made. In the meantime, the developments in molecular biology and biochemistry, coupled with the accomplishment of efficient and relatively safe fetal blood sampling techniques, have made antenatal diagnosis possible. This and the introduction of carrier detection programs in high-risk populations have opened the possibility of controlling this group of fatal disorders at a population level. Although no definitive cure has been developed, better management of these patients has resulted. Consequently, the prognosis for survival has improved progressively from about 10 years in 1960, to around 16 years by 1970, to an "open-ended" prognosis by 1980.

From June 7th through the 11th, 1981, molecular biologists, geneticists, biochemists, hematologists, and pediatricians met in Forte Village, S. Margherita di Pula, Cagliari, Sardinia, to present new data and to review the most recent developments in the thalassemia field. The program got off to a good start with the presentation on the historical perspectives and modern concerns of thalassemia syndromes.

A number of fascinating papers were presented at the session dedicated to molecular biology, specifically on the arrangement of globin structural genes, the molecular mechanisms of α-, β-, $\delta\beta$-thalassemias, the different expression of the two α-globin structural genes, the structure, function and metabolism of the different globin mRNA, the molecular basis of clinical heterogeneity, and DNA polymorphic restriction sites linked to human globin structural loci. Another session was devoted to consideration of the polymorphism of hemoglobin F and hemoglobin switching in clonal culture and animal models.

A round table on thalassemia types observed in different parts of Italy showed the extraordinary heterogeneity of these genetic anemias.

Selected clinical and pathophysiologic aspects, such as the clinical phenotype of sickle cell β°- or β^{+}-thalassemia interaction and the problems related to hypoxemia and the mechanism of red blood cell membrane damage, were also discussed.

The present status of management was presented with particular emphasis on the supertransfusion regimen, methods to decrease the iron burden, such as splenectomy and the transfusion of young red blood cells, the chelation treatment with desferrioxamine and the emerging physical and emotional problems created by the improved prognosis. The question of whether or not marrow grafts from HLA-identical donors should now be considered was also widely discussed. A high point of the conference was the session on prevention. In selected high-risk populations, such as Sardinians, Cypriots, and Italians from the Ferrara region, it has been possible to reduce the incidence of the homozygous state through carrier screening and antenatal diagnosis. The fascinating progress made in the field of antenatal diagnosis, either by direct or indirect method of DNA analysis of amniotic fluid cells, was included in this session.

This volume contains the formal papers presented at this conference. It represents a compilation of the present state-of-the-art and the status of current thinking, in the various areas discussed above.

We thank Doctor Yuet Wai Kan for his continuing advice and counsel and would like to acknowledge the great dedication and assistance of the secretaries Miss Rita Loi, Lucia Mocci, Raimonda Porcu, and Marisa Amat in all phases of the conference and publication of the volume.

The staff of the 2nd Pediatric Clinic and the 1st Department of Internal Medicine, in particular: Dr. Stefano De Virgiliis, Dr. Renzo Galanello, Dr. Aldo Pintus, and Dr. Piero Montaldo were extemely helpful.

Financial support from the March of Dimes Birth Defects Foundation, Department of Public Health of the Sardinian Region, National Research Council, Committee on Biology and Medicine, National Research Council Program of Preventive Medicine: project M.E.E., "A. Businco" Oncological-Hospital, Council of the Sardinian Region and Cagliari Town-Council, Centro di Cura S. Michele, many pharmaceutical and laboratory instrument companies, and banks made the conference possible.

Finally, the editors express their gratitude to Natalie Paul and her staff, who provided the expert editorial assistance to ensure the publication of these proceedings.

The Editors

INTRODUCTION

The History of Thalassemia

Hermann Lehmann, CBE, FRS

The history of thalassemia dates back to a much earlier time than the formal recognition of the disease. It is established that the ancient Greeks knew of a childhood disorder associated with pallor and geophagia. Such references, as well as certain bone changes in prehistoric remains, and for that matter even in more recent finds, may well be the outcome of other hemolytic anemias rather than the thalassemias. Geophagia is associated more with deficiency anemias, and there are a wide variety of possible causes of spongy bone structure other than thalassemia. Indeed, one may doubt that, under the severe selective pressure of natural selection up to and within living memory in the so-called developed countries and to this very day in developing countries, children with thalassemia ever lived long enough to produce the specific bone changes of thalassemia.

My own experience with sickle cell anemia in Uganda, 1947–1949, may be to the point. We were unable to discover more than a very few cases of sickle cell anemia. The sequence of events was that the incidence of sickle cell anemia was at first overestimated because patients with anemia and a positive sickle cell test tended to be classified as having sickle cell anemia. Naturally, as the sickle incidence in East Africa is high and, as there were many anemic patients, sickle cell anemia was thought to be very frequent. When the nature of these anemias, mostly hookworm and malarial anemias, became worked out and the familial background of sickle cell anemia was appreciated, the number of patients with proven sickle cell anemia dwindled to a proportion well below the expected number of homozygotes. This changed when the Lambottes and Vandepitte directed the search to infants, but it was only when electrophoresis was added to the diagnostic procedures that it became apparent that in a population with an infant and child mortality of 500 or more per 1,000 infants born, there were many cases of homozygous sickle cell anemia who died before clinical symptoms and signs, even such as dactylitis, could suggest this diagnosis.

This almost Hegelian progress of thesis → antithesis → synthesis, of overestimate → underestimate → correct assessment was, in the case of sickle anemia assisted by two clean-cut laboratory procedures — the sickle cell test and hemoglobin electrophoresis on the one hand, and on the other by the comparatively simple situation in Central Africa of deciding between three definite states: AA, AS, and SS.

Birth Defects: Original Article Series, Volume 18, Number 7, pages 1–11
© 1982 March of Dimes Birth Defects Foundation

In the history of thalassemia the background was much more complicated and only gradually did the laboratory feed essential information into the maelstrom of the emerging clinical and laboratory sciences. Thalassemia became more complex the more searchingly it was studied and, as we now know it, is a group of different genetic disorders. Indeed it may even be doubtful whether we can make a truly firm division of the hemoglobinopathies into "Abnormal Hemoglobins" and "Thalassemias." Certainly the hemoglobins Portland, H, Barts, Lepore, and Constant Spring belong to the disorders of biosynthesis, and the reduction of rate of production of the abnormal β-chains of the perfectly ordinary β-chain variant hemoglobin Woolwich is not different from that seen in β^{+}-thalassemia.

The modern history of thalassemia rightly dates back to the recognition by von Jaksch almost a hundred years ago in Prague of a non-leukemic, ie a red cell anemia with nucleated red cells in the circulating blood in a 14-month-old infant with splenomegaly who died before it reached the age of 2. Whether this condition referred to as "von Jaksch anemia" was a case of thalassemia is difficult to say. Thalassemia certainly exists in Central Europe, and, though it is rare, there could be every reason why an unusual case should have found its way into von Jaksch's clinic. In Berlin, I have recently been shown a case described first in 1969 by Teichmann and Kleihauer of (clinically intermedia) homozygous thalassemia in a patient from Wroclaw (formerly Breslau), the daughter of unrelated German-Silesian parents. Silesia is not far from Prague.

It was, however, this recognition of an anemia related to the red cells and presumably hemolytic in nature which was a first step.

There were now two different developments, one in the USA and the other in Europe. In Detroit, in 1925, Cooley described children with splenic anemia whom he considered to be affected by von Jaksch anemia, a severe lethal anemia with specific pathognomonic bone changes and increased osmotic resistance of the red cells, which to this day is a full description of β-thalassemia major, except that the familial aspect of the disorder is not mentioned.

There are a number of excellent reviews of observations at about this time in Europe leading to the recognition of thalassemia as such.

Observations following von Jaksch were made, notably in Italy and Greece, and were recognizing, under various names, what we now call thalassemia minor. They described splenomegaly but differentiated it (as von Jaksch had done) from the splenomegaly of leukemia. The anemia was hemolytic and had a familial element, but, in contrast to the spherocytic anemia of acholuric jaundice, the red cells had an increased osmotic resistance to hypotonic salt solutions. The three names associated with this phase are Rietti, Greppi, and Micheli. In 1925 in Ferrara, Rietti had described an association of hemolytic anemia with increased osmotic resistance. It was a very definite step because it contradicted a dogma by Eppinger of "no hemolytic familial anemia without decreased osmotic resistance." Greppi not only noted the specific appearance of the red cells, microcytosis, and mild polycythemia, but contributed particularly to the observation of a relatively high number of red cells. Micheli contributed to the recognition of the abnormal shapes, among them the poikilocytes and elliptocytes, and also recognized that this condition was different from the microcythemia of iron deficiency, though it shared with it the resistance to hemolysis by salt solutions of low concentration. Campinopetros in Greece and Angelini in Italy became very definite about the familial nature of this anemia and a link was being formed to the anemia described in the United States by Cooley.

It is not possible to clearly partition credit to individuals for historical developments shaping the concept of thalassemia as we know it today. In Italy, Silvestroni and Bianco belong both to the Rietti-Greppi-Micheli period and to the next, in which Cooley anemia became thalassemia major, the Rietti-Greppi-Micheli disease became thalassemia minor, and both thalassemias, major and minor, were related to a single genetic cause. Reviews by Marmont and Bianchi in 1948 and Chini and Valeri in 1949 cover this period in which the European and the American workers joined up in a single purpose. I refer also to the excellent review by Chernoff in 1959 and the scholarly book by Bannerman in 1961.

The term thalassemia for Mediterranean anemia was introduced by Whipple and Bradford in 1932. It seems that there is some confusion about the use of the word "thalatta" or "thalassa" for the Mediterranean Sea. It was to be appreciated that the ancient Greeks did apply thalatta to what we now know as the Mediterranean Sea, as well as using it as a general description of what was to them an expanse of water. Thus, "thalassemia" or "thalassanemia" is quite correct as a translation of the term "Mediterranean anaemia." It seems that Whipple remembered that Xenophon's men shouted thalatta when they reached the Black Sea. But they used that as a general term — "the sea." Thalatta meant both sea in general and, because the great sea known to the ancient Greeks was the Mediterranean Sea, it also referred specifically to that great body of water. The Black Sea was pontos euxinos, and if they had wanted to call out that name they would have done so. They would have shouted "Black Sea" or "pontos euxinos," but they did not! "Thalassemia" may be a misnomer for several reasons. For example, it should have been thalassanemia, because thalassemia to a Greek means "Sea in the Blood." Also the Mediterranean, as we now know, is by no means the sole or even the most important focus of the disorder. However, thalassemia was quite appropriate when it was desired to relate the disorder to the Mediterranean.

In the United States, in 1944 and in 1948, Valentine and Neel linked the observations of Dameshek (target cell anemia) in 1941 and 1943, Strauss and collaborators in 1941, Wintrobe's important notes in his 1942 textbook, and Smith in 1943 with those from Italy by Gatto (1942, 1947 and 1948) and Silvestroni's and Bianco's (1946) microcytemia to give us the standard mendelian inheritance pattern of β-thalassemia as we know it today. Silvestroni and Bianco

(1944-1945) had found an interaction of Cooley anemia with sickle cell disease. In 1949 Pauling, with Singer and Itano, had shown that sickling was due to an abnormal hemoglobin. From then on dates the attention given to the nature and state of the hemoglobin in thalassemia, and to this day the thalassemic disorder is considered to be a hemoglobinopathy. From the discovery of sickle cell hemoglobin and the recognition of the inheritance pattern of microdrepanocytic anemia (sickle cell thalassemia) dates the firm recognition of thalassemia as a hemoglobinopathy.

We must, however, not leave the year 1949 without turning our attention once more to Italy, where that great originator Haldane, on a visit to his friend Montalenti in 1949, discussed the high incidence of thalassemia in some populations in spite of the invariable death of homozygotes before they reached the age of puberty. He proposed that this was due to a benefit conferred on heterozygotes by natural selection. It is often thought that Haldane had fetal hemoglobin (Hb F) in mind, whose raised level in thalassemia might be beneficial to heterozygotes. This is not so. Though Vecchio in 1946 had made some observations on Hb F in thalassemia, it was not until 1951 that Liquori put this aspect on a sound basis. Haldane in 1948 and 1949 thought that the microcytosis might be of advantage in malnutrition or infectious diseases — possibly malaria. It is unlikely that he even knew of Vecchio's observation.

It was known from the days of von Körber (1864) that the hemoglobin of the newborn differed from that of the adult. It became clear in the early 1950s that thalassemics had more of that fetal hemoglobin in their cells than non-thalassemics, and that, correspondingly, they produced less normal (called adult) hemoglobin. This was supported at first by a series of technical advances in the recognition of Hb F, which were based on spectral properties related to a higher tryptophan content. Much of our knowledge of fetal hemoglobin in thalassemia to this day has been contributed by T.H.J. Huisman who, as a young man worked with J.H.P. Jonxis, whose name (with that of Brinkman) figures prominently in the literature of that period on fetal hemoglobin of man and animals. Hb F estimation based on its resistance to alkaline denaturation was made available as a simple routine technique by Singer and Chernoff in 1951. Hb F was not only raised in sickle cell anemia when Hb S replaced adult hemoglobin (Hb A), but also in thalassemia when Hb A in some cases was not produced at all. There were a number of theories, but the most fruitful was that by Rich in 1952, who defined thalassemia as a failure of Hb A production.

The hemoglobins of adult man are three, adult hemoglobin (Hb A) which comprises more than 90% of the pigment in adults; fetal hemoglobin which is present as the major hemoglobin at birth, and declines over the first few months of life to a level of about 1%; and a mysterious minor fraction, Hb A_2, very similar to adult hemoglobin, amounting to about 3%. Schroeder showed that the hemoglobin molecule is composed of different subunits, each one having a heme. Ingram then showed that these subunits formed two pairs of unlike chains.

$$A = \alpha_2\beta_2$$
$$F = \alpha_2\gamma_2$$
$$A_2 = \alpha_2\delta_2$$

Thus, the three hemoglobins are composed of four polypeptide chains, each containing a heme — two α and two non α-chains. The α-chains are 141 amino acid residues long, and the non α-chains are composed of 146 residues. The α-chains are, as it were, interchangeable. If one labels radioactively normal adult hemoglobin (Hb A) and mixes the labeled protein $\alpha_2^*\beta_2^*$with unlabeled sickle cell hemoglobin in which the β-chains differ by one amino acid from the normal β-chain ($\alpha_2\beta^S{}_2$), and dissociates the two hemoglobins into its subunits α_2^*; α_2, β_2^*; $\beta^S{}_2$, and recombines them again, the sickle cell hemoglobin will now contain labeled α-chains: $\alpha^*{}_2\beta^S{}_2$

There are two γ-chains, differing from each other by having either glycine or alanine at position 136 of their 146 residues. They are the $^G\gamma$ and the $^A\gamma$-chains. A variant of the $^A\gamma$-chain which at position 75 has a threonine instead of an isoleucine was found here in Sardinia: Hb F Sardinia. It is widely distributed and in some areas amounts to up to 20% of the $^A\gamma$-chains. It is often called the $^T\gamma$-chain, but it does not represent a third Hb F locus in addition to the $^G\gamma$ and $^A\gamma$ loci. The δ- and the β-chains differ by 12 residues. The α-chains are all alike structurally.

The three hemoglobins develop one after the other in uterine and postnatal life

$$F \rightarrow A \rightarrow A_2$$

and are preceded by prefetal hemoglobins with prefetal non α-chains:- ϵ, and prefetal α-chains: ζ. These give rise to the embryonic hemoglobins

	hemoglobin Gower	$\alpha_2\,\epsilon_2$
and	hemoglobin Portland	$\zeta_2\gamma_2$

Thus, there are the prefetal hemoglobins $\zeta_2\gamma_2$ and $\alpha_2\epsilon_2$, and also $\zeta_2\epsilon_2$ followed by fetal hemoglobin $\alpha_2{}^G\gamma_2$, $\alpha_2{}^A\gamma_2$, followed by the adult hemoglobins A, $\alpha_2\beta_2$ and A_2, $\alpha_2\delta_2$. It became clear that, in thalassemia, adult hemoglobin could not be formed in adequate quantity, and for a time there was a controversy whether thalassemia arose from yet another abnormal hemoglobin which could not be recognized by the then available methods of analysis — largely electrophoresis, or whether there was a true absence of Hb A as such without any formation of globin at all — a failure of normal biosynthesis. The latter had been suggested by Rich, but there were many attempts to discover an abnormal hemoglobin. In some cases the Hb A was not completely absent and the inability to produce Hb A was only partial. It was found however that this "thalassemic" Hb A was structurally normal. It now became established that there were α- and β-chain abnormal hemoglobins. Microdrepanocytosis, the interacting state arising from simultaneous inheritance of thalassemia and sickling, was already known. Classic Cooley anemia affected the adult hemoglobin $\alpha_2\beta_2$ but not hemoglobins F ($\alpha_2\gamma_2$) and A_2 ($\alpha_2\delta_2$). To the contrary, these two hemoglobins were raised above the normal level either absolutely or relatively in proportion to Hb A. This suggested that the defect concerned the β-chain and that Cooley anemia was, as it were, a β-thalassemia. It explained the interaction of Cooley anemia with sickle cell hemoglobin which had an abnormality in the β-chain, and with all other β-chain abnormal hemoglobins when they were inherited together with β-thalassemia: Hb E - thalassemia, Hb C - thalassemia, Hb D - thalassemia, etc. However, there were other hemoglobins which did not interact with β-thalassemia and these turned out to be variants with their abnormality in the α-chain. What is more, there were thalassemias without a raised Hb A_2 and Hb F, and there was a surplus of β-chains as shown by presence of a β tetramer β_4, Hb H.

In 1959, Ingram and Stretton proposed that just as there were α- and β-chain abnormal hemoglobins, so could thalassemia affect either the α- or the β-chain part of Hb A, and that this would give rise to two classes of thalassemia: β-thalassemia, with raised Hb A_2 and F interacting with β-chain abnormal hemoglobins such as Hb S, and α-thalassemia, which could cause a surplus of noncombined β-chains and γ-chains, Hbs β_4 and γ_4 (Hb H and Hb Barts). There was a controversy at the time. I owe the disentanglement of what one might find difficult to understand to Weatherall's recent (1980) review in Wintrobe's "History of Hematology (Blood, Pure and Eloquent)." Pauling had proposed that thalassemia perhaps arose from an abnormal gene that produced a globin that could not bind its heme, ie that there was structure rate relation, and that the structure of this hypothetic globin resulted in low or nil synthesis. Ingram and Stretton added the proposal that the defect might not be caused by a mutation in the globin structure, but in the nonstructural DNA involved in the biosynthetic process. The discussion was really less about the concepts than about the priority of the hypotheses. We now know that both hypotheses are correct — the tap defect explains the majority of thalassemias but there are also thalassemic states due to a structure-biosynthesis rate effect: Hb K Woolwich is an example.

Abnormal hemoglobins continued to contribute to the understanding of the thalassemic process, and any further developments were strictly related to either the α-chain or the β-chain locus of hemoglobin production. Indeed in due course it was shown by Deisseroth that the genes for the two types of chain were on different chromosomes, No. 16 for α and No. 11 for β. For the details of the arrangement on chromosome 11, the fusion hemoglobins Lepore (δ/β) and Kenya (${}^{A}\gamma/\beta$) provided tentative evidence — later confirmed by gene mapping — that the sequence on the chromosome was ${}^{G}\gamma$, ${}^{A}\gamma$, δ and β.

The α-thalassemias with their unstable hemoglobin H instigated the search by

Fessas for similar unstable combinations of α-chains in β-thalassemia. He found these inclusion bodies in the bone marrow of patients with β-thalassemia. "Fessas bodies" consisting of unstable free (mostly dimeric) α-chains and Hb H inclusion bodies consisting of free tetrameric β-chains are important causes of the disease process in β- and α-thalassemia. Free α-chains in β-thalassemia and free β-chains in α-thalassemia damage the red cells and cause hemolysis. They arise from a disproportion of either α-chain or β-chain production. Here again, technical progress had been foremost in arriving at these conclusions. A simplified separation of hemoglobin into α- and β-chains was introduced by Clegg, Naughton, and Weatherall. This permitted globin biosynthesis in reticulocytes in the presence of labeled amino acids to be followed by subsequent separation of the labeled globin-chains and a determination of α/β globin synthesis ratio: > 1 in β-thalassemia and < 1 in α-thalassemia. A most satisfying observation was that a combination of α- and β-thalassemia was a less severe condition than either α- or β-thalassemia alone. This clearly showed that it was the disproportion of α/β globin ratio, rather than the mere fall of globin production, which was the most important cause of the clinical disorder.

The study of α-thalassemia was made difficult by the fact that there did not exist a simple mendelian pattern for the inheritance of Hb H disease. There existed some α-thalassemias which were very mild, with only slightly abnormal hematologic parameters and occasionally Hb H inclusion bodies in a few red cells but without enough Hb H to be shown on electrophoresis, and others with typical Hb H disease — splenomegaly — anemia and numerous inclusion bodies demonstrable in the erythrocytes as well as plenty of Hb H seen on electrophoresis. Parents of Hb H disease patients usually did not have Hb H disease, and while one of them showed the mild thalassemic status just mentioned, the other had no thalassemic stigmata at all.

In Thailand, Supananakorn and Wasi studying this situation found that a third type of α-thalassemia had to be added. From family studies it could be concluded that the symptomless parent of an offspring with hemoglobin H disease also carried a gene related to α-thalassemia. It caused no symptoms in its owner, but, in conjunction with a gene of the other parent with a mild α-thalassemia syndrome, it would cause the fullblown hemoglobin H disease. They named three types of α-thalassemia: Hb H disease, α-thalassemia type 1, the mild but recognizable α-thalassemia trait, and α-thalassemia type 2, a symptomless "silent" α-thalassemia as far as its carrier is concerned. The addition of α-thalassemia type 1 to α-thalassemia type 2 caused Hb H disease. There was yet another type of failure to produce α-chains, discovered by Lie-Injo Luan Eng in Indonesia, but now seen all over South East Asia and from time to time in some Mediterranean countries also. A hydrops fetalis not due to Rhesus disease or other causes of infants' red cell hemolysis had red cells without any α-chains. Nearly all the hemoglobin was fetal hemoglobin without α-chains - γ_4 or hemoglobin Barts.

Hence the condition was named hemoglobin Barts hydrops fetalis. A small amount of the primitive hemoglobin Portland $\zeta_2\gamma_2$ was also present. On examining the parents, it was found that both of them had α-thalassemia type 1. Thus, homozygotes for α-thalassemia type 1 had Barts hydrops fetalis, and double heterozygotes for α-thalassemia type 1 and type 2 had hemoglobin H disease. The different types, including the "silent" α-thalassemia, could be recognized at birth, according to the level of free γ-chains, ie γ-chains which had failed to find α-chains as partners to form fetal hemoglobin, $\alpha_2\gamma_2$. These γ-chains combined to form γ_4 (Hb Barts).

α-Thalassemia and types of severity:

	Severity	At Birth
1. Type 2	silent	3% Hb Barts
2. Type 1	mild	6% Hb Barts
3. Hb H disease	significant	15% Hb Barts
4. Hydrops fetalis	lethal	90% Hb Barts

It was already known that the γ-chain locus is duplicated. Thanks to the superb analysis of Hb F by Schroeder and Huisman, we know that there are two γ-chain genes producing, differing by one in their 146 residues each: $^{G}\gamma$ and $^{A}\gamma$. There was no such evidence for the α-chain, but if one assumed that, although all α-chains were chemically alike, they might yet be the product of two rather than one single gene, then the inheritance pattern of α-thalassemia could be interpreted as following a simple mendelian pattern. Evidence came forward also for this concept from a comparison of α- and β-chain abnormal variants and from the interaction of some α-chain abnormal hemoglobins such as hemoglobin Q with α-thalassemia. For a long time it was pointed out that heterozygotes for α-chain abnormal hemoglobins had a lesser proportion of the abnormal hemoglobin in their cells than heterozygotes for β-chain abnormal variants. This was related to the greater restraint on their structure because they had to function and combine equally well with γ-, β-, and δ-chains.

When one compared, however, hemoglobin variants with homologous mutations in the α- and β-chain, respectively, it was noted that the proportion of the abnormal hemoglobin was a quarter for the α variant and half for the β-chain variant. For nonpathologic hemoglobins it was 50% for the β mutant and 25% for the homologous α-chain abnormal hemoglobin. This suggested that the β-chain mutation affected all the available β-chain on one chromosome, but that the α-chain mutation affected only one-half, ie that there were two α-chain genes per chromosome and that an α-chain mutation altered only one of these two, and hence altered only one of four genes in the heterozygote, the β-chain mutation affecting one of two.

With two α-chain genes per chromosome there would then be four degrees of thalassemia in contrast to the two β-thalassemias: minor and major. In β-

thalassemia minor, the one β-chain gene on one of the 2 chromosomes per person would be affected, and in β-thalassemia major this would apply to both chromosomes. α-Thalassemia could affect one or two genes per chromosome or one, two, three, or four per individual.

Classification of α-thalassemia based on two α-chain genes per chromosome:

α-thalassemia type 2	1α-thalassemia
α-thalassemia type 1	2α-thalassemia
Hb H disease	3α-thalassemia
Hydrops fetalis	4α-thalassemia

The symptomless α-thalassemia would be the outcome of inaction of one of four, the mild but definite α-thalassemia trait represents the inactivity of two genes, hemoglobin H disease that of three, and would thus be the combination of the other two. The homozygous state for α-thalassemia type 1, or the failure of both genes on both chromosomes, would then cause a complete absence of α-chains, the α-chainless hydrops fetalis.

Family studies of interaction between α-chain abnormal hemoglobins such as Hb Q and α-thalassemia added a third dimension to these concepts. Only by assuming that the α-chain abnormal hemoglobin Q was not the sole occupier of the α-gene locus on a parent's chromosome could it be understood that the child of a Hb Q trait carrier and another parent with α-thalassemia type 1 could have Hb H disease with only Hb Q and no Hb A. This required that the Hb Q trait carrier had, on the chromosome on which the gene for Hb Q was transmitted, another locus — a locus for α-thalassemia which, together with α-thalassemia type 1, caused Hb H disease.

The next stage in the α-thalassemia story is the discovery of the abnormal α-chain hemoglobin Constant Spring by Weatherall and colleagues. This is a chain elongation hemoglobin that is underproduced and results in a kind of α^+-thalassemia rather like hemoglobin K Woolwich was a kind of β^+-thalassemia. A combination of thalassemia type 1 and of Constant Spring trait resulted in a Hb H disease and homozygotes had α-thalassemia type 1, ie 2 functioning and 2 malfunctioning α genes which required that, besides the gene for the α-chain variant Constant Spring, there was a normal α-chain gene on the same chromosome.

Hybridization of complementary DNA prepared from patients with Hb H disease by Y.W. Kan eventually confirmed that only a quarter of the expected α-globin genes could be found, ie that Hb H disease is derived from the loss of 75% of man's α-chain genes.

We come now to the exciting events of the last six years when gene mapping explored the thalassemias no longer at the level of the study of clinical symptoms, hematologic parameters, family studies, biosynthesis in reticulocytes, but at the fountain of the disorder or disorders — the structure and sequence of the

DNA. This is a mighty saga of the present and has yet to become history. Many, if not most, of the heroes of this new period are with us here in Cagliari tonight, and they will tell us of their discoveries in the course of this meeting. Recently, there has been the story of the difference between nuclear and protoplasmic mRNA, and we shall see how this leads to the understanding of β^{+}-thalassemia!

While research on the nature of thalassemia continued there has been, since the days of Haldane's theory of its persistence on the basis of balanced polymorphism, a search for the nature of this balance. Could it be that heterozygotes, as it is now proved for sickle cell trait, are relatively protected against death by malaria? One of the most convincing population studies has come from here in Sardinia where it has been shown that otherwise identical populations had a high incidence of thalassemia in the coastal regions, which were until recently malarious, but not in the mountains where the disease has never been prevalent. In vitro studies have shown that fetal hemoglobin is not easily digested by the parasite, but that the often only slight increase of that pigment in thalassemia minor could protect the cell against the malaria parasite is not yet generally accepted. There is certainly no increase of fetal hemoglobin in α-thalassemia. Hemoglobin H, being an unstable hemoglobin, could possibly generate antimalarial superoxide, but could it be that the worldwide high incidence of the one α-chain gene thalassemia is related not to malaria, whose geographic contribution it follows so closely, but to the β-chain abnormal hemoglobins S, C, and E, and to β-thalassemia? The severity of sickling, the intracellular levels of Hb E and of Hb C are all reduced by the additional presence of α-thalassemia. As I have mentioned already, the course of β-thalassemia is favorably influenced by α-thalassemia. Thus, a high incidence of α-thalassemia may not at all be related directly to the equally high incidence of malaria, but rather to the antimalarial β-chain variants and β-thalassemia, whose damage to the red cell is countered by mild α-thalassemia.

Before I close I would like, however, to make two more points, one historical and one general.

The historical consideration I want to put before you is that the methods and approaches of old have led further than we perhaps realize in 1981 in the exhilaration of today's thalassemia research.

If gene mapping had not helped us at all we would yet know what the sequence of the genes on the β chromosome would have to be from the abnormal hemoglobins Lepore and Kenya: namely $^{G}\gamma\ ^{A}\gamma\ \delta\ \beta$. We might even have made an inspired guess that the ϵ gene would have to precede the γ-chain genes "upstream," as you call it nowadays. The sequence in downstream direction corresponds to the appearance in the ontogeny of the various chains: $^{G}\gamma$ is higher than $^{A}\gamma$ at birth and $^{A}\gamma$ then increases until fetal hemoglobin makes room for the δ and β globins.

The chain elongation hemoglobins taught us to think in terms of stop codons either being eliminated by single point mutations or by unequal intracodon crossovers altering the reading of the mRNA, or of stop codons being introduced where there should be codons for amino acids. The anti Lepore δ-(β/δ)-β sequence arising from unequal crossing-over of chromosomes within neighboring $\delta\beta$ areas led us to predict the existence of the triple α gene. There are more examples. Let us therefore with our present excitement not neglect the old approaches. Cytology, clinical biochemistry, bedside studies, and family studies will continue to be a rich field for research on thalassemia.

The second reminder which I want to put before you is that the hemoglobinopathies are not the only genetic disorders in the world. We must investigate them not only for their own sake but also see them as trail blazers in molecular pathology as a whole. Surely the lessons which you will be teaching us over the next three days must have a bearing on muscular disorders, on immunologic problems, possibly even on cancer, and diseases of the mind?

I owe to Professor R.W. Carrell a most fitting quotation which he recently discovered in the Physiological Reviews of October 1925. Sir Joseph Barcroft wrote there more than half a century ago: " . . . such variations have a significance of their own . . . for there are many things which are true of hemoglobin that may also be true of all the other proteins of the body; in the case of hemoglobin they may be discovered because the globin possesses a label the heme on which the story writes itself and may be read by all who have eyes to see. Once that story has been read completely methods may be devised for the discovery of its applicability to proteins generally and in the revelation of this story . . . may lie the significance of hemoglobin . . ."

It took 150 years for typhoid to change from a disease of delirium (typhos) to one of specific intestinal ulceration, then to be caused by a specific Salmonella, and then again to become curable by chloromycetin. We have come a long way from von Jaksch, and there has been an increasing speed in describing and defining the thalassemic disorders to discover their etiology at various levels. We have now reached blood transfusion, chelation therapy of iron overload, and, particularly triumphantly successful under Professor Cao here in Sardinia, prenatal diagnosis. Dare one hope that besides improvements in all these three measures, before long, thanks to your important and thrilling achievements, genetic surgery will bring us the ultimate goal of a cure?

GUIDE TO FURTHER READING

Bannerman RM: "Thalassemia. A Survey of Some Aspects." New York: Grune & Stratton, 1961. (375 references)

Chernoff AI: The distribution of the thalassemia gene: A historical review. Blood 14:899–912, 1959. (190 references)

Chini V, Valeri CM: Mediterranean hemopathic syndromes. Blood 4:989–1013, 1949. (87 references)

Marmont A, Bianchi V: Mediterranean anemia. Clinical and haematological findings, and pathogenic studies in the milder form of the disease. Acta Haematol 1:4–28, 1959. (277 references)

Weatherall DJ: Toward the understanding of the molecular biology of some common inherited anemias: The story of thalassemia. In Wintrobe MM (ed): "Blood, Pure and Eloquent." New York: McGraw-Hill Co, 1980, pp 373–414. (127 references)

MOLECULAR BIOLOGY AND GENETICS OF THALASSEMIA SYNDROMES

The Clinical and Genetic Heterogeneity and Interactions of the α- and β-Thalassemias

D.J. Weatherall, MD, L. Pressley, MB, D.R. Higgs, MB, W.G. Wood, PhD, J.B. Clegg, PhD, and J. Wainscoat, MB

In this chapter we shall review the heterogeneity of α- and β-thalassemias and present some preliminary data on the interactions of these two conditions in patients with the intermediate forms of β-thalassemia.

Current data regarding the fine structure of the human α- and non-α-gene clusters, on which much of the present work is based, are summarized by Proudfoot et al [1] and Weatherall and Clegg [2].

THE α-THALASSEMIAS

At the phenotypic level the α-thalassemias produce several well-defined clinical disorders [2]. These include the hemoglobin Barts hydrops syndrome, hemoglobin H disease, and 2 different carrier states, the more severe and easily recognizable form, α-thalassemia 1 or α°-thalassemia, and the "silent" carrier state, α-thalassemia 2 or α^{+}-thalassemia. The homozygous state for α-thalassemia 1 produces the hemoglobin Barts hydrops syndrome, and the compound heterozygous state for α-thalassemia 1 and 2 results in hemoglobin H disease.

Alpha-thalassemia 1 is better called α°-thalassemia since it describes an α-thalassemia determinant which results in the complete absence of output from the α-globin genes on chromosome 16. Alpha-thalassemia 2 should really be called α^{+}-thalassemia since it is associated with a reduced output of α-chains.

It is now clear that both α-thalassemia 1 and 2 are caused by a very heterogeneous series of molecular defects. It follows, therefore, that the main clinical disorders which result from the interaction of these determinants, ie the hemoglobin Barts hydrops syndrome and hemoglobin H disease, are themselves very heterogeneous at the molecular level. Unfortunately, much of this information has been obtained so recently that it has not yet been possible to determine whether the different genetic interactions which produce these conditions are associated with distinguishable clinical phenotypes.

Birth Defects: Original Article Series, Volume 18, Number 7, pages 15–27
© 1982 March of Dimes Birth Defects Foundation

The α-Thalassemia 1 Determinants

The heterozygous state for α-thalassemia 1 is easy to recognize. The hematologic changes are very similar to those of heterozygous β-thalassemia, with significantly reduced MCH and MCV values. The α/β-chain synthesis ratio is reduced to about 0.6-0.7, and the α/β-globin messenger RNA ratio is clearly distinguishable from normals or α-thalassemia 2 heterozygotes [3].

Using the techniques of soluble cDNA/DNA hybridization, it was found that the α-thalassemia 1 determinant results from the loss of both the linked α-chain genes on chromosome 16 [4,5]. Using restriction endonuclease analysis of DNA of homozygotes for α-thalassemia 1 or from individuals with hemoglobin H disease, it has been possible to examine the extent of these deletions. These studies indicate that there is considerable heterogeneity of the defects which result in the α-thalassemia 1 phenotype; to date at least 4 different sized deletions have been identified.

The 2 α genes are linked to 2 ζ genes with an inactive α locus, the $\psi\alpha$ gene, in between [6]. The deletion which causes the α-thalassemia 1 phenotype in Thai patients involves both the α-globin genes but leaves both ζ genes intact. On the other hand, in a Greek infant with the Hb Barts hydrops syndrome a deletion of about 17.4 kb was found which involved both α-globin genes, the $\psi\alpha$ gene and the 3′ ζ-globin gene. Since this infant was producing significant amounts of hemoglobin Portland ($\zeta_2\gamma_2$), these observations provide direct evidence that the 5′ ζ-globin genes are functional [7,8]. A similar deletion has been found in a Cypriot case of hemoglobin Barts hydrops fetalis [9]. A third variety of deletion has been found in a Greek patient with hemoglobin H disease [10]. This appears to involve the loss of a piece of the α-globin gene about 5.2 kb in length. It starts within the 3′ (right hand) gene and extends downstream to involve the 5′ gene but not the two ζ genes.

A further type of genetic determinant which produces the α-thalassemia 1 phenotype was first described by Orkin et al [11]. When DNA is digested with the restriction enzyme Eco R1, the α genes are normally found on a fragment 22.2 kb in length. An α-thalassemia 1 determinant was found in several individuals with hemoglobin H disease which gave a fragment 2.6 kb in length. More recently, Orkin and Michelson [12] have isolated this fragment, cloned it in a suitable phage, and sequenced the DNA of the fraction obtained in this way. They found that it contains part of a single α-globin gene which appears to start at codon 57. Further analysis indicates that this α-thalassemia determinant has arisen by a large deletion involving all of the 3′ α-globin gene and part of the 5′ α-globin gene up to codon 57. Judging by the size of the original fragment obtained by Eco R1 digestion, this must be a very extensive deletion, probably involving both the ζ-globin genes. If this is the case, homozygotes for this determinant would not be able to synthesize any embryonic hemoglobin.

It seems likely that these different sized deletions of the α-globin genes have resulted from unequal crossing-over as occurred, for example, to produce the Lepore hemoglobins [7]. The finding of hemoglobin Portland ($\zeta_2\gamma_2$) in infants with the hemoglobin Barts hydrops syndrome who are homozygous for some of these determinants is of great interest. Since hemoglobin Barts is physiologically useless, it seems likely that these infants are able to survive to term by using hemoglobin Portland as an oxygen carrier. During normal fetal development hemoglobin Portland synthesis ceases in early fetal life. In the presence of these different deletions of the α-globin gene cluster, there is persistent embryonic hemoglobin (ie ζ chain) synthesis. The situation seems closely analogous to that observed with deletions of the δ- and β-chain gene cluster which cause HPFH. It follows, therefore, that deletions which, as well as involving the α-globin genes, involve both ζ-globin genes, will be incompatible with fetal survival.

The α-Thalassemia 2 Determinants

In 1977, Kan and his colleagues [13] showed that individuals with hemoglobin H disease are missing 3 out of the normal 4 α-globin genes. Since it had already been demonstrated that all the genes are deleted in the hemoglobin Barts hydrops syndrome, and since hemoglobin H disease was thought to result from the compound heterozygous state for α-thalassemia 1 and 2, this suggested that the α-thalassemia 2 determinant must result from the loss of one of the linked pair of α-globin genes per haploid genome.

If the normal α-globin gene haplotype (ie gene complement on a single chromosome) is written $\alpha\alpha$, the α-deletion form of α-thalassemia 2 can be written $-\alpha$. Extensive studies of the Jamaican and American Negro populations [14,15] and some Mediterranean and Oriental populations [11,16] have indicated that the form of α-thalassemia 2 which results from a single α-gene deletion is widespread. Studies of American Negroes [15] and of Jamaicans [17] indicate that approximately 23-25% of these populations are heterozygous for the deletion form of α-thalassemia 2 ($-\alpha$) and about 2% are homozygous ($-\alpha/-\alpha$) for this determinant. These findings have clarified the nature of α-thalassemia in Africans. In these populations, many individuals have been encountered who have the phenotype of the severe form of α-thalassemia (α-thalassemia 1), and yet hemoglobin H disease is extremely rare and the hemoglobin Barts hydrops syndrome has not been reported. It is now clear that individuals of African background with the blood changes of α-thalassemia 1 are nearly always homozygous for the deletion form of α-thalassemia 2 ($-\alpha/-\alpha$). Since the output of each of the α-globin genes appears to be more or less equal [3], the phenotypic expression of two α-globin genes is the same whether they are both on one chromosome or on opposite pairs of homologous chromosomes, ie whether they have the genotype $-\alpha/-\alpha$ or $-/\alpha\alpha$. Hence, unlike the situation in β-thalassemia, deletions are a common basis for α-thalassemia [18].

Gene mapping analysis indicates that there is also heterogeneity in the molecular basis for the production of deletion forms of α-thalassemia 2. The most common mechanism seems to have been unequal crossing-over which has resulted in loss of parts of both the 5′ and 3′ α-globin genes with the production of a single gene [16,17,19]. However, a Chinese subject has been found with a different type of deletion which involves the 5′ α-globin gene [20]. This deletion, which seems less common than the one mentioned above, has resulted from crossing-over at a different site. A consequence of unequal crossing-over between mispaired α-chain genes is that one of the chromosomes produced should have three α genes on it, just as the anti-Lepore chromosome has 3 non-α-globin genes [21]. Quite recently, examples of the $\alpha\alpha\alpha$ haplotype resulting from both types of crossing-over have been discovered [22-24]. The clinical consequences of having five α-globin genes, ie chromosomes with the arrangement $\alpha\alpha$ and $\alpha\alpha\alpha$, seem to be minimal. There are no hematologic abnormalities and globin-chain synthesis is almost balanced, although it is clear that all 5 genes are expressed since there is an increased α/β-globin messenger RNA ratio [23]. Clearly, the slight excess of α chains produced can be dealt with by the proteolytic enzymes of the red cell precursors. It is possible that this genotype may behave as a mild form of β-thalassemia (?silent β-thalassemia) and might interact with true β-thalassemia to produce a mild form of β-thalassemia intermedia.

Not all α-thalassemia 2 determinants result from gene deletions. Using soluble hybridization techniques Kan et al [13] reported a nondeletion form of α-thalassemia 2 in a Chinese family. Nondeletion forms of α-thalassemia of this type have been found in many populations [11,16]. It is becoming clear that there is considerable heterogeneity within this group of α-thalassemias. Thus, although some nondeletion determinants behave phenotypically as an α-thalassemia 2, recent work [25] in the Eastern Saudi Arabian population indicates that there is a nondeletion form of α-thalassemia which causes a greater deficiency of α-chain production and which, in the homozygous state, produces typical hemoglobin H disease. A third form of the condition has been recognized in the authors' laboratory, in which relatively large amounts of ?inactive α-globin mRNA are produced [26].

The phenotype of α-thalassemia 2 can also result from the inheritance of one of the α-chain termination mutants, such as hemoglobin Constant Spring [27]. This group of hemoglobin variants results from single base mutations in the α-chain termination codon so that instead of the α chains being 141 amino acid residues long they have an extra 30 residues at their C terminal end due to "read-through" of α-globin messenger RNA which is not normally translated. The reason for the grossly inefficient synthesis of these chain termination mutants appears to be instability of their messenger RNAs [28]. Why the "reading through" of normally untranslated α-globin messenger RNA sequences causes this instability is not yet understood.

THE β-THALASSEMIA

The β-thalassemias show considerable heterogeneity. They can be broadly divided into β^+-thalassemia in which there is some β-chain synthesis and β°-thalassemia in which there is a complete absence of β-chain production. Recent work indicates that both forms of the condition are very heterogeneous at the molecular level.

β^+-Thalassemia

The homozygous state for β^+-thalassemia usually produces a transfusion-dependent form of thalassemia major. However, this is not always the case and there is considerable clinical heterogeneity which almost certainly reflects a diversity of molecular forms of the condition. For example, in the severe Mediterranean form of β^+-thalassemia there is a very low level of β-chain synthesis, whereas in the milder Negro forms there is considerably more β-chain production. Evidence for the existence of several distinct forms of β^+-thalassemia is reviewed by Weatherall and Clegg [2].

Recently, some progress has been made in establishing the molecular basis for the β^+-thalassemias. Most of them are associated with a reduced output of β-globin messenger RNA. At least in some cases this may result from a defect in processing of the nuclear messenger RNA precursor to its definitive cytoplasmic form [29,30]. Maquat and her colleagues [30] have speculated that the underlying genetic lesions are at splicing signal regions or within the introns of the β-globin genes. Recent structural analysis of the β-globin genes indicates that this is indeed the case [31,32].

β°-Thalassemia

The homozygous state for β°-thalassemia usually results in a transfusion-dependent disorder, although some patients with the disorder have the clinical phenotype of thalassemia intermedia [33].

The β°-thalassemias are very heterogeneous at the molecular level. In most cases, globin-gene mapping has shown no abnormality. An exception was found in DNA obtained from 3 Afro-Asians. Although these children appear to be homozygous for a β°-thalassemia, they are in fact compound heterozygotes for a β°-thalassemia determinant associated with a normal β-globin gene map and one in which there is an 0.6 kb deletion at the 3′ end of the β gene [18,34]. More recently, the β gene from one of these patients has been cloned and its structure determined. The 0.6 kb deletion has removed the terminal third of the large intervening sequence, the entire 3′ coding block, and about 150 base pairs past the end of the β-globin gene [35].

The technique of cDNA/mRNA hybridization has also produced evidence for heterogeneity of the β°-thalassemias. In some cases there appears to be no β-globin messenger RNA transcribed [36-42], while in others some is detectable. Old et al [41] analyzed β-globin messenger RNA in peripheral blood samples of β°-thalassemics from a wide variety of racial groups. Three patterns were defined; 1) no β-globin messenger RNA detectable, 2) significant amounts of apparently full-length but nonfunctional β-messenger RNA, and 3) structurally abnormal β-messenger RNA. The molecular basis for these conditions has yet to be determined.

Chang and Kan [43] have determined the nucleotide sequence of the nonfunctional β-messenger RNA from a Chinese patient with β°-thalassemia. They have shown that the AAG codon for lysine at position β^{17} has changed to the chain termination codon UAG, thus leading to premature chain termination with the production of a short 16 residue N-terminal fragment of the β chain. The same workers went on to confirm these findings by translating the defective β-globin messenger RNA in a cell-free system using a UAG tyrosine suppressor tRNA; full-length β-globin genes were synthesized [43].

In addition to these cases of β°-thalassemia with nonfunctional β-globin messenger RNA, 2 groups have reported cases in which β-messenger RNA could be detected only in the nuclei of bone marrow cells. [44]. This suggests that some forms of β°-thalassemia may result from defects of processing β-globin RNA precursor.* Finally, there is the Ferrara form of β°-thalassemia in which it appears that β-globin messenger RNA is present, but β-globin chain synthesis only occurs in the presence of a factor obtained from a soluble cell fraction from normal red cells [45,46]. This condition has not been found in any other racial group.

Clearly the β°-thalassemias are remarkably heterogeneous at the molecular level. It seems very likely that more nonsense mutations of the type described by Chang and Kan [43] will be defined. As pointed out by Chang et al [47], 25 different single base mutations in the β-globin gene could result in termination codons. Thus, assay with suppressor tRNAs may be a useful screening method for detecting this type of lesion in β°-thalassemia.

Further Diversity of the β-Thalassemias

Some progress has been made in defining forms of the β-thalassemias in which there are normal hemoglobin A_2 levels in heterozygotes. In one type, the

*See also Bank et al, this volume. Several different splicing mutations have now been found in β-thalassemia.

hematologic findings in carriers are normal and yet there is imbalanced globin-chain synthesis; this determinant can interact with high hemoglobin A_2 β-thalassemia to produce a form of thalassemia intermedia [48,49]. In another variety, the hematologic changes in heterozygotes are indistinguishable from those of high hemoglobin A_2 β-thalassemia; this determinant interacts with the latter to produce a transfusion-dependent disorder [49]. There is some evidence that the second variety of normal hemoglobin A_2 β-thalassemia may in fact represent the compound heterozygous state for both δ- and β-thalassemia [50]. These varieties of β-thalassemia with normal hemoglobin A_2 levels are of considerable importance from the point of view of genetic counseling, since hematologically they resemble the α-thalassemia carrier states. Recent gene mapping studies in the authors' laboratory have shown no abnormalities of δ and β genes in these conditions.

There seem to be yet more distinct types of β-thalassemia. For a complete review the reader is referred to the monograph of Weatherall and Clegg [2].

PRELIMINARY STUDIES OF THE INTERACTION OF α- AND β-THALASSEMIA

Thalassemia intermedia is a clinical term used to describe a group of conditions ranging in severity from a disorder similar to the transfusion-dependent major forms of thalassemia to a symptomless anemia which is only slightly more severe than that of heterozygous carriers. Several different genetic interactions can produce this clinical picture including the combination of α-thalassemia with homozygous $\beta°$- or β^{+}-thalassemia. This results in relatively less globin-chain imbalance and hence a milder degree of ineffective erythropoiesis than usually occurs in these conditions. [2,50].

Since both α- and β-thalassemia occur at a high frequency in many countries, and because programs for the antenatal diagnosis of β-thalassemia are being set up in these populations, it is clearly important to establish which varieties of α-thalassemia can modify the homozygous state for β-thalassemia and so produce the phenotype of β-thalassemia intermedia. We have studied 5 Cypriot patients with β-thalassemia intermedia and their families who were referred to us for clinical evaluation [51].

The results are summarized in Table 1. In *Family S,* the mother's DNA gave only the 10.5 kb band after digestion with Bam H1 and she is therefore homozygous for the deletion form of α-thalassemia 2 ($-\alpha/-\alpha$) as well as being a β-thalassemia carrier. Her daughter, who is homozygous for β^{+}-thalassemia, has both 14 kb and 10.5 kb Bam H1 α-specific bands showing that she is heterozygous for α-thalassemia 2 ($-\alpha/\alpha\alpha$). Similarly, the probands in *Families G* and *H* are also homozygous for β^{+}-thalassemia and heterozygous for the deletion form of α-thalassemia 2 ($-\alpha/\alpha\alpha$). which they each received from a parent with the

TABLE 1. Findings in 5 Families in Which the Propositus Has a Mild Form of β^+-Thalassemia

Family	Family Member	Hb gm/dl	MCV fl	MCH pg	Hb F %	Hb A_2 %	α/β Total cpm	α bands Bam H1	α Genotype	Thalassemia genotype
S	Father	14.1	67	21	5.6	5.4	2.4	14.0	$\alpha\alpha/\alpha\alpha$	Heterozygous β^+-thal.
	Mother	13.3	77	24	2.2	4.5	0.7	10.5	$-\alpha/-\alpha$	Heterozygous β^+-thal.
										Homozygous α-thal. 2
	Propositus	8.3	73	23	82.5	2.7	—	14.0	$-\alpha/\alpha\alpha$	Homozygous β^+-thal.
								10.5		Heterozygous α-thal. 2
G	Father	14.1	69	22	0.8	5.7	1.1	14.0	$-\alpha/\alpha\alpha$	Heterozygous β^+-thal.
								10.5		Heterozygous α-thal. 2
	Mother	11.8	64	21	0.8	5.0	2.6	14.0	$\alpha\alpha/\alpha\alpha$	Heterozygous β^+-thal.
	Propositus	7.6	79	24	54.1	4.3	—	14.0	$-\alpha/\alpha\alpha$	Homozygous β^+-thal.
								10.5		Heterozygous α-thal. 2
H	Father	14.8	70	24	1.0	5.1	1.1	14.0	$-\alpha/\alpha\alpha$	Heterozygous β^+-thal.
								10.5		Heterozygous α-thal. 2
	Mother	11.8	66	21	1.2	3.5	1.7	14.0	$\alpha\alpha/\alpha\alpha$	Heterozygous β^+-thal.
	Propositus	8.1	86	26	55.0	4.6	—	14.0	$-\alpha/\alpha\alpha$	Homozygous β^+-thal.
								10.5		Heterozygous α-thal. 2
C	Father	13.0	62	20	1.0	4.0	2.2	14.0	$\alpha\alpha/\alpha\alpha$	Heterozygous β^+-thal.
	Mother	12.8	69	22	1.1	5.0	1.1	14.0	$\underline{\alpha\alpha}^T/\alpha\alpha$	Heterozygous β^+-thal.
										Heterozygous α-thal.[a]
	Propositus	7.1	72	21	54.3	9.4	—	14.0	$\underline{\alpha\alpha}^T/\alpha\alpha$	Homozygous β^+-thal.
										Heterozygous α-thal.

E	Grandfather (*I-1*)	14.7	73	24	2.7	5.4	1.3	—	—	Heterozygous β^+-thal. Heterozygous α-thal.
	Grandmother (*I-2*)	13.9	81	27	1.3	2.5	0.8	—	—	Heterozygous α-thal.
	Father (*II-1*)	14.6	79	25	4.7	5.3	0.8	14.0 10.5	$\underline{\alpha\alpha}^T/-\alpha$	Heterozygous β^+-thal. Compound heterozygous α-thal.[b]
	Mother (*II-2*)		55		3.2	6.4	2.7	14.0	$\alpha\alpha/\alpha\alpha$	Heterozygous β^+-thal.
	Propositus	8.2	57	17	69.1	4.9	—	14.0	$\underline{\alpha\alpha}^T/\alpha\alpha$	Homozygous β^+-thal. Heterozygous α-thal.

[a]Presumed nondeletion α-thalassemia ($\alpha\alpha^T/$).

[b]Presumed to have deletion and nondeletion forms of α-thalassemia [51].

phenotype of heterozygous β-thalassemia, but who has balanced globin-chain synthesis and a single α gene deleted ($-\alpha/\alpha\alpha$).

In *Family E,* the propositus has a normal α-gene map but his father has both 14.0 and 10.5 kb α-specific bands and is therefore heterozygous for a deletion form of α-thalassemia 2 ($-\alpha/\alpha\alpha$). However, he has an α/β-globin chain synthesis ratio of 0.8, somewhat lower than that normally seen in individuals doubly heterozygous for β-thalassemia and α-thalassemia 2. This suggests that he may have a second α-thalassemia 2 lesion. This is likely to be on the chromosome yielding the 14.0 kb band with the α probe, and would have to be of the nondeletion type. The findings in the father's parents (who were not available for subsequent DNA analysis) provide evidence for a second α-thalassemia determinant. The grandfather *(I-1)* has an α/β-chain synthesis ratio of 1.3, suggesting that he is a compound heterozygote for α-thalassemia and β-thalassemia. The grandmother *(I-2)* has an α/β-synthesis ratio typical of α-thalassemia trait. The fact that the father *(II-1)* carries the same β-thalassemia gene as the grandfather *(I-1)* but has a much lower α/β ratio strongly suggests that he is doubly heterozygous for both deletion and nondeletion α-thalassemia genes and that the propositus has inherited the nondeletion determinant.

In *Family C,* gene mapping data show no abnormality in the DNA of the propositus or either parent but the mother has a balanced α/β-chain synthesis ratio showing that she has α-thalassemia. Thus, she must be heterozygous either for an α-thalassemia 1 deletion determinant or a nondeletion determinant, which she has presumably passed on to her son. The latter interpretation seems more likely because ζ gene analysis, which may be used to identify the presence of α-thalassemia 1 determinants, shows no evidence for the deletion which gives rise to the α-thalassemia 1 disorder in Mediterranean populations.

Since antenatal diagnosis is now being applied widely to the problem of β-thalassemia in populations in which there is also a high incidence of α thalassemia, it is obviously important to determine whether the presence of a single α-thalassemia determinant can ameliorate the course of homozygous β^+- or β°-thalassemia. These preliminary studies suggest that this may be the case, but it will be necessary to analyze a series of transfusion-dependent homozygous β^+- and β°-thalassemics and compare the incidence of α-thalassemia in that group with a large series of patients with mild homozygous β^+- or β°-thalassemia to confirm this and to fully define the clinical spectrum of these interactions. The presence of the deletion forms of α-thalassemia can be detected by restriction enzyme analysis, but because there is no way of identifying the nondeletion forms of α-thalassemia by this method, extensive family studies will be required to analyze the possible interactions between this type of α-thalassemia determinant and β-thalassemia.

A preliminary analysis of a study being carried out by the authors in collaboration with Professor Antonio Cao and Dr. Elizabeth Letsky suggests that deletion forms of α-thalassemia may have a significant effect in ameliorating homozygous β^+- and β°-thalassemia.

REFERENCES

1. Proudfoot NJ, Shander MHM, Lanley JL, Gefter ML, Maniatis T: Structure and in vitro transcription of human globin genes. Science 209:1329, 1980.
2. Weatherall DJ, Clegg JB: "The Thalassaemia Syndromes," 3rd Ed. Oxford: Blackwell Scientific Publications, 1981.
3. Hunt DM, Higgs DR, Old JM, Clegg JB, Weatherall DJ, Marsh GW: Determination of α thalassemia phenotypes by messenger RNA analysis. Br J Haematol 45:53, 1980.
4. Ottolenghi S, Lanyon WG, Paul J, Williamson R, Weatherall DJ, Clegg JB, Pritchard J, Pootrakul S, Wong HB: The severe form of α thalassaemia is caused by a haemoglobin gene deletion. Nature 251:389, 1974.
5. Taylor JM, Dozy A, Kan YW, Varmus HE, Lie-Injo LE, Ganeson J, Todd D: Genetic lesion in homozygous α thalassemia (hydrops foetalis). Nature 251:392, 1974.
6. Lauer J, Shen C-KJ, Maniatis T: The chromosomal arrangement of human α-like globin genes: Sequence homology and α-globin gene deletions. Cell 20:119, 1980.
7. Pressley L, Higgs DR, Clegg JB, Weatherall DJ: Gene deletions prove that the 5′ ζ locus is functional. Proc Natl Acad Sci USA 77:3586, 1980.
8. Kattamis C, Metaxatou-Mavromati A, Tsiarta E, Metaxatou C, Wasi P, Wood WG, Pressley L, Higgs DR, Clegg JB, Weatherall DJ: The haemoglobin Bart's hydrops syndrome in Greece. Br Med J 2:268, 1980.
9. Sophocleous T, Higgs DR, Aldridge B, Trent RJ, Clegg JB, Weatherall DJ: The molecular basis for the haemoglobin Bart's hydrops fetalis syndrome in Cyprus. Br J Haematol 47:153, 1981.
10. Pressley L, Higgs DR, Aldridge B, Metaxatou-Mavromati A, Tsiarta E, Kattamis C, Wood WG, Clegg JB, Weatherall DJ: Characterisation of a new α thalassemia defect due to a partial deletion of the α globin gene complex. Nucleic Acids Res 8:4889, 1980.
11. Orkin SH, Old JM, Lazarus H, Altay C, Gurgey A, Weatherall DJ, Nathan DG: The molecular basis of α thalassemias: Frequent occurrence of dysfunctional α loci among non-Asians with Hb H disease. Cell 17:33, 1979.
12. Orkin SH, Michelson A: Partial deletion of the α globin structural gene in human α thalassemia. Nature 286:538, 1980.
13. Kan YW, Dozy AM, Trecartin R, Todd D: Identification of a non-deletion defect in α thalassemia. N Engl J Med 297:1081, 1977.
14. Higgs DR, Pressley L, Old JM, Hunt DM, Clegg JB, Weatherall DJ, Serjeant GR: Negro α-thalassemia is caused by a deletion of a single α-gene. Lancet 2:272, 1979.
15. Dozy AM, Kan YW, Embury SH, Mentzer WC, Wang WC, Lubin B, Davis JR, Koenig HM: Alpha globin gene organization in Blacks precludes the severe form of α thalassemia. Nature 280:605, 1979.
16. Kan YW, Dozy AM, Stamatoyannopoulos G, Hadjiminas MG, Zachariades Z, Furbetta M, Cao A: Molecular basis of hemoglobin-H disease in the Mediterranean. Blood 54:1434, 1979.
17. Higgs DR, Pressley L, Clegg JB, Weatherall DJ, Serjeant GR: α Thalassemia in Black populations. Johns Hopk Med J 146:300, 1980.
18. Orkin SH, Old JM, Weatherall DJ, Nathan DG: Partial deletion of β-globin gene DNA in certain patients with β° thalassemia. Proc Natl Acad Sci USA 76:2400, 1979.
19. Phillips JA, Scott AF, Smith KD, Young KD, Lightbody KL, Jiji RM, Kazazian HH: A molecular basis for hemoglobin-H disease in American Blacks. Blood 54:1439, 1979.

20. Embury SH, Lebo RV, Dozy AM, Kan YW: Organization of the α-globin genes in the Chinese α-thalassemia syndromes. J Clin Invest 63:1307, 1979.
21. Baglioni A: The fusion of two peptide chains in hemoglobin Lepore and its interpretation as a genetic deletion. Proc Natl Acad Sci USA 48:1880, 1962.
22. Goossens M, Dozy AM, Embury SH, Zachariades Z, Hadjiminas MG, Stamatoyannopoulos G, Kan YW: Triplicated α globin loci in humans. Proc Natl Acad Sci USA 77:518, 1980.
23. Higgs DR, Old JM, Pressley L, Clegg JB, Weatherall DJ: A novel α globin gene arrangement in man. Nature 284:632, 1980.
24. Trent RJ, Higgs DR, Clegg JB, Weatherall DJ: A new triplicated α-globin gene arrangement in man. Br J Haematol (In press).
25. Pressley L, Higgs DR, Pembrey ME, Clegg JB, Weatherall DJ: A new genetic basis for hemoglobin H disease. N Engl J Med 303:1383, 1980.
26. Higgs DR, Pressley L, Aldridge B, Clegg JB, Weatherall DJ, Cao A, Hadjiminas MG, Kattamis C, Metaxatou-Mavromati A, Rachmilewitz EA, Sophocleous T: Genetic and molecular diversity in nondeletion Hb H disease. Proc Natl Acad Sci USA 78:5833, 1981.
27. Weatherall DJ, Clegg JB: The α chain termination mutants and their relationship to the α thalassemias. Philos Trans R Soc Lond [Biol] 271:411, 1975.
28. Hunt DM, Higgs DR, Clegg JB, Weatherall DJ: Haemoglobin Constant Spring has an unstable α chain messenger RNA. Br J Haematol (In press).
29. Nienhuis AW, Turner P, Benz EJ: Relative stability of α- and β-globin messenger RNAs in homozygous β^+ thalassemia. Proc Natl Acad Sci USA 74:3960, 1977.
30. Maquat LE, Kinniburgh AJ, Beach LR, Honig GR, Lazerson J, Ershler WB, Ross J: Processing of human β-globin mRNA precursor mRNA is defective in three patients with β^+ thalassemia. Proc Natl Acad Sci USA 77:4287, 1980.
31. Spritz RA, Jagadesswaran P, Choudary P, Biro PA, Elder JT, deRiel JK, Manley JL, Gefter ML, Forget BG, Weissman SM: Base substitution in an intervening sequence of a β^+ thalassemic human globin gene. Proc Natl Acad Sci USA 78:2455, 1981.
32. Westway D, Williamson R: An intron nucleotide sequence variant in a cloned β^+-thalassemia globin gene. Nucleic Acids Res 9:1777, 1981.
33. Weatherall DJ, Clegg JB, Wood WG, Old JM, Higgs DR, Pressley L, Darbre PD: The clinical and molecular heterogeneity of the thalassemia syndromes. Ann NY Acad Sci 344:83, 1980.
34. Flavell RA, Bernards R, Kooter JH, de Boer E, Little PFR, Annison G, Williamson R: The structure of the human β-globin gene in β-thalassemia. Nucleic Acids Res 6:2749, 1979.
35. Orkin SH, Kolonder R, Michelson A, Husson R: Cloning and direct examination of a structurally abnormal human beta° thalassemia globin gene. Proc Natl Acad Sci USA 77:3558, 1980.
36. Forget BG, Baltimore D, Benz EJ, Housman D, Lebowitz P, Marotta CA, McCaffrey RP, Skoultchi A, Swerdlow PS, Vernon IM, Weissman SM: Globin messenger RNA in the thalassemia syndromes. Ann NY Acad Sci 232:76, 1974.
37. Forget BG, Hillman DG, Cohen-Solal M, Prensky W: Beta globin messenger RNA in β° thalassemia. Blood 48:998, 1976.
38. Housman D, Skoultchi A, Forget BG, Benz EJ: Use of globin cDNA as a hybridisation probe for globin mRNA. Ann NY Acad Sci 241:280, 1974.
39. Ottolenghi S, Lanyon WG, Williamson R, Weatherall DJ, Clegg JB, Pitcher CS: Human globin gene analysis for a patient with $\beta^\circ/\delta\beta^\circ$ thalassemia. Proc Natl Acad Sci USA 72:2294, 1975.
40. Tolstoshev P, Mitchell J, Lanyon G, Williamson R, Ottolenghi S, Comi P, Giglioni B, Masera G, Modell B, Weatherall DJ, Clegg JB: Presence of gene for β globin in homozygous β° thalassaemia. Nature 260:95, 1976.
41. Old JM, Proudfoot NJ, Wood WG, Longley JI, Clegg JB, Weatherall DJ: Characterization of β-globin mRNA in the β° thalassemias. Cell 14:289, 1978.

42. Benz EJ, Forget BG, Hillman DG, Cohen-Solal M, Pritchard J, Cavallesco C: Variability in the amount of β globin mRNA in $\beta°$ thalassemia. Cell 14:299, 1978.
43. Chang JC, Kan YW: $\beta°$ thalassemia, a nonsense mutation in man. Proc Natl Acad Sci USA 76:2886, 1979.
44. Comi P, Giglioni B, Barbarano L, Ottolenghi S, Williamson R, Novakova M, Amsera G: Transcription and post-transcriptional defects in $\beta°$ thalassemia. Eur J Biochem 79:617, 1977.
45. Conconi F, Rowley PT, del Senno L, Pontremoli S, Volpato S: Induction of β-globin synthesis in the β-thalassemia of Ferrara. Nature 238:83, 1972.
46. Conconi F, del Senno L: The molecular defect of Ferrara β-thalassemia. Ann NY Acad Sci 232:54, 1974.
47. Chang JC, Kan YW, Trecartin RF, Temple GF: Nonsense mutation as a cause of $\beta°$ thalassemia. Ann NY Acad Sci 344:113, 1980.
48. Schwartz E: The silent carrier of beta thalassemia. N Engl J Med 281:1327, 1969.
49. Kattamis C, Metaxatou-Mavromati A, Wood WG, Nash JR, Weatherall DJ: The heterogeneity of normal Hb A_2-β thalassemia in Greece. Br J Haematol 42:109, 1979.
50. Bianco I, Graziani B, Carboni C: Genetic patterns in thalassemia intermedia (constitutional microcytic anemia). Familial and biosynthetic studies. Hum Hered 27:257, 1977.
51. Weatherall DJ, Pressley L, Wood WG, Higgs DR, Clegg JB: The molecular basis for mild forms of homozygous β thalassemia. Lancet 1:527, 1981.

The Arrangement of the Human Globin Genes*

Robert Williamson, PhD

INTRODUCTION

The progress in this field has been so great that it is difficult to recall that as recently as 10 years ago direct analysis of the human globin genes was not yet possible. The advances of the past decade rely on the preparation of gene-specific probes. A gene-specific probe is a nucleic acid sequence which is able to hybridize only with a particular gene and its near relatives. In the case of the human globin genes, scientists are fortunate in that it is possible to isolate globin messenger RNA (mRNA) from reticulocytes, one of the few tissues that can be obtained from patients in reasonable amounts without trauma.

The globin mRNA is itself a globin gene-specific probe if labeled to high specific activity using the enzyme phosphokinase, but the terminal radioactive phosphate can be removed by adventitious phosphatases; therefore, this system does not work well quantitatively. The first gene-specific probe that was widely used was complementary DNA (cDNA) copied from globin mRNA using the viral enzyme RNA-dependent DNA polymerase (''reverse transcriptase'') with an oligo(T) primer. It is useful to note that such a probe is not only specific for the globin genes themselves, but also for mRNA and its precursor nuclear transcript. Thus, a single-stranded probe will always be complementary to (and a suitable probe for) genomic DNA, but only a ''negative'' single strand probe can be used to probe RNA transcripts of a gene.

Using cDNA, it was shown that the globin gene numbers are as predicted from genetic data [1]. However, reticulocyte mRNA contains not only globin mRNA—approximately 5-10% of the total mRNA codes for other proteins. Moreover, the globin mRNA itself is a mixture of at least two major species (alpha and beta) and two minor species (delta and gamma); it also became clear

*Supported by the U.K. Medical Research Council and NIH grant #1RO1AM20125-01A1.

Birth Defects: Original Article Series, Volume 18, Number 7, pages 29–33
© 1982 March of Dimes Birth Defects Foundation

that, as there are two α- and two γ-globin genes, there is no certainty that each of these sequences is not a mixture of two species. Attempts were made to purify cDNA specific for a single globin gene, starting with thalassemic mRNAs and then prehybridizing to cDNA under defined kinetic conditions. In our experience, it was rare to obtain a cDNA that was greater than 90% pure.

The preparation of recombinant molecules in bacterial plasmids and phage, followed by purification, by cloning and rapid growth, and by isolation, allowed the preparation of unlimited amounts of gene-specific probes for any identifiable sequence which could be obtained as an mRNA. Moreover, the availability of cDNA clones also allowed the isolation of long genomic DNA recombinants cloned in phage or cosmid, whose organization and sequence could be studied in detail. Finally, any clone can now be isolated from a single individual, and the structure and function of the globin genes studied to determine the limits of normal variation and the causes of dysfunction in thalassemia and sickle cell disease.

GLOBIN GENE CLONES

Human globin cDNA clones in bacterial plasmids were isolated simultaneously by Wilson et al [2], and Little et al [3]. In each case, sequences corresponding to the three major globin genes, alpha, beta, and gamma, were obtained by transcribing cDNA from total human reticulocyte mRNA, double-stranding the cDNA enzymatically, tailing the double stranded cDNA to insert it into plasmid, and transfecting *E. coli* with the recombinant plasmids obtained. The clones obtained did not contain the full length cDNA sequences, which is not surprising considering that these were the first human coding genes isolated using these techniques.

The DNA sequence of the recombinants proved that each could code for the appropriate globin protein chain. Southern's blot hybridization analysis [4] in combination with restriction enzymes singly and in pairs elucidates the general organization of both the α-globin and β-globin gene families [5,6].

There are two structural genes for α-globin on chromosome 16, and both appear to be functional in the normal person. They are separated by 3.7 kilobase pairs (kb), and each contains 2 introns. There is also a single functional ζ-globin gene, active in early embryonic life, and a second ζ-pseudogene which differs from the functional gene only by a single base change, but one which introduces a premature termination codon into the protein coding sequence. The ζ-pseudogene is located between the functional ζ-gene and the two α-genes. The total α-globin gene cluster spans approximately 25 kb.

The β-globin gene cluster is somewhat larger, with a total length of approximately 55 kb. There is a single gene for the ϵ-globin which is active during the first 2 months of fetal life, two γ-globin genes which are active from midfetal life to birth, and a single δ- and a single β-globin gene. Once again the gene order from 5′- to 3′- is the same as the ontogenic order, and the "groups" of genes are separated by longer lengths of DNA than pairs within groups. There are pseudogenes in the β-globin gene locus, and repetitive sequences have been mapped relative to the structural genes. At least 6 repetitive sequences occur, including 5 related to the "Alu family," which may play an important role in gene activation [7].

A general picture of globin gene organization can be obtained by using restriction site analysis on human DNA, but fine gene mapping relies upon the isolation of long genomic DNA clones and the determination of their nucleotide sequence. This has been carried out for genes from several normal individuals, and from some affected by thalassemia [6,8,9]. The coding regions do not appear unusual in codon usage, but it is apparent that there must be some mechanism by which the genome is able to "compare" the two γ-globin gene sequences with each other, as there is a high degree of conservation of the DNA sequence even in the third position of the codon, where a change would not affect the protein sequence. Various explanations have been put forward, in particular, a mechanism for unequal crossing-over known as gene conversion [9].

It is also of interest to note that Jeffreys has examined a number of different individuals for polymorphisms in restriction sites flanking the globin genes [10]. He concludes that there is approximately one base difference in every hundred base pairs in this region of the genome, and that these single base polymorphisms for the most part are random and nonselected [10].

INITIATION AND TERMINATION OF TRANSCRIPTION

With the determination of the fine structure of the regions surrounding and within the structural genes, it is possible to define the "signals" that control the initiation and termination of transcription. The initiation site for transcription has been mapped by studying nuclear globin pre-mRNA, and it is clear that transcription starts at the same nucleotide as does the 5′-terminus of the polysomal mRNA [5,11]. There are 3 DNA signals that appear to be of importance in determining the site and rate of initiation: the "CCAAT box" 70 nucleotides 5′- to the initiation site, the "TATA box" 30 nucleotides 5′- to the initiation site, and the "CAP site" at which initiation occurs. The most essential of these is apparently the TATA box; the other 2 sequences regulate rate and fidelity of initiation, but only the TATA box is an unambiguous requirement.

There is a possibility that transcription does not terminate at a specific site, but continues until finishing randomly 3′- to the mRNA terminus. The invariant sequence AATAAA occurs approximately 10 bases before the poly(A) addition site, but it may act as a signal to an enzyme processing the pre-mRNA rather than as a terminator of transcription [12].

Transcription is studied, not only by analogy and comparison, but also directly in cell-free systems [11]. Such systems reflect in vivo transcription in specificity of initiation, but rarely terminate correctly. Also, the differentiation-specific controls which determine which genes are transcribed in a given tissue do not operate in the in vitro systems; globin genes are transcribed quite happily in extracts from HeLa cells, though of course not in intact HeLa cells.

Since there is no linkage between α-globin and β-globin gene loci, it was assumed that the two major globin gene families are not on the same chromosome. This was proven to be correct when DNA from rodent-human hybrid cells containing only a single or limited number of human chromosomes were hybridized to globin gene-specific probes, and confirmed using chromosome sorting [13,14]. The β-globin gene locus is on chromosome 11 (at 11p12) and the α-globin gene locus on chromosome 16 (at 16p).

The ease of cloning has also led to attempts to study the evolution of the globin genes. It is really quite remarkable that intron position is conserved not only among mammalian hemoglobins, but even in plant leghemoglobin, indicating that the general structure of the globin genes has been conserved over hundreds of millions of years [15]. However, the separation of the α- and β-globin gene families is a relatively recent phenomenon, eg in *Xenopus* these genes are closely linked.

CONCLUSIONS

There remain many outstanding questions. It is remarkable that we still have no clue as to the DNA sequences which are involved in control of the switch from embryonic to fetal to adult gene transcription. We also do not know the organization of the globin genes in chromatin, or in the nucleus of the cell. It is quite possible that genes which appear to be remote in our 2-dimensional representation of DNA are adjacent in the cell. This could be equally true in the α- and β-globin genes, or the β- and γ-globin genes. Advances in methods both for studying gene function in vitro and for analyzing the structure of interphase chromosomes are required before we can truly understand the organization of even those human genes most studied—those coding for the globins.

ACKNOWLEDGMENTS

I thank my colleagues, and in particular Peter Little and Dick Flavell, for many helpful discussions.

REFERENCES

1. Williamson R: Direct measurement of the number of globin genes. Br Med Bull 32:246, 1976.
2. Wilson JT, Wilson JB, DeRiel JK, Villa-Komaroff L, Efstratiadis A, Forget BG, Weissman SM: Insertion of synthetic copies of human globin genes into bacterial plasmids. Nucleic Acids Res 5:563, 1978.
3. Little PFR, Curtis P, Coutelle C. Van den Berg J, Dalgleish R, Malcolm S, Courtney M, Westaway D, Williamson R: The isolation of recombinant plasmids containing human α-, β- and γ-globin cDNA fragments. Nature 273:640, 1978.
4. Southern EM: Detection of specific sequences among DNA fragments separated by gel electrophoresis. J Mol Biol 98:503, 1975.
5. Dahl HH, Flavell RA, Grosveld FG: The use of genomic libraries for the isolation and study of eukaryotic genes. In Williamson R (ed): "Genetic Engineering 2." London: Academic Press, 1981, p 49.
6. Efstratiadis A, Posakony JW, Maniatis T, Lawn RM, O'Connell C, Spritz RA, DeRiel JK, Forget BG, Weissman SM, Slightom JL, Blechl AE, Smithies O, Baralle FE, Shoulders CC, Proudfoot NJ: The structure and evolution of the human β-globin gene family. Cell 21:653, 1980.
7. Coggins LW, Grindlay GJ, Vass JK, Slater AA, Montague P, Stinson MA, Paul J: Repetitive DNA sequences near three human β-type globin genes. Nucleic Acids Res 8:3319, 1980.
8. Westaway D, Williamson R: An intron nucleotide sequence variant in a cloned β^+-thalassaemia globin gene. Nucleic Acids Res 9:1777, 1981.
9. Slightom JL, Blechl AE, Smithies O: Human fetal $^G\gamma$- and $^A\gamma$-globin genes: Complete nucleotide sequences suggest that DNA can be exchanged between these duplicated genes. Cell 21:627, 1980.
10. Jeffreys AJ: DNA sequence variants in the α-, β-, δ- and γ-globin genes of man. Cell 18:1, 1979.
11. Wickens MP, Laskey RA: Expression of cloned genes in cell-free systems and in microinjected *Xenopus* oocytes. In Williamson R (ed): "Genetic Engineering 1." London: Academic Press, 1981, p 103.
12. Hofer E, Darnell JE: The primary transcription unit of the mouse β-major globin gene. Cell 23:585, 1981.
13. Deisseroth A, Nienhuis A, Turner P, Velez R, Anderson WF, Lawrence J, Creagan R, Kucherlapati R: Localization of the human α-globin structural gene to chromosome 16 in somatic cell hybrids by molecular hybridization assay. Cell 12:205, 1977.
14. Lebo RV, Carrano AV, Buckhardt-Schultz K, Dozy AM, Yu L-C, Kan YW: Assignment of human γ-, δ- and β-globin genes to the short arm of chromosome 11 by chromosome sorting and DNA restriction analysis. Proc Natl Acad Sci USA 76:5804, 1979.
15. Jeffreys A: Recent studies of gene evolution using recombinant DNA. Supra #5, p 1.

Molecular Pathology of α-Thalassemia*

Stephen A. Liebhaber, MD, and Yuet Wai Kan, MD

THE α-THALASSEMIA SYNDROMES

Four clinical states of increasing severity are recognized in the α–thalassemia syndromes: the silent carrier state, α-thalassemia trait, hemoglobin H disease (Hb H), and fetal hydrops associated with homozygous α-thalassemia [1]. Initially, these four clinical syndromes were attributed to two different genetic defects, the α-thalassemia-1 and the α-thalassemia-2 genotypes [2]. The former genotype suppresses α-globin chain production more severely than the latter. The silent carrier state is due to heterozygosity for the α-thalassemia-2 genotype; α-thalassemia trait is caused by heterozygosity for the α-thalassemia-1 genotype, or homozygosity for the α-thalassemia-2 genotype [3]. The compound heterozygous state of α-thalassemia-1 and α-thalassemia-2 produces Hb H disease. Homozygosity for α-thalassemia-1 results in the lethal hydrops fetalis.

During the past several years, new methods of DNA analysis have helped define the exact molecular defect in many of these disorders. We now know that several different mutations in the α-globin genes adversely affect α-globin gene function and produce the α-thalassemia phenotype. These defects include partial as well as complete α-globin gene deletion and single nucleotide mutations. The cause of defective α-globin gene expression in several subsets of α-thalassemia remains undefined.

NORMAL α-GLOBIN GENES

The duplicated human α-globin genes are located approximately 3,700 basepairs (bp) (1,000 bp = 1 kilobase = 1 kb) apart on chromosome 16 [4-6] (Fig. 1). The more 3′ (rightward) locus according to the direction of transcription is known as the α1-globin gene and the 5′ (leftward) locus as α2. The pseudo α-globin gene, which is 75% homologous to the α-globin gene, lies 5′ to the α2-

*Supported in part by grants from NIH (AM 16666) and the March of Dimes Birth Defects Foundation. Y.W.K. is an investigator of the Howard Hughes Medical Institute.

Birth Defects: Original Article Series, Volume 18, Number 7, pages 35–44
© 1982 March of Dimes Birth Defects Foundation

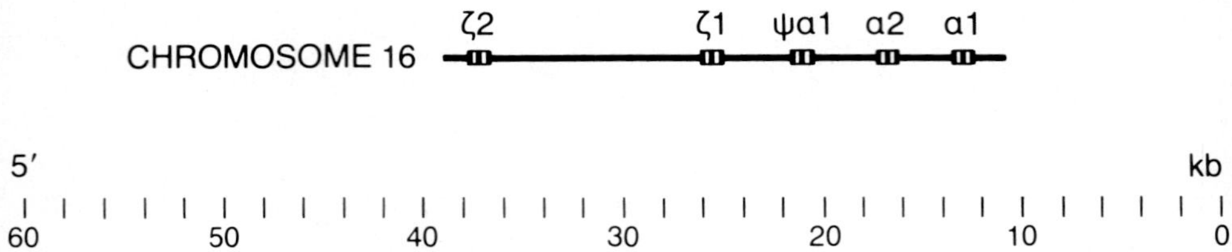

Fig. 1. Diagram of the human α-globin gene cluster. The ψ α1- and ζ-globin genes are nonfunctional. The genes are expressed during development in a 5′ to 3′ direction. The scale indicates distances in kilobases (kb).

gene locus [7]. Sequence analysis of this pseudogene indicates that it is nonfunctional [8]. Two embryonic α-like genes, ζ1 and ζ2, lie upstream from the pseudo α-gene. A termination codon at amino acid position number 6 renders the ζ1-globin gene nonfunctional [9]. Thus there is only one functional ζ-globin gene, ζ2, on the chromosome [10].

The nucleotide sequences of both α-globin structural genes have been determined [11-13] (Fig. 2). As with most eukaryotic genes, the coding sequences are not colinear with their respective mRNA, but are interrupted by two intervening sequences, also called introns. α-Globin has two introns: the first, which lies between amino acids 30 and 31, is 117 nucleotides long; the second, located between amino acid 99 and 100, is 149 nucleotides long in α2 and 156 in α1. While the proteins encoded by both α-globin loci are identical, the DNA sequences vary somewhat in the second intervening sequence and extensively in the 3′ noncoding region following the termination codon.

MOLECULAR MECHANISM OF α-THALASSEMIA

The heterogeneous molecular mechanisms that produce the α-thalassemia syndromes are summarized in Table 1. The most common mechanism is deletion of DNA segments that contain either one α-globin locus or both loci and result in the α-thalassemia-2 and α-thalassemia-1 genotypes, respectively. In addition to the deletion-type α-thalassemias, several α-thalassemia lesions have now been defined in which the impairment of α-globin gene function does not stem from gross deletion. These are categorized as nondeletion α-thalassemias.

DELETION-TYPE α-THALASSEMIA

Several different deletions that produce the α-thalassemia-1 genotype have been identified. Two of these deletions remove completely both α-globin loci and are probably caused by unequal crossing-over of homologous chromosomes

```
cccgggctccgcgccagccaatgagcgccgcccggccgggcgtgcccccgcgccccaagcataaaccctgg

                                                            1
                                                            Val Leu Ser
cgcgctcgcggcccggcACTCTTCTGGTCCCCACAGACTCAGAGAGAACCCACCATG   GTG CTG TCT

                        10                                      20
Pro Ala Asp Lys Thr Asn Val Lys Ala Ala Trp Gly Lys Val Gly Ala His Ala
CCT GCC GAC AAG ACC AAC GTC AAG GCC GCC TGG GGT AAG GTC GGC GCG CAC GCT

                                30
Gly Glu Tyr Gly Ala Glu Ala Leu Glu Arg
GGC GAG TAT GGT GCG GAG GCC CTG GAG AGG  tgaggctccctcccctgctccgacccgggc

tcctcgcccgcccggacccacaggccaccctcaaccgtcctggccccggacccaaaccccacccctcactc

                    32                          40
                    Met Phe Leu Ser Phe Pro Thr Thr Lys Thr Tyr Phe Pro
tgcttctccccgcagg    ATG TTC CTG TCC TTC CCC ACC ACC AAG ACC TAC TTC CCG

                    50                                      60
His Phe Asp Leu Ser His Gly Ser Ala Gln Val Lys Gly His Gly Lys Lys Val
CAC TTC GAC CTG AGC CAC GGC TCT GCC CAG GTT AAG GGC CAC GGC AAG AAG GTG

                            70                                      80
Ala Asp Ala Leu Thr Asn Ala Val Ala His Val Asp Asp Met Pro Asn Ala Leu
GCC GAC GCG CTG ACC AAC GCC GTG GCG CAC GTG GAC GAC ATG CCC AAC GCG CTG

                                    90
Ser Ala Leu Ser Asp Leu His Ala His Lys Leu Arg Val Asp Pro Val Asn Phe
TCC GCC CTG AGC GAC CTG CAC GCG CAC AAG CTT CGG GTG GAC CCG GTC AAC TTC

99
Lys
AAG  gtgagcggcgggccgggagcgatctgggtcgagggcgagatggcgccttcctcgcagggcagagg
                                                               t

atcacgcgggttgcgggaggtgtagcgcaggcggcggctgcgggcctgggccctcggccccactgaccctc
                                                    -------g
                100                                     110
                Leu Leu Ser His Cys Leu Leu Val Thr Leu Ala Ala His Leu
ttctctgcacag    CTC CTA AGC CAC TGC CTG CTG GTG ACC CTG GCC GCC CAC CTC

                        120                                     130
Pro Ala Glu Phe Thr Pro Ala Val His Ala Ser Leu Asp Lys Phe Leu Ala Ser
CCC GCC GAG TTC ACC CCT GCG GTG CAC GCC TCC CTG GAC AAG TTC CTG GCT TCT

                                140
Val Ser Thr Val Leu Thr Ser Lys Tyr Arg OC
GTG AGC ACC GTG CTG ACC TCC AAA TAC CGT TAA   GCTGGAGCCTCGGTGGCCATGCTTCT
                                                            A   G T C  C

TGCCCCTTGGGCCTCCCCCAGCCCCTCCTCCCCTTCCTGCACCCGTACCCCCGTGGTCTTTGAATAAAGT
     GC          AA G G            C T      G CC TT  -

CTGAGTGGGCGGCagcctgtgtgtgcctgggtttttccctcagcaaacgtgccaagcatgggcgtggaca
                                 c c  tg  ccgg   t      ca    ag   ttt

gct
c
```

Fig. 2. Nucleotide sequence of the human α1- and α2-globin genes. The α1-globin gene is completely displayed and the differences found in the α2-gene are indicated.

TABLE 1. Defined Molecular Mechanisms in α-Thalassemia

α-thalassemia-2 (decreased function of a single α-globin locus)
1. Deletions of a single α-globin locus (-α).
2. Termination codon mutation in the α2-locus; eg Hb Constant Spring ($\alpha^{c.s.}\alpha$).
3. Intron mutation affecting processing of α2-globin mRNA precursor.
4. Single amino acid substitution preventing α1-β1-formation.
α-thalassemia-1 (decreased function of both α-globin loci in cis)
1. Deletions of both α-loci (--); no α-globin chains present in the homozygous state.

that malalign between the pseudo-α-globin gene on one chromosome and the ζ2-globin gene on another. The extent of the deletion varies according to the point of cross-over [10]. One deletion, characterized in a Greek subject, is produced by a cross-over that occurs 5′ to the ζ1-globin gene. The resultant chromosome contains only the ζ2-gene; the ζ1-, pseudo-α-, α2-, and α1-genes are deleted. A second type of cross-over occurs at a point 3′ to the ζ1-gene, and the resultant chromosome bears the ζ2- and ζ1-genes, but no pseudo-α-, α1- or α2-genes. Two other deletions which result from different mechanisms remove the entire α2-globin gene and the 5′ portion of the α1-locus to amino acid 56 of the α1-locus [14]. In one case, the deletion is quite extensive and involves the ζ2-gene; in the other, the α2-locus and the 5′ part of the α1-locus are deleted. Both cause loss of function of both α-globin genes [15].

The α-thalassemia-2 genotype, in which only one functional α-globin gene remains on the chromosome, is most frequently caused by gene deletion (Fig. 3). Two deletion mechanisms that involve unequal cross-over between malaligned chromosomes have been defined [5,7,16]. In the so-called "leftward" deletion, a stretch of DNA just 3′ to the pseudo-α-globin gene malaligns with a homologous region 3′ to the α2-locus of the other chromosome. Unequal crossing-over in this region removes a 4.2-kb DNA fragment that contains the α2-globin locus. The "rightward" deletion involves misalignment between the homologous region that embraces the α1- and α2-globin loci. Unequal crossing-over deletes a 3.7-kb DNA fragment and again yields a chromosome that contains only one α-globin locus (Fig. 3).

The reciprocal products of the unequal exchange that produces the rightward and leftward deletions are chromosomes that contain three α-globin loci. Triplicated α-globin loci generated both from rightward and leftward cross-overs have been identified by restriction endonuclease mapping [17-19]. The rightward cross-over mechanism appears to be far more common than the leftward and has been found in people of African, Mediterranean, and Asian origin. The leftward

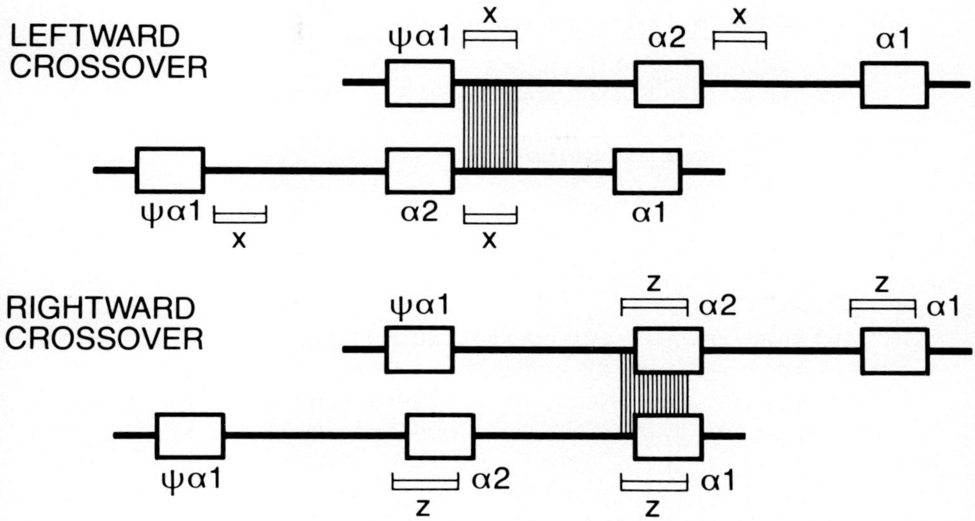

Fig. 3. Two types of chromosomal malalignment and unequal cross-over that produce the single α-globin locus. The homologous regions are designated X and Z. Vertical lines show the border of crossing-over.

cross-over, both for the single α-globin locus and the triple loci, has so far been defined only in the Asian population. The significantly lower frequency of the triple α-chromosome, as compared to the single α-chromosome, suggests that the latter offers a selective advantage.

POPULATION GENETICS OF DELETION-TYPE α-THALASSEMIA

The frequency of the single α-globin locus produced by deletion is high; in certain populations it exceeds the normal genotype with the duplicated α-loci [20]. The distribution of α-thalassemia appears to follow that of malaria, and may be related to the protection it offers against this disease [21].

The geographic distribution patterns of the various α-thalassemia syndromes can be explained by comparing the frequencies of the α-thalassemia-1 and α-thalassemia-2 genotypes (Table 2). Both genotypes occur with approximately equal frequency in Asians and combine to produce all four α-thalassemia syndromes (D. Todd, personal communication). In Mediterraneans, on the other hand, the frequency of the α-thalassemia-2 genotype is much higher than the α-thalassemia-1 genotype [22]. Hence, in this population, α-thalassemia trait is usually due to homozygosity for the α-thalassemia-2 gene; Hb H disease occurs because of the high frequency of the α-thalassemia-2 chromosome coupled with

TABLE 2. Distribution of α-Thalassemia in World Populations

	Haplotype		Common Genotype for α-Thal Trait	Hb H Disease	Homozygous α-Thalassemia
	-α	--		--/-α	--/--
Asian	Present	Present	--/$\alpha\alpha$	Present	Present
African	Frequent	Very rare	-α/-α	Rare	Absent
Greek Cypriot	Common	Not common	-α/-α	Present	Rare
Sardinian	Frequent	Rare	-α/-α	Rare	Absent

the rarer α-thalassemia-1 chromosome; and homozygous α-thalassemia-1 is rarely seen. In Africans, the α-thalassemia-2 gene is common and the α-thalassemia-1 gene is rare. Hence, Hb H disease is unusual, and homozygous α-thalassemia-1 (fetal hydrops) has never been described [23].

NONDELETION α-THALASSEMIA

Alpha-thalassemia can also be caused by lesions that do not involve gross α-globin gene deletion. The first such lesion recognized was a termination codon mutation found in Hb Constant Spring [24]. A single nucleotide mutation alters the termination codon of the α2-gene (UAA $\rightarrow$ CAA) so that α-globin mRNA translation continues until the next termination codon is reached 93 nucleotides (31 amino acids) later in the normally untranslated 3′ noncoding region of the mRNA. The Constant Spring chain thus contains 172 amino acids instead of the normal 141. Only very small quantities of this mutant chain are produced, possibly because of its instability [25], and the instability of the mRNA that encodes it [26]. The mutant α-globin Constant Spring chain comprises approximately 1% of total α-globin in heterozygotes for this mutation. The net effect on α-globin production is loss of globin from the α-Constant Spring gene, which in an otherwise normal genetic setting, results in the α-thalassemia-2 genotype. The Constant Spring mutation is prevalent in Southeast Asia. Termination codon mutations have also been described in other populations. These and several other similar types of mutations can result in depressed production of abnormal α-globin proteins [27-29].

Another so-called nondeletion α-thalassemia found in the Mediterranean population is due to a small deletion that affects the α2-locus [30]. Five basepairs are deleted from the first intervening sequence, just one nucleotide past the 5′ splice junction. This lesion affects the invariant GT sequence at the intron-exon junction (which is essential for splicing out the intergenic sequences). The mRNA is abnormally spliced and the reading frame is shifted, causing early termination.

The improperly processed mRNA from this gene presumably is destroyed in the nucleus as no mRNA from this locus is found in the reticulocyte.

A third type of nondeletion α-thalassemia is due to a posttranslational mechanism which results from a single amino acid substitution [31,32]. A leucine (Leu) to proline (Pro) mutation in the α2-globin gene disrupts the major α1-β1 contact points and impedes the formation of α1-β1 dimers. The heterozygous state of the resultant syndrome resembles α-thalassemia trait. When combined with α-thalassemia due to deletion of both α-globin genes, this nondeletion lesion produces Hb H disease.

α-GLOBIN GENE EXPRESSION

Since both the α1- and α2-loci normally encode α-globin chains of identical amino acid sequences, it has been previously impossible to identify the defective genes in the α-thalassemia syndromes. However, the relative levels of expression of the two α-globin loci can now be determined by assaying the level of α1- and α2-globin mRNA in the reticulocytes and bone marrow. One and one-half to three times more mRNA originates from the α2-globin locus than the α1-locus [26,33]. Since most α-globin mutants are present at 25% in mature reticulocytes, the amount of α-globin chains synthesized by both loci must be identical [34]. The disparity in mRNA levels may be related to differences in mRNA metabolism or in the translation rate of the two mRNA species.

Measuring the proportion of α1- to α2-globin mRNA has increased our understanding of certain α-thalassemia syndromes. mRNA transcripts from both the leftward and rightward α-thalassemia-2 genotypes contain the 3′ end of the α1-locus (Fig. 4). Thus the cross-over that results in the rightward deletion must occur upstream from the 3′ noncoding region of the α1-globin gene [26,32]. One patient heterozygous for the triple α-chromosomes had more than the normal quantity of α2-globin mRNA [26], indicating that the extra α-globin locus (α2) is active in mRNA transcription.

The discriminatory α-globin mRNA assays can be used to identify defective genes and determine the nature of the defect in the nondeletion α-thalassemias. For example, in a patient with Hb H Constant Spring, α2-globin mRNA (ie mRNA encoding the Constant Spring protein) was seen in the bone marrow, but not in the reticulocytes [26], implying that the Constant Spring mRNA is unstable. In the patient with the splicing site abnormality in the α2-gene, no α2-globin mRNA was detected in reticulocytes, confirming the lack of function of this gene [33]. In the patient with the posttranslational defect, the α1- to α2-ratio was normal [35]. Further application of this approach may help identify and classify nondeletion α-thalassemia in other populations.

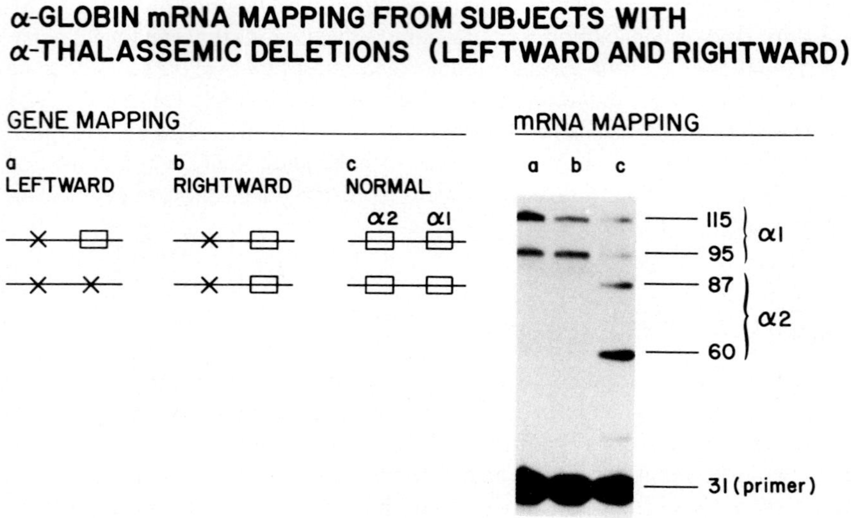

Fig. 4. Analysis of the function of the α-globin genes. The principle of the cDNA assay is detailed in reference 26. The mRNA from the $\alpha 2$-locus generates two bands of 60 and 87 nucleotides; mRNA from the $\alpha 1$-locus produces two bands of 95 and 115 nucleotides. Only $\alpha 1$-mRNA is detected in both the rightward and leftward cross-overs.

CONCLUSION

Several different mutational events can decrease α-globin production and result in α-thalassemia. As in the β-thalassemia syndromes, these lesions are heterogeneous, and many other mutations will undoubtedly be uncovered. The severity of the α-thalassemia phenotype correlates inversely with the number of actively functioning α-globin genes. While the most commonly identified cause of loss of α-globin gene function is gene deletion, other etiologies such as small deletions and point mutations are clearly important. The frequency and variety of these nondeletion α-thalassemia genotypes can be investigated by a combination of α-globin mRNA analysis discriminatory for the two α-globin loci, and fine structure analysis of identified dysfunctional genes.

ACKNOWLEDGMENTS

We thank Dr. Bernard Forget for supplying the pJW101, and Jennifer Gampell for editorial comments.

REFERENCES

1. Weatherall DJ, Clegg JB: "The Thalassemia Syndromes," 3rd Ed. Oxford, England: Blackwell, 1980.
2. Wasi P, Na-Nakorn S, Suingdumrong A: Haemoglobin H disease in Thailand: A genetical study. Nature 204:907–908, 1964.
3. Lehmann H: Different types of alpha-thalassaemia and significance of haemoglobin Bart's in neonates. Lancet 2:78–80, 1970.
4. Orkin S: The duplicated human α-globin genes lie close together in cellular DNA. Proc Natl Acad Sci USA 75:5950–5954, 1978.
5. Embury SH, Lebo RV, Dozy AM, Kan YW: Organization of the α-globin genes in the Chinese α-thalassemia syndromes. J Clin Invest 63:1307–1310, 1979.
6. Deisseroth A, Nienhuis A, Turner P, Velez R, Anderson WF, Ruddle F, Lawrence J, Creagan R, Kucherlapati R: Localization of the human α-globin structural gene to chromosome 16 in somatic cell hybrids by molecular hybridization assay. Cell 12:205–218, 1977.
7. Lauer J, Shen C-KJ, Maniatis T: The chromosomal arrangement of human α-like globin genes: Sequence homology and α-globin gene deletions. Cell 20:119–130, 1980.
8. Proudfoot NJ, Maniatis T: The structure of a human α-globin pseudogene and its relationship to α-globin gene duplication. Cell 21:537–544, 1980.
9. Proudfoot N, Shander M, Woude SV, Maniatis T: The structure and transcription of normal and abnormal human globin genes. J Supramol Struc Cell Biochem (Suppl) 5:381, 1981.
10. Pressley L, Higgs DR, Clegg JB, Weatherall DJ: Gene deletions in α-thalassemia prove that the 5′ ζ locus is functional. Proc Natl Acad Sci USA 77:3586–3589, 1980.
11. Liebhaber SA, Goossens M, Kan YW: Cloning and complete nucleotide sequence of human 5′-α-globin gene. Proc Natl Acad Sci USA 77:7054–7058, 1980.
12. Michelson AM, Orkin SH: The 3′ untranslated regions of the duplicated human α-globin genes are unexpectedly divergent. Cell 22:371–377, 1980.
13. Liebhaber SA, Goossens M, Kan YW: Homology and concerted evolution at the α1 and α2 loci of human α-globin. Nature 290:26–29, 1981.
14. Orkin SH, Michelson A: Partial deletion of the α-globin structural gene in human α-thalassemia. Nature 286:538–540, 1980.
15. Pressley L, Higgs DR, Aldridge B, Metaxatou-Mavromati A, Clegg JB, Weatherall DJ: Characterisation of a new thalassaemia 1 defect due to a partial deletion of the α-globin gene complex. Nucleic Acids Res 8:4889–4898, 1980.
16. Embury SH, Miller JA, Dozy AM, Kan YW, Chan V, Todd D: Two different molecular organizations account for the single α-globin gene of α-thalassemia-2 genotype. J Clin Invest 66:1319–1325, 1980.
17. Goossens M, Dozy AM, Embury SH, Zachariades Z, Hadjiminas M, Stamatoyannopoulos G, Kan YW: Triplicated α-globin loci in humans. Proc Natl Acad Sci USA 77:518–521, 1980.
18. Higgs DR, Old JM, Pressley L, Clegg JB, Weatherall DJ: A novel α-globin gene arrangement in man. Nature 284:632–635, 1980.
19. Lie-Injo LE, Herrera AR, Kan YW: Two types of triplicated α-globin loci in humans. Nucleic Acids Res 9:3707–3717, 1981.
20. Brittenham G: Genetic model for observed distribution of proportions of haemoglobin in sickle-cell trait. Nature 268:635–636, 1977.
21. Friedman MJ: Oxidant damage mediates variant red cell resistance to malaria. Nature 280: 245–247, 1979.
22. Pirastu M, Lee KY, Dozy AM, Kan YW, Stamatoyannopoulos G, Hadjiminas MG, Zachariades Z, Angius A, Furbetta M, Rosatelli C, Cao A: Alpha-thalassemia in two Mediterranean populations. Blood (In press)

23. Dozy AM, Kan Y, Embury SH, Mentzer WC, Wang WC, Lubin B, Davis JR Jr, Koenig HM: α-Globin gene organisation in blacks precludes the severe form of α-thalassemia. Nature 280:605–607, 1979.
24. Milner PF, Clegg JB, Weatherall DJ: Haemoglobin-H disease due to a unique haemoglobin variant with an elongated alpha-chain. Lancet 1:729–732, 1971.
25. Kan YW, Todd D, Dozy AM: Haemoglobin Constant Spring synthesis in red cell precursors. Br J Haematol 28:103–107, 1974.
26. Liebhaber SA, Kan YW: Differentiation of the mRNA transcripts originating from the α1- and α2-globin gene in normals and α-thalassemics. J Clin Invest 68:439–446, 1981.
27. Clegg JB, Weatherall DJ, Contopoulou-Griva I, Caroutsos K, Poungouras P, Tsevrenis H: Haemoglobin Icaria, a new chain-termination mutant which causes α thalassaemia. Nature 251:245–247, 1974.
28. De Jong WW, Khan PM, Bernini LF: Hemoglobin Koya Dora: High frequency of a chain termination mutant. Am J Hum Genet 27:81–90, 1975.
29. Bradley TB, Wohl RC, Smith GJ: Elongation of the α-chain in a Black family: Interaction with Hb G Philadelphia. Clin Res 23:131, 1975.
30. Orkin SH, Goff SC, Hechtman RL: An intervening sequence splice junction mutation in man. Proc Natl Acad Sci USA 78:5041–5045, 1981.
31. Kan YW, Dozy AM, Trecartin R, Todd D: Identification of a nondeletion defect in α-thalassemia. N Engl J Med 297:1080–1084, 1977.
32. Goossens M, Lee KY, Liebhaber SA, Kan YW: Globin structural mutant $\alpha^{125Leu \rightarrow Pro}$: A novel cause of α thalassemia. Nature (In press)
33. Orkin S, Goff S: The duplicated human α-globin genes: Their relative expression as measured by RNA analysis. Cell 24:345–351, 1981.
34. Nute P: Multiple hemoglobin α-chain loci in monkeys, apes and man. Ann NY Acad Sci 241:39–60, 1974.
35. Liebhaber SA, Kan YW: α-Thalassemia caused by an unstable α-globin mutant. Submitted for publication.

The Gene Defects in the β-Thalassemias*

Arthur Bank, MD, Michael Baird, PhD, M. Catherine Driscoll, MD, Robert G. Pergolizzi, PhD, and Sally E. Spence, PhD

The β-thalassemias are a heterogeneous group of human anemias characterized by decreased or absent β-globin synthesis [1, 2]. Recent molecular biology techniques have permitted the analysis of gene defects in these disorders. These new methods have permitted the precise delineation of the nucleotide defects in DNA in several different types of patients with these disorders. To date, patients with β°-thalassemia have been shown to have several different kinds of defects: 1) deletion of the 3′ end of the β-globin gene [3, 4], and 2) termination codons due to amber mutations at various positions of the β-globin gene. These have included defects at codons 17 and 39 [5, 6]. Recently, we have defined defects at the splice junction of the large intervening sequence (IVS 2) of the β-globin gene associated with β°-thalassemia phenotype as well [7]. In β^+-thalassemia, a single nucleotide defect within the small intervening sequence (IVS 1) of the β-globin gene has been described [8, 9]. This defect creates a false splice junction within IVS 1, which is used to splice out a smaller than normal portion of the IVS 1 during the process of RNA metabolism in the nucleus; this results in an abnormal β-globin mRNA precursor and decreased β-globin synthesis. This paper will summarize the defects reported to date in β^+- and β°-thalassemia, and will give details about recent results in our laboratory in two different kinds of β°-thalassemia. In addition, we will describe new polymorphisms in the β-globin genes which may be useful in the antenatal diagnosis of the β-thalassemias, and in following the evolution of β-thalassemia genes.

MATERIALS AND METHODS

Restriction Endonuclease Analysis

Restriction enzyme analysis is carried out as described previously, using high molecular weight DNA derived from white blood cells, lymphocyte cell lines, or spleen material [10]. The DNA is separated on agarose gels on the basis of size,

*This work was made possible by NIH-AM-25274 grant, New York Community Trust 6-40664 grant, and NIH-CA-21768 grant.

Birth Defects: Original Article Series, Volume 18, Number 7, pages 45–50
© 1982 March of Dimes Birth Defects Foundation

and subjected to cleavage with specific restriction enzymes. Probes used in the studies reported here were directed at specifically detecting IVS 2 sequences. To do this, we used the 0.92 kilobase (kb) β-IVS 2-containing fragment of the β-globin gene isolated in our laboratory [7, 11]. After cleavage of the pBR 322 plasmid containing this fragment with Eco RI and Bam HI, the specific probe was isolated by sucrose density gradient centrifugation separation; this and other probes were labeled with P^{32} [11]. A 4.4 kb Pst probe, which contains the entire β-globin gene including approximately 2 kb of 5′ and 3′ flanking nucleotide sequences was also used [11]. A specific probe for the δ-globin gene was obtained by isolating δ-IVS sequences from a pBR 322 plasmid containing the 0.95 kb fragment.

Cloning

Genes from two different patients with β^+-thalassemia were isolated by creating a charon 4A library of DNA fragments [12]. In these studies, partial Eco RI digestion was used to obtain fragments of between 15 and 20 kb in size [11]. Clones were obtained which contained β-globin genes. These clones subsequently were subcloned into pBR 322 [11], and appropriate regions sequenced by either Maxam-Gilbert sequencing [13] or dideoxynucleotide analysis and sequencing as described by Sanger et al [14].

RESULTS

Termination Codon in a β°-Gene

DNA from a patient with a β^+-thalassemia phenotype was used to clone β-globin genes. One of the two β-globin genes was isolated from a charon 4A library and subcloned [11]. The β-globin gene was completely sequenced from 200 nucleotides 5′ to the cap site through the three coding regions and two IVS, and past the 3′ poly A addition site in the untranslated region 3′ to the gene [15]. The only change from normal detected in this gene was a single nucleotide change at position 39: a change leading from codon CAG, which codes for glutamine to a codon TAG, which is a nonsense, amber, or termination codon [15]. This result indicates that this patient most likely is doubly heterozygous for β^+- and β°-thalassemia, and we have isolated and sequenced a β°-thalassemia gene. The other gene in this patient is an obligate β^+-thalassemia gene, and should be of great interest. It is currently being isolated. A formal alternative to this hypothesis is that human cells may contain suppressor mutations, and we have isolated a β^+-thalassemia gene in a patient with a suppressor mutation, which permits the biosynthesis of β-globin from this amber mutation-containing sequence.

Splice Junction Mutations in the β-Globin Gene

We have used restriction analysis to detect a subgroup of patients with β°-thalassemia who have defects at the 5′ splice junction of IVS 2. The enzyme Hph I was found to recognize the specific sequence at this 5′ splice junction, including the highly conserved GGT sequence found in this region. A variety of DNAs from different ethnic groups with β°-thalassemia were analyzed using the enzyme Hph I [7]. With a β-IVS 2 DNA probe, the normal fragment found in normal cellular DNA is 0.9 kb in size. When there is a change in the sequence at the 5′ end of IVS 2, this 0.9 kb fragment is lost, and is replaced by a 1.0 kb fragment. Subsequent double digestions have confirmed that the site of the change which causes the larger than normal Hph I fragment in these patients is at the 5′ end of IVS 2. Figure 1 shows DNAs from patients with β°-thalassemia who are either homozygous or heterozygous for this change. These latter patients have both the normal 0.9 kb fragment as well as the abnormal 1.0 kb fragment. These patients are of Greek and Italian extraction, which indicates that this defect is widespread in Mediterranean populations. The initial patients homozygous for this defect were of Iranian and Italian origins [7].

β^+-Thalassemia

We have isolated another β-globin gene-containing clone from a patient with β^+-thalassemia. This clone's DNA contains no defects in any of the coding regions or in IVS 1. IVS 2 is currently being completely sequenced, and there are preliminary data indicating that changes in IVS 2 are present [16].

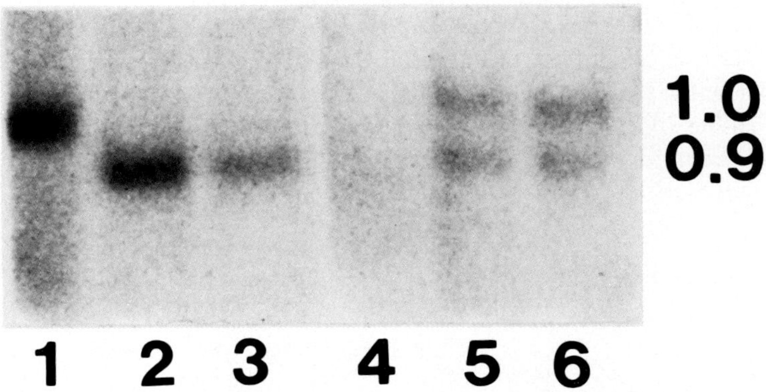

Fig. 1. Restriction analysis of human cellular DNA with Hph I. The 0.9 kb normal band, and the abnormal 1.0 kb bands are seen as described in the text. Lane 1, DNA from a patient with β°-thalassemia, homozygous for 5′ splice junction defect; Lane 2, a normal; Lane 3, normal Hph I pattern, from a patient homozygous for β°-thalassemia; Lane 5, a heterozygote for β-thalassemia; and Lane 6, a homozygote for β-thalassemia.

New Polymorphisms in the β-Globin Gene

Recently, we have screened several populations with an enzyme Asu I, which recognizes the sequence 5′ GGNCC 3′ [17]. When the β-IVS 2 probe is used, a 0.8 kb fragment is usually found to contain the entire β-IVS 2 in normal DNA. However, we have found that approximately 10% of patients in an Israeli population without thalassemia, have a polymorphism in this gene which leads to the loss of an Asu I site and a 1.0 kb fragment generated. Over 30% of patients have a similar polymorphism in β^+- and β°-thalassemia. Although this polymorphism does not appear to be very tightly linked to the β-thalassemia gene, it can be used in combination with other polymorphisms and family data for the antenatal diagnosis of thalassemia, and to follow the evolution of specific gene defects in the β-thalassemias. Using a δ-IVS 2 probe, a polymorphism in the δ-gene locus has also been detected with Asu I. A 3.0 kb fragment is found to occur in a minority of patients who are either normal or have thalassemia, while a 1.1 kb fragment is detected in normals [17].

DISCUSSION

New techniques in molecular biology have permitted a more precise analysis of the DNA defects in patients with β^+- and β°-thalassemia (Table 1). These studies have revealed a marked heterogeneity of nucleotide changes in these disorders, leading to similar phenotypes. In β°-thalassemia, deletions at the 3′ end of the β-globin gene, termination codon defects, and defects at the 5′ splice junction of IVS 2 have all been associated with the β°-thalassemia phenotype. The discovery that a single nucleotide change at a splice junction can cause absent function of the β-globin locus [7] is the first evidence in eukaryotes that splice junction integrity is required for normal gene function. Other defects in β°-thalassemia may be caused by other changes in IVS 1 or IVS 2, other nonsense codons, or defects in the 5′ or 3′ flanking regions of these genes, which may affect either initiation of transcription of these genes or normal processing of their transcripts.

TABLE 1. Gene Defects in Thalassemias

β^+-Thalassemia	- Mid-IVS I Change
	- ? Other Mid IVS OR 5′ OR 3′ Flanks
β°-Thalassemia	- Premature Termination Mutations
	- Codon 17
	- Codon 39
	- Other Termination Codons
	- Splice Junction Defects
	- 5′ IVS II Junction
	- Structural Gene Deletions

In the β^+-thalassemias, defects with β-IVS 1 appear to cause the β^+-thalassemia phenotype by producing a new false splice junction within the β-IVS 1, which leads to an abnormal β-globin mRNA produce [8, 9]. Studies of intact bone marrow cells of patients with β^+-thalassemia have indicated that large molecular weight β-globin mRNA-containing molecules accumulate in the nuclei of some patients with β^+-thalassemia, and support this concept [18-20]. We have recently begun to analyze a gene from a patient with β^+-thalassemia, whose defects appear to be localized entirely within β-IVS 2, except for a single codon change, a third base change at codon 2 [16]. It will be of great interest to determine if these changes within β-IVS 2 can produce the β^+-thalassemia phenotype. Again, other defects within both the IVS 1 and IVS 2, as well as in the 5′ or 3′ flanking regions of these genes, may be expected to cause β^+-thalassemia by either leading to decreased transcription of β-globin mRNA precursors or abnormal processing of these precursors. Further studies using both nuclear and whole cell systems will be necessary to distinguish between these possibilities. However, the availability on cloned DNA fragments representing the entire β-globin gene complex and developing cell culture systems for expressing these isolated genes [21,22] should make these studies feasible in the near future.

REFERENCES

1. Bank A, Mears JG, Ramirez F: Disorders of human hemoglobin. Science 207:486, 1980.
2. Weatherall DJ, Clegg JB: "The Thalassemia Syndromes," 3rd Ed. Oxford, England: Blackwell, 1979.
3. Orkin SH, Old JM, Weatherall DJ, Nathan DG: Partial deletion of β globin DNA in certain patients with $\beta°$ thalassemia. Proc Natl Acad Sci USA 76:2400, 1979.
4. Flavell RA, Bernards R, Kooter JM, De Boer R: The structure of the human β globin gene in β^+ thalassemia. Nucleic Acids Res 6:2749, 1979.
5. Chang JC, Kan YW: $\beta°$ thalassemia, a nonsense mutation in man. Proc Natl Acad Sci USA 76:2888, 1979.
6. Trecartin RF, Liebhaber SA, Chang JC, Lee KY, Kan YW, Furbetta M, Angius A, Cao A: $\beta°$ thalassemia in Sardinia is caused by a nonsense mutation. J Clin Invest 68:1012, 1981.
7. Baird M, Driscoll MC, Schreiner H, Sciarratta GV, Sansone G, Niazi G, Ramirez F, Bank A: A nucleotide change at a splice junction in the human β globin gene is associated with $\beta°$ thalassemia. Proc Natl Acad Sci USA 78:4218, 1981.
8. Spritz RA, Jagadeeswaran P, Choudary PV, Biro PA, Elder JT, deRiel JK, Manley JL, Gefter ML, Forget BG, Weissman SM: Base substitution in an intervening sequence of a β^+ thalassemic human globin gene. Proc Natl Acad Sci USA 78:2455, 1981.
9. Westaway D, Williamson R: An intron nucleotide sequence variant in a cloned β^+ thalassemia globin gene. Nucleic Acids Res 9:1777, 1981.
10. Mears JG, Ramirez F, Leibowitz D, Nakamura F, Bloom A, Konotey-Ahulu F, Bank A: Changes in restricted human cellular DNA fragments containing globin gene sequences in the thalassemias and related disorders. Proc Natl Acad Sci USA 75:1222, 1978.
11. Burns AL, Spence S, Kosche KA, Ramirez F, Mears JG, Schreiner H, Miller C, Baird M, Leibowitz D, Giardina P, Markenson A, Bank A: Isolation and characterization of cloned DNA: The δ and β globin genes in homozygous β^+ thalassemia. Blood 57:140, 1981.

12. Maniatis T, Hardison RC, Lacy E, Lauer J, O'Connell C, Quon D, Sim UK, Efstratiadis A: The isolation of structural genes from libraries of eucaryotic DNA. Cell 15:686, 1978.
13. Maxam AM, Gilbert W: A new method for sequencing DNA. Proc Natl Acad Sci USA 74:560, 1977.
14. Sanger FE, Coulson AR, Barelle BG, Smith AJH, Roe BA: Cloning in single stranded bacteria phage as an aid to rabbit cDNA sequencing. J Mol Biol 143:161, 1981.
15. Pergolizzi RG, Spritz RA, Spence SE, Goossens M, Kan YW, Bank A: Two cloned β thalassemia genes are associated with amber mutations at codon 39. Nucleic Acids Res 9:7065, 1981.
16. Spence SE, Pergolizzi RG, Donovan-Peluso M, Kosche KA, Dobkin CS, Bank A: Five nucleotide changes in the large intervening sequence of a β globin gene in a β^+ thalassemia patient. Nucleic Acids Res 10:1283, 1982.
17. Driscoll MC, Baird M, Rachmilewitz EA, Bank A: A new polymorphism in the human β globin gene useful in antenatal diagnosis. J Clin Invest 68:915, 1981.
18. Maquat LE, Kinniburgh AJ, Beach LR, Honig GR, Lazerson J, Ershler WB, Ross J: Processing of human β globin mRNA is defective in three patients with β^+ thalassemia. Proc Natl Acad Sci USA 77:4287, 1980.
19. Kantor JA, Turner PH, Nienhuis AW: β thalassemia: Mutations which affect processing of the β globin mRNA precursor. Cell 21:149, 1980.
20. Benz EJ, Scarpa AL, deRiel JK, Tonkonow BL, Ritchey AK, Forget GB: Globin messenger RNA metabolism in normal and thalassemic erythroblasts. In Stamatoyannopoulos G, Nienhuis AW (eds): "Organization and Expression of Globin Genes." New York: Alan R Liss, 1981, p 269.
21. Gluzman Y: SV40 transformed simian cells support the replication of early SV40 mutants. Cell 23:175, 1981.
22. Mellon P, Parker V, Gluzman Y, Maniatis T: Identification of DNA sequences required for transcription of the human α_1 globin gene using a new SV40 host vector system. Cell 27:279, 1981.

Globin mRNA Metabolism and Gene Structure in β^+-Thalassemia*

Bernard G. Forget, MD, Edward J. Benz, Jr., MD, Richard A. Spritz, MD, and Sherman M. Weissman, MD

INTRODUCTION

The thalassemia syndromes are characterized by quantitatively deficient synthesis of either α- or β-globin chains of Hb A ($\alpha_2\beta_2$) in the erythroid cells of affected individuals [reviewed in Refs. 1,2]. Our current understanding of the molecular basis of the thalassemias has been recently reviewed [3-5]. In homozygous $\beta°$-thalassemia there is complete absence of β-globin chain synthesis, associated with either the complete absence of β-mRNA or with the presence of small amounts of apparently nonfunctional β-globin mRNA. In β^+-thalassemia, the most common type of β-thalassemia, decreased amounts of β-globin chains are produced. These β-globin chains appear normal by peptide mapping analysis, and the small amounts of β-globin produced are associated with correspondingly low levels of β-globin mRNA in the erythroid cells of affected individuals. This mRNA appears to be qualitatively normal as assessed by its ability to direct globin synthesis in cell-free protein synthesizing systems, and by its ability to hybridize completely to a cDNA copy of normal β-globin mRNA. In all likelihood, β^+-thalassemia results from a defect in the level of globin gene transcription, globin mRNA processing, mRNA transport, mRNA stability, or some combination of these processes. In fact, an increasing body of experimental evidence [6,7] strongly suggests that posttranscriptional defects in the processing of precursor mRNA molecules are responsible for β^+-thalassemia.

We have studied the process of β-globin gene transcription in normal and β^+-thalassemic individuals using a number of different approaches. We have incubated intact bone marrow cells of normal and β^+-thalassemic individuals with a radioactive precursor to RNA (^{3}H-uridine), quantitated the relative amounts of newly synthesized α- and β-globin mRNA molecules initially transcribed from

*Supported in part by grants from the NIH, the March of Dimes Birth Defects Foundation, The Charles E. Culpeper Foundation, and the Cooley's Anemia Foundation, Inc.

Birth Defects: Original Article Series, Volume 18, Number 7, pages 51–59
© 1982 March of Dimes Birth Defects Foundation

the genes, and analyzed directly the amount of β-precursor mRNA synthesized and accumulated in the nuclei of erythroid precursor cells by using a specific molecular hybridization probe for the intervening sequence of the β-globin gene. In pulse-chase experiments, we also studied the relative stabilities of nascent α- and β-globin mRNA molecules in normal and β^+-thalassemic subjects. Using another approach to the problem, we isolated, by recombinant DNA technology, the β-globin gene from a β^+-thalassemic subject and studied its transcription in vitro as well as its fine structure by nucleotide sequence analysis.

RESULTS AND DISCUSSION

In Vivo Studies of Globin Gene Transcription Using Intact Bone Marrow Cells

Bone marrow cells were obtained from 6 individuals with homozygous β^+-thalassemia and 4 control subjects with erythroid hyperplasia due to hemolytic anemia of various etiologies. The cells were incubated in the presence of ^{3}H-uridine for 20 – 30 minutes, then total cellular RNA was extracted. In some experiments, the cells were removed by centrifugation from the radioactive medium, then resuspended in medium containing an excess of nonradioactive uridine, and incubated for an additional 24 hours (pulse-chase experiment). The labeled RNA extracted from the cells was then analyzed by molecular hybridization assays to determine: 1) the ratio of labeled α- to β-mRNA sequences corresponding to the sequences of the mature cytoplasmic globin mRNA molecule; 2) the ratio of intervening sequence copies to coding mRNA copies in newly synthesized ^{3}H-labeled β-mRNA molecules; and 3) the ratio of labeled α- to β-mRNA coding sequences after a 24-hour chase period. The molecular hybridization probes that we used in these assays consisted of the following: 1) cloned recombinant DNA plasmids containing cDNA copies of α- and β-globin mRNA [8], originally obtained by reverse transcription of mature α- and β-mRNAs using the enzyme viral reverse transcriptase; and 2) a probe to specifically quantitate those sequences in the β-pre-mRNA that correspond to the large intervening sequence (IVS-2) found within the β-globin structural gene; this probe was constructed by subcloning, in a plasmid, the Bam HI-Eco RI restriction endonuclease fragment that contains the IVS-2 of the β-globin gene [9].

The general hybridization method has been described in detail elsewhere [10]. In summary, it consisted in binding excess amounts of nonradioactive plasmid DNA containing the globin cDNAs or the β-IVS-2 DNA to millipore filters. The filters were then incubated with appropriate amounts of the ^{3}H-labeled RNA, extracted from the bone marrow cells, for sufficient periods of time to allow complete hybridization of any homologous molecules. The filters were then washed extensively to remove nonspecifically bound RNA, and the residual radioactivity bound to the filters, representing specific hybridization of coding or intervening sequences in nascent mRNA or pre-mRNA molecules, was quantitated in a liquid scintillation counter. The results of these experiments are listed in Table 1 and illustrated graphically in Figure 1.

It can be seen from Table 1 and Figure 1 that in all cases studied, approximately equal amounts of nascent α- and β-mRNA molecules were synthesized in both normal and β^+-thalassemic individuals: the β/α-ratio of radioactive RNA binding to cloned globin cDNA ranged between 0.7 and 1.3. Therefore, in all of the β^+-thalassemic subjects that we studied there was no defect in the initial transcription of the β-globin gene into nascent β-mRNA molecules containing sequences corresponding to the mature mRNA. In the 2 cases that were studied by pulse-chase experiments however, the ratio of β- to α-mRNA radioactivity decreased dramatically to levels similar to that found in the steady-state mRNA in the individual's cell cytoplasm, whereas in normal individuals the ratio remained constant (Fig. 1). These results indicate that in these 2 individuals, there is either a defect in the processing of the precursor mRNA molecules to mature mRNA, or a defect in the stability of the mRNA once it is processed to its mature form. To distinguish between these 2 possibilities, the amount of ^{3}H-RNA corresponding to β-gene IVS-2 was quantitated in relation to the amount of ^{3}H-labeled RNA corresponding to mature β-globin mRNA (or cDNA). The results in Table 1 indicate that in 4 of the 6 β^+-thalassemic patients the β-IVS-2/β-cDNA ratio was significantly higher than in nonthalassemic erythroid cells. This suggests that in these patients there is a defect in the processing of the IVS-2 sequences in the precursor β-mRNA molecules to yield mature β-mRNA molecules. However, in 2 β^+-thalassemic patients (patients 5 and 6), there was no such accumulation of IVS-2 sequences in the ^{3}H-labeled RNA. These patients appear therefore not to have a defect in the processing of IVS-2. In a pulse-chase experiment, however, the ^{3}H β/α-mRNA ratio of one of these patients (no. 5) decreased dramatically after 24 hours, suggesting instability of nascent β-mRNA molecules in the patient's erythroid cells.

TABLE 1. Results of Hybridization of ^{3}H-Uridine Labeled Bone Marrow RNA to Globin cDNA or β-Globin IVS-2 DNA Probes

		β/α-ratio		β-IVS-2/β-ratio	
Patient		Pulse	Chase	Pulse	Chase
Nonthalassemic		0.67-1.3	0.58-0.9	0.06-0.12	0.01-0.03
β^+-thalassemic	1	0.91	0.41	1.08	0.23
	2	1.09	—	1.0	—
	3	0.87	—	0.41	—
	4	0.93	—	0.21	—
	5	0.79	0.17	0.11	0.05
	6	0.81	—	0.08	—

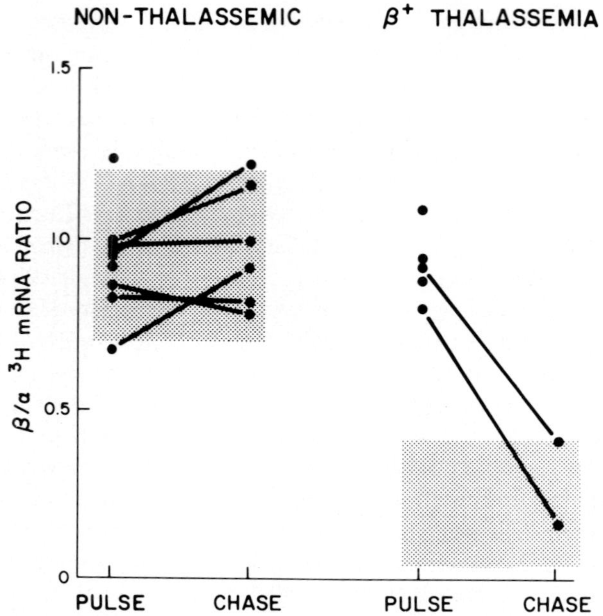

Fig. 1. Results of analysis of ^{3}H-uridine labeled bone marrow RNA by molecular hybridization to unlabeled α- and β-globin cDNA plasmids. The shaded areas indicate the range of steady-state total β/α-mRNA ratios obtained by hybridizing the RNA samples to ^{3}H-labeled α- and β-globin cDNA. (From Benz EJ Jr et al: Post-transcriptional defects in β-globin mRNA metabolism in β-thalassemia: Abnormal accumulation of β mRNA precursor sequences. J Clin Invest 68:1529, 1982, with permission.)

Structural and Transcriptional Analysis of a Cloned β^{+}-Thalassemic Globin Gene

In order to determine the molecular basis of the abnormal posttranscriptional metabolism of β-globin mRNA in β^{+}-thalassemia, we isolated, by recombinant DNA technology, clones of β-globin gene fragments from a patient with β^{+}-thalassemia (patient 6 in Table 1). Detailed restriction endonuclease analysis revealed no difference between the cloned DNA fragments from this thalassemic individual and similar β-globin gene fragments from a normal individual (data not shown). These results indicated that the structural gene itself and its flanking DNA do not contain any major deletions or other sequence rearrangements that could be detected by such an analysis.

The 5′ (5.2 kb) Eco RI fragment obtained from the β^{+}-thalassemic DNA was transcribed in a cell-free transcription system in vitro that contains RNA polymerase II activity [11]. An RNA transcript was obtained that was similar in yield and in size to that obtained from similar transcription of a normal β-globin gene fragment (data not shown). These results therefore confirm the in vivo study shown in Table 1 that indicated normal transcriptional activity of this patient's β^+-thalassemic globin genes. The defect in RNA metabolism associated with this gene must therefore be the result of a posttranscriptional phenomenon.

In order to determine the nature of the posttranscriptional defect associated with this gene, we carried out nucleotide sequence analysis of the gene. Approximately 2,000 nucleotides were sequenced including all of the structural gene with its 2 intervening sequences, and 100 – 200 nucleotides of the flanking DNA to either side of the structural gene. The nucleotide sequence obtained was compared to that of a normal β-globin gene by Lawn et al [12]. Only one nucleotide difference was observed between the β-globin genes of the 2 individuals [13]. This one base substitution was found in the small intervening sequence (IVS-1), 22 nucleotides from the 3′-junction between this IVS and the adjacent coding sequence (Fig. 2). It should be stressed that our nucleotide sequence analysis revealed no abnormalities at the junction points between intervening sequences and coding sequences in these globin gene fragments, no abnormalities in the 5′- and 3′-untranslated sequences corresponding to the β-mRNA, and no abnormalities in the 5′-flanking sequences thought to be important or responsible for the initiation of transcription of the gene.

Examination of the region of the base substitution in the small IVS of this β^+-thalassemic gene reveals a finding that might mediate a posttranscriptional defect in mRNA metabolism in this patient and possibly explain the molecular basis of β^+-thalassemia. Specifically, the base change creates in the β^+-thalassemic globin gene a hexanucleotide sequence which is identical, in all but one nucleotide, with the hexanucleotide sequence situated at the 3′-junction between the IVS-1 and the adjacent coding region; the one nucleotide that differs has been found to be variable in other non-α-globin genes in man [14]. More important, the base

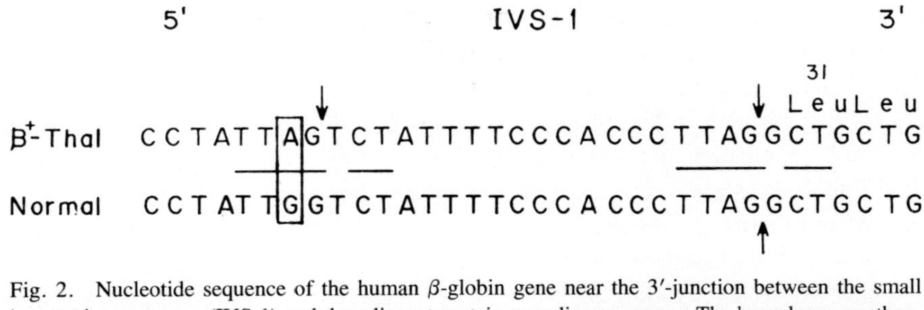

Fig. 2. Nucleotide sequence of the human β-globin gene near the 3′-junction between the small intervening sequence (IVS-1) and the adjacent protein-encoding sequence. The homologous authentic and putative internal 3′-splice regions are indicated by the solid lines and the potential sites of intron excision are indicated by the arrows. The single nucleotide change in the β^+-thalassemic DNA sequence is indicated by the box. Normal β-globin mRNA codon position 31 is numbered. (Adapted from Ref. 13.)

change of A to G creates an AG dinucleotide in this sequence, and it is now recognized that the dinucleotide AG constitutes the necessary 3′-splicing signal for the excision of intervening sequences. In Figure 2, the hexanucleotide region of sequence homology is shown by the horizontal line and the potential splicing sites following AG nucleotides are shown by arrows.

We postulate that the base substitution in the β^+-thalassemic globin gene may create an alternative splicing site for processing of the β-mRNA precursor molecules. A model of our hypothesis is illustrated in Figure 3. A given β-mRNA precursor molecule could be spliced in 2 ways, either normally, as shown in the lower portion of Figure 3, or abnormally, as shown in the upper portion of the figure. The abnormal splicing pathway would not be expected to cause a defect in the metabolism or processing of IVS-2 sequences in this patient and, in fact, ^{3}H-uridine labeling of the bone marrow cells of this individual does not show accumulation of IVS-2 sequences. The abnormal alternative splicing pathway, however, would lead to the synthesis of a mRNA molecule containing an additional 19 nucleotides derived from the 3′-end of the IVS-1. The nucleotide sequence of this abnormal region of the β-mRNA, in the expected reading frame, would be as follows:

30					35	
Ser	Leu	Phe	Ser	His	Pro	Term
—AGT	CTA	TTT	TCC	CAC	CCT	TAG —

This abnormal β-mRNA would therefore contain a nonsense codon following amino acid position 35 that should cause premature termination of translation of the mRNA at that point. It is also interesting to note that the downstream sequence of the mRNA, put out of phase by the insertion of the additional 19 nucleotides, contains a number of additional in-phase termination or nonsense codons. It has been previously shown by Chang and Kan [15] that one form of β°-thalassemia is caused by a nonsense mutation in the coding region of β-mRNA. This mutation would not necessarily be expected, in itself, to lead to a decreased accumulation of β-globin mRNA in the cell. However, it is well established that β-mRNA levels in such β°-thalassemic patients are quite low: 5 – 15% of normal. β-Globin mRNAs that contain nonsense mutations must therefore be unstable and decay more rapidly than normal β-globin mRNA. Hence, our theory postulates that the deficient β-globin mRNA that is observed in β^+-thalassemia probably represents the normal β-mRNA that accumulates through the normal splicing pathway (lower portion of Fig. 3). The mRNA that results from the abnormal processing pathway (upper portion of Fig. 3) contains a nonsense mutation and therefore is presumably unstable and rapidly degraded in the cell.

Our theory has one additional corollary: all things being equal, approximately

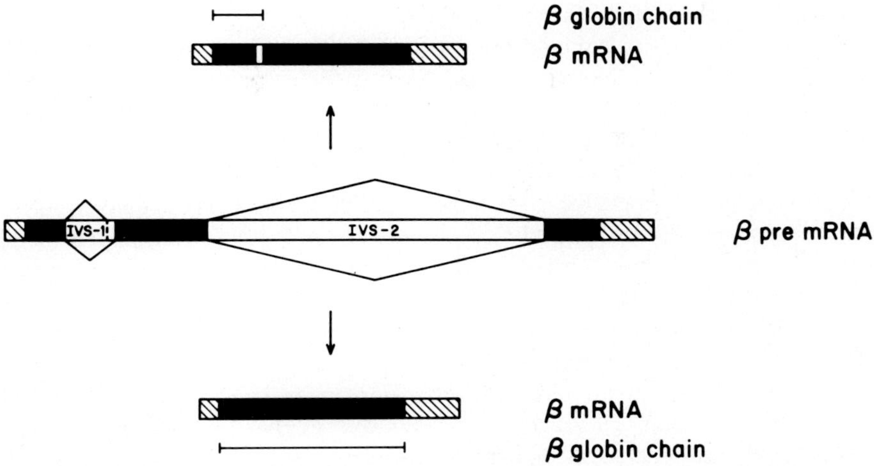

Fig. 3. Model of alternative splicing of precursor β-mRNA molecules as a result of the base substitution within IVS-1 of the β^+-thalassemic gene. See text for detailed explanation. (From Forget BG et al: *In vivo* and *in vitro* transcription of normal and abnormal human globin genes.In Weatherall DJ, Fiorelli G, Gorini S (eds): "Advances in Red Blood Cell Biology." New York: Raven Press, 1982, pp 155-163, with permission.)

50% of the precursor β-globin mRNA molecules in β^+-thalassemia should be processed normally, and 50% should be processed abnormally. However in β^+-thalassemia, the β-globin mRNA level in reticulocytes is not 50% of normal but only 10 – 20% of normal. If our theory, as illustrated in Figure 3, is correct, then the presence of only 10 – 20% of normal β-mRNA implies that there is preferential splicing of the β^+-thalassemic precursor β-mRNAs at the alternative or abnormal splicing site rather than at the normal splicing site. As a result, one would observe a more marked deficiency of normally spliced β-mRNA sequences than would normally be expected if splicing occurred only randomly at one site versus the other. Confirmation of our theory will require the demonstration of RNA sequences that contain the abnormal additional nucleotides in β^+-thalassemic erythroid cells. Results of preliminary experiments in our laboratory indicate that the predicted abnormal mRNA can in fact be detected [16]. The recent finding of the same mutation in another individual with β^+-thalassemia [17] also supports our hypothesis that the base substitution that we have identified is directly related to the molecular defect in β^+-thalassemia.

SUMMARY AND CONCLUSIONS

Our results indicate that in all cases of β^+-thalassemia studied there does not appear to be a defect in the initial transcription of the β-globin gene into precursor β-mRNA molecules. In all subjects studied, newly synthesized β-globin mRNA molecules were synthesized in normal amounts relative to nascent α-globin mRNA molecules. In 4 of the 6 cases studied, there appeared to be a defect in the processing of nascent molecules into mature mRNA molecules as evidenced by abnormal accumulation of RNA molecules containing transcripts of the large intervening sequence (IVS-2) of the β-globin gene. In the other 2 cases, processing of the large IVS appeared to be normal, but the stability of the newly synthesized β-globin mRNA appeared to be decreased. A β-globin gene was cloned from one of these latter 2 patients, and the only structural abnormality of the gene that was detected by nucleotide sequence analysis consisted of a single nucleotide base substitution within the body of the small intervening sequence (IVS-1) of the gene. The base change generates at that point a nucleotide sequence very similar to the normal splicing signal present at the 3′-extremity of the small intervening sequence. Therefore, we believe that the base change causes β^+-thalassemia by mediating alternative splicing of β-precursor mRNA molecules and leads to the synthesis of abnormal β-globin mRNA molecules that might be unstable in the cell.

ACKNOWLEDGMENTS

We thank E. Coupal, R. Ezekiel, A. Scarpa, and V. Vellucci for skilled technical assistance, and N. Grinnell for assistance in preparation of the manuscript.

REFERENCES

1. Weatherall DJ, Clegg JB (eds): "The Thalassemia Syndromes," 3rd Ed. Oxford: Blackwell Scientific Publications, 1981.
2. Bunn HF, Forget BG, Ranney HM: "Human Hemoglobins." Philadelphia: WB Saunders, 1977, p 140.
3. Forget BG: Molecular genetics of human hemoglobin synthesis. Ann Intern Med 91:605, 1979.
4. Bank A, Mears JG, Ramirez F: Disorders of human hemoglobin. Science 207:486, 1980.
5. Benz EJ Jr, Forget BG: The thalassemia syndromes: Models for the molecular analysis of human disease. Annu Rev Med 33:363, 1982.
6. Kantor JA, Turner PH, Nienhuis AW: β-thalassemia: Mutations which affect processing of the β globin mRNA precursor. Cell 21:149, 1980.
7. Maquat LE, Kinniburgh AJ, Beach LR, Honig GR, Lazerson J, Ershler WB, Ross J: Processing of the human β globin mRNA precursor to mRNA is defective in three patients with β^+-thalassemia. Proc Natl Acad Sci USA 77:4287, 1980.
8. Wilson JT, Wilson LB, deRiel JK, Villa-Komaroff L, Efstratiadis A, Forget BG, Weissman SM: Insertion of synthetic copies of human globin genes into bacterial plasmids. Nucleic Acids Res 5:563, 1978.
9. Lawn RM, Fritsch EF, Parker RC, Blake G, Maniatis T: The isolation and characterization of linked δ and β globin genes from a cloned library of human DNA. Cell 15:1157, 1978.
10. Benz EJ Jr, Scarpa AL, Tonkonow BL, Pearson HA, Ritchey AK: Post-transcriptional defects in β globin mRNA metabolism in β-thalassemia: Abnormal accumulation of β mRNA precursor sequences. J Clin Invest 68:1529, 1982.

11. Manley JL, Fire A, Cano A, Sharp PA, Gefter ML: DNA-dependent transcription of adenovirus genes in a soluble whole cell extract. Proc Natl Acad Sci USA 77:3855, 1980.
12. Lawn RM, Efstratiadis A, O'Connell C, Maniatis T: The nucleotide sequence of the human β globin gene. Cell 21:647, 1980.
13. Spritz RA, Jagadeeswaran P, Choudary PV, Biro PA, Elder JT, deRiel JK, Manley JL, Gefter ML, Forget BG, Weissman SM: Base substitution in an intervening sequence of a β^+-thalassemic human globin gene. Proc Natl Acad Sci USA 78:2455, 1981.
14. Efstratiadis A, Posakony JW, Maniatis T, Lawn RM, O'Connell C, Spritz RA, deRiel JK, Forget BG, Weissman SM, Slightom JL, Blechl AE, Smithies O, Baralle FE, Shoulders CC, Proudfoot NJ: The structure and evolution of the human β globin gene family. Cell 21:653, 1980.
15. Chang JC, Kan YW: $\beta°$-Thalassemia, a nonsense mutation in man. Proc Natl Acad Sci USA 76:2886, 1979.
16. Fukumaki Y, Ghosh PK, Benz EJ Jr, Reddy VB, Lebowitz P, Forget BG, Weissman SM: Abnormally spliced messenger RNA in erythroid cells from patients with β^+-thalassemia and monkey cells expressing a cloned β^+-thalassemic gene. Cell 28:585, 1982.
17. Westaway D, Williamson R: An intron nucleotide sequence variant in a cloned β^+-thalassemia globin gene. Nucleic Acids Res 9:1777, 1981.
18. Forget BG, Benz EJ Jr, Spritz RA, Weissman SM: *In vivo* and *in vitro* transcription of normal and abnormal human globin genes. In Weatherall DJ, Fiorelli G, Gorini S (eds): "Advances in Red Blood Cell Biology." New York: Raven Press, 1982 pp 155-163.

Ferrara $\beta°$-Thalassemia

Francesco Conconi, MD, Francesco Bernardi, BS,
Giovanna Marchetti, BS, Carla Perrotta, BS, and Laura Del Senno, BS

Several hereditary abnormalities of the red blood cell have been described in the Po River delta; a β^+- and a $\beta°$-thalassemia [1]; a nondeletion α-thalassemia [2]; mutations of the β-globin chain (Hb Hasharon [3]; O Indonesia [4]; J-Rovigo [5]); G6PD deficiency of Mediterranean type [6], and alterations of the pyridoxal phosphate metabolism [7].

$\beta°$-thalassemia is the most common red cell abnormality of the region. We will present in separate paragraphs the information available on this form of thalassemia.

THE GENE FOR β-GLOBIN IS PRESENT

Restriction enzyme analysis has been carried out in Ferrara $\beta°$-homozygous subjects using several enzymes [8]. The results obtained for the thalassemic DNA are identical to those for control DNA, thus excluding the presence of extensive deletions in or adjacent to the coding regions of the β-globin gene in Ferrara $\beta°$-thalassemia. Identical results have been obtained by B. Forget and co-workers (personal communication).

β-GLOBIN mRNA SEQUENCES ARE DETECTABLE

cDNA/mRNA hybridization studies have demonstrated the presence in erythroid cells of β-globin mRNA sequences in amounts ranging from 2 to 12% [9]. The melting profile of the Ferrara β-mRNA-β-cDNA hybrids is indistinguishable from the normal one. Similar findings have been obtained by Forget and Hillman [10]. Incomplete hybridization of Ferrara β-globin mRNA-β-cDNA has been reported by Ramirez et al [11].

Birth Defects: Original Article Series, Volume 18, Number 7, pages 61–63
© 1982 March of Dimes Birth Defects Foundation

Hb A is UNDETECTABLE

The absence of Hb A and β-globin synthesis has been established by means of several chromatographic techniques, employed separately or in combination. The amount of β-globin synthesis relative to α-globin, if any, is less than 0.1% [12].

β-GLOBIN SYNTHESIS OCCURS AFTER BLOOD TRANSFUSION

A characteristic of Ferrara β°-thalassemia is the appearance in intact cells of β-globin synthesis following blood transfusion [12,13]. This phenomenon is unique for this type of thalassemia and does not appear in β°-subjects from other Italian regions (Sicily, Sardinia) treated with the identical transfusion therapy and examined in our laboratory, as well as in other laboratories.

CELL-FREE TRANSLATION OF FERRARA β-GLOBIN mRNA ISOLATED FROM HOMOZYGOUS β°-SUBJECTS

The translatability of β-globin mRNA in Ferrara thalassemia was proposed in 1972, based on the results obtained in homologous cell-free translation (Ferrara ribosomes incubated with normal hemolysate) [14]. Heterologous cell-free translation has been carried out more recently using mRNA from transfused and untransfused subjects in a rabbit reticulocyte system. The results are consistent with the synthesis of authentic β-globin molecules [12].

INFORMATION FROM FERRARA β°-THALASSEMIA HETEROZYGOTES

In hybridization studies the amount of β-globin mRNA sequences relative to α-mRNA has been shown to be higher in Ferrara than in other thalassemic heterozygotes, including two δ β. In addition, in younger reticulocytes the imbalance of α- to β-globin synthesis is smaller than in adult cell fractions.

The findings obtained in Ferrara β°-heterozygotes indicate an instability of β-globin mRNA.

CONCLUSION

In Ferrara β°-thalassemia, the gene for β-globin is present and transcribed. Since β-mRNA sequences are present in the cytoplasm, β-mRNA splicing and processing take place. β-globin mRNA translation, undetectable in β°-homozygous subjects before transfusion, occurs in intact cells after transfusion, and in homologous and heterologous cell-free systems.

The instability of β-mRNA, demonstrated in heterozygotes, cannot give rise to a β°-thalassemia and is therefore secondary. A specific inhibition of β-mRNA translation could explain the decay of β-globin mRNA (due to lack of ribosomal protection) in heterozygotes, and the absence of translation of β-globin mRNA in homozygotes.

REFERENCES

1. Del Senno L, Bernardi F, Busin M, Marchetti G, Perrotta C, Conconi F, Cappellozza G, Vullo C: Genotipi α e β talassemici nel delta del Po. Atti del VI° Congresso Internazionale della "Associazione Nazionale per la lotta contro le microcitemie in Italia (Roma)," 1980, p 135.
2. Del Senno L, Bernardi F, Buzzoni D, Marchetti G, Perrotta C, Conconi F: Molecular characteristics of a nondeletion α-thalassemia of the Po river delta. Eur J Biochem 116:127, 1981.
3. Del Senno L, Bernardi F, Marchetti G, Perrotta C, Conconi F, Vullo C, Salsini G, Cristofori G, Cappellozza G, Bellinello F, Bedendo B, Mercuriati M: Organization of α-globin genes and mRNA translation in subjects carrying haemoglobin Hasharon (α 47 Asp → His) from the Ferrara region (Northern Italy). Eur J Biochem 111:125, 1980.
4. Del Senno L, Bernardi F, Bruno MR, Buzzoni D, Casoni I, Marchetti G, Mariuzzi GM, Alberti R, Perrotta C, Conconi F: Reduced levels of variant α-globins in β thalassemia. Haematologica 64:278, 1979.
5. Alberti R, Mariuzzi GM, Artibani L, Bruni E, Tentori L: A new haemoglobin variant: J-Rovigo α-53 (E-2) Alanine → aspartic acid. Biochem Biophys Acta 342:1, 1974.
6. Gandini E, Menini C, De Filippis A, Dell'Acqua GB: Deficit di G6PD eritrocitaria. Studio della distribuzione nella provincia di Ferrara e del rapporto con malaria e talassemia. Acta Genet Med Gemellol (Roma) 3:271, 1969.
7. Anderson BB, Perry GM, Clements JE, Vullo C, Cristofori G: Red cell metabolism of pyridoxine in controls and β thalassemia in Ferrara, Northern Italy. Biomedicine 35:147, 1981.
8. Del Senno L, Conconi F, Little PFR, Williamson R: Restriction enzyme analysis of the β-globin gene in DNA from thalassemic subjects from Ferrara. Biochem Biophys Res Commun 91:548, 1979.
9. Ottolenghi S, Comi P, Giglioni B, Williamson R, Vullo C, Del Senno L, Conconi F: Direct demonstration of β-globin mRNA in homozygous Ferrara β° thalassaemia patients. Nature 266:231, 1977.
10. Forget BG, Hillman DG: β-globin mRNA in Ferrara β° thalassaemia. Nature 269:356, 1977.
11. Ramirez F, O'Donnell JV, Marcks PA, Bank A, Musumeci S, Schillirò G, Pizzarelli G, Russo G, Luppis B, Gambino R: Abnormal or absent β mRNA in β° Ferrara and gene deletion in δ β thalassaemia. Nature 263:471, 1976.
12. Conconi F, Bernardi F, Buzzoni D, Casoni I, Del Senno L, Marchetti G, Perrotta C: β-globin messenger RNA in Ferrara β° thalassemia. Ann NY Acad Sci 344:120, 1980.
13. Conconi F, Del Senno L, Ferrarese P, Menini C, Borgatti L, Vullo C, Labie D: Appearance of β-globin synthesis in erythroid cells of Ferrara β° thalassaemic patients following blood transfusion. Nature 254:256, 1975.
14. Conconi F, Rowley PT, Del Senno L, Pontremoli S, Volpato S: Induction of β-globin synthesis in β thalassemia. Nature (New Biol) 238:83, 1972.

$\delta\beta$-Thalassemia and HPFH*

Sergio Ottolenghi, MD, Barbara Giglioni, BS, Roberto Taramelli, MD, Paola Comi, BS, and Alessandro Massimo Gianni, MD

$\delta\beta$-Thalassemia and hereditary persistence of Hb F (HPFH) are a group of inherited syndromes characterized by the persistent expression of γ-globin genes in adult age; this is in contrast to the more common β-thalassemias in which γ-globin genes are usually kept repressed at a level similar to that in normal cells. We recently observed some new interesting cases of $\delta\beta$-thalassemia and HPFH, and now wish to discuss the relationship between the molecular defect in DNA and the persistent activity of γ-globin genes.

A variety of $\delta\beta$-thalassemic and HPFH defects have already been characterized in several laboratories; with the exception of $\delta\beta°$-thalassemia from Sardinia [1] and Greek type HPFH [2, 3], large deletions are found in these syndromes [reviewed in ref. 4]. This had been predicted originally by Huisman et al [5] on the basis of the comparison of Hb F production in carriers of Hb Lepore and Hb Kenya, both arising from the fusion of the 3′ end of the β-globin gene with the 5′ end of the $^A\gamma$- or δ-globin genes, respectively, with concomitant deletion of the intergene area. The persistent activity of γ-globin genes is thought to occur, in heterozygotes, only on the chromosome affected by the deletion [5]; the same was also demonstrated recently in $\delta\beta$-thalassemia [1]. The mechanism whereby this effect occurs is unknown; the above-mentioned comparison between the (presumed) deletion in Hb Kenya and that in Hb Lepore suggested, however, the sequences are present in the $^A\gamma$ - δ-intergene area, whose deletion is responsible for the abnormal γ-globin gene activity. Apparently, involvement of DNA 3′ to the β-globin gene is not essential for this effect. Studies [6–8] in the common southern Italian type (from Sicily and Calabria) of $\delta\beta$-thalassemia indicate that the $^A\gamma$ - δ-intergene area is not affected by the deletion, and that the low level of

*Supported in part by CNR grants Progetto Finalizzato Medicina Preventiva no. 80.01133.83 (to S.O.), and Progetto Finalizzato Crescita Neoplastica no. 79.00634.96 (to A.M.G.). R.T. was supported by an AV Rusconi fellowship.

Birth Defects: Original Article Series, Volume 18, Number 7, pages 65–67
© 1982 March of Dimes Birth Defects Foundation

persistent activity of γ-globin genes observed in this condition must therefore be ascribed either to the loss of distant sequences 3′ to the β-globin gene [8] or to disruption of a critical structure, possibly in the δ-globin gene region [6, 9].

On the other hand, the level of Hb F production in HPFH is much higher than in $\delta\beta$-thalassemia; while the role, if any, of sequences 3′ to the β-globin gene cannot be evaluated at present, due to the lack of suitable mapping data; the critical DNA region postulated on the basis of Hb Kenya studies might be identified by comparison of $\delta\beta$-thalassemias and HPFH. A recently studied Spanish $\delta\beta$-thalassemic case [1] shows that the additional loss of ~ 3 kb of DNA 5′ to the δ-globin gene does not affect the phenotype significantly (Fig. 1); however, in HPFH, deletions (when observed) always extend beyond (~ 1 kb or more) the 5′ end point of the Spanish deletion. We wish to suggest that sequences essential for the correct regulation of globin gene expression are retained in Spanish $\delta\beta$-thalassemia, but are lost in HPFH; this defines their location approximately (Fig. 1).

Although deletions have been demonstrated in many $\delta\beta$-thalassemias and HPFH, in at least two cases no evidence was found for gross rearrangements in the globin gene cluster (although only heterozygotes were available for this study, a fact that limits the sensitivity of the analysis). In Sardinian $\delta\beta$-thalassemia, the whole globin cluster is apparently intact, yet genetic data suggest that the β-globin gene is inactive, while the $^{A}\gamma$ (and to a more limited extent the $^{G}\gamma$-gene) are kept active [1]. A similar situation is also observed in the Greek type HPFH [2, 3], although in this case the β-globin gene is probably active. These cases suggest that small changes in critical areas may be sufficient

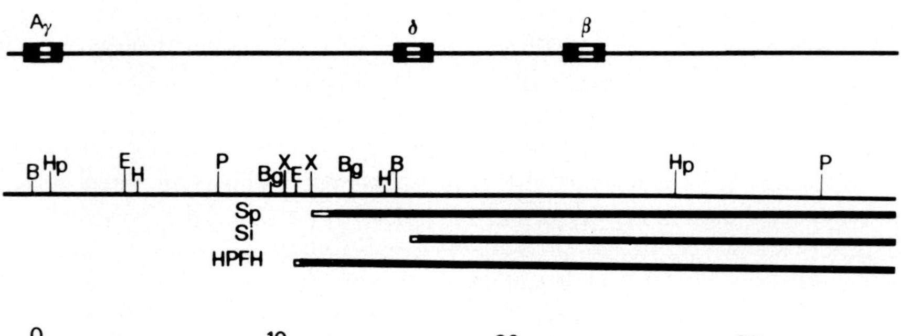

Fig. 1. Comparison of deletions in Spanish and Italian $\delta°\beta°$-thalassemia, and in a Negro HPFH [7]. Black boxes indicate the extent of deletions; the 5′ end point of the deletion is within white boxes. B (Bam HI), Hp (Hpa I), E (Eco RI), H (Hind III), P (Pst I), Bg (BGI II), X (Xba I), indicate restriction enzyme sites in the $\delta°\beta°$-thalassemic map. Kb: kilobase pairs; Sp: Spanish $\delta\beta$-thalassemia; Si: southern Italian $\delta\beta$-thalassemia.

to alter γ-globin gene regulation, and that deletions per se might have no effect except to remove, or displace, small critical DNA regions. There is essentially no information as to the location of the defect in these two types of persistence of Hb F. It is also unclear whether the effect is *in cis* only, or also *in trans*. However, preliminary gene mapping studies on a southern Italian patient, phenotypically very similar to Greek patients with HPFH, show abnormalities in the γ-globin region, suggesting close linkage of the defect to the globin cluster [10]. In addition, typical patterns of polymorphic Hind III and Bam HI sites appear to be linked to the Sardinian $\delta\beta$-thalassemic defect in the few patients studied so far by our group; this will provide opportunities for the future identification and characterization of these interesting mutant genes by molecular cloning.

REFERENCES

1. Ottolenghi S, Giglioni B, Taramelli R, Comi P, Mazza U, Saglio G, Camaschella C, Izzo P, Cao A, Galanello R, Gimferrer E, Baiget M, Gianni AM: Molecular comparison of $\delta\beta$-thalassemia and hereditary persistence of fetal hemoglobin DNAs: Evidence of a regulatory area? Proc Natl Acad Sci USA 79:2347–2351, 1982.
2. Tuan D, Murnane MJ, DeRiel JK, Forget BG: Heterogeneity in the molecular basis of hereditary persistence of fetal haemoglobin. Nature 285:335–337, 1980.
3. Bernards R, Flavell RA: Physical mapping of the globin gene deletion in hereditary persistence of foetal haemoglobin (HPFH). Nucleic Acids Res 8:1521–1534, 1980.
4. Jones RW, Old JM, Trent RJ, Clegg JB, Weatherall DJ: Major rearrangement in the human β-globin gene cluster. Nature 291:39–44, 1981.
5. Huisman THJ, Schroeder WA, Efremov GD, Duma H, Mladenovski B, Hyman CB, Rachmilevitz EA, Bouver N, Miller A, Brodie A, Shelton JB, Apell G: The present status of the heterogeneity of fetal hemoglobin in β-thalassemia. Ann NY Acad Sci 232:107–124, 1974.
6. Ottolenghi S, Giglioni B, Comi P, Gianni AM, Polli E, Acquaye GTA, Oldham JM, Masera G: Globin gene deletions in HPFH $\delta°\beta°$ thalassemia and Hb Lepore disease. Nature 278:654–656, 1979.
7. Fritsch EF, Lawn RM, Maniatis T: Characterisation of deletions which affect the expression of fetal globin genes in man. Nature 279:598–603, 1979.
8. Bernards K, Kooter SM, Flavell RA: Physical mapping of the globin gene deletion in (delta beta) degrees—Thalassemia. Gene 6:265–280, 1979.
9. Bank A, Mears G, Ramirez F: Disorders of human hemoglobin. Science 207:486–493, 1980.
10. Ottolenghi S, Giglioni B, Taramelli R, Comi P, Mazza U, Saglio G, Camaschella C, Izzo P, Cao A, Galanello R, Gimferrer E, Baiget M, Gianni AM: Heterogeneity of $\delta\beta$ thalassemia and HPFH in Mediterranean population: Gene mapping studies. In Stamatoyannopoulos G, Nienhuis AW (eds): "Organization and Expression of Globin Genes." New York: Alan R Liss, 1981, pp 287–298.

Molecular Defects in β-Thalassemia

Arthur W. Nienhuis, MD, Timothy Ley, MD, Guglielmina Pepe, MD, Joseph Tam, PhD, and Judith Kantor, PhD

Reduced synthesis of structurally normal β-globin, the characteristic phenotype of genetic mutations which cause β-thalassemia, reflects a quantitative deficiency of β-globin mRNA in patients who have these mutations [1,2]. Accumulation of globin mRNA in normal erythroid cells is dependent on a relatively high level of transcription of the globin genes, efficient processing of the globin mRNA precursors, and marked stability of the mature globin mRNAs [3]; mutations which affect any of these processes can cause a quantitative deficiency of globin mRNA. In this paper, we review the approaches which we have taken to define the mutations which cause β-thalassemia.

β-GLOBIN GENE STRUCTURE

Development of the techniques of Southern blotting whereby DNA fragments, generated by complete digestion of genomic DNA with a particular restriction endonuclease, are resolved on an agarose gel, transferred to a nitrocellulose filter, and annealed to a specific gene probe [4], provides an approach to the analysis of globin gene structure in patients with β-thalassemia. We and others [5–7] have applied this experimental strategy to the analysis of globin genes in many such patients. A complete knowledge of the β-globin gene region had been developed by molecular cloning of DNA fragments containing the β-like globin genes and by restriction endonuclease mapping of genomic DNA [8–12]. Thus, comparison of the various restriction fragments of thalassemic DNA samples to the normal fragments containing the β-globin gene was very feasible.

The structure of the β-globin genes in most patients is normal (Fig. 1). The precision of this methodology in detecting mutations is relatively low. Complete deletion of the β-globin gene (eg in patients with pancellular hereditary persistence of fetal hemoglobin [13,14]) is readily detected (Fig. 1A, lane 2). Also, deletions as small as 50 base pairs would be detected in small fragments, such as the 0.9 kilobase (kb) Bam HI-Eco RI β-globin intron fragment depicted in Figure 1B. However, in a fragment of several kilobases, a deletion would have to be

Birth Defects: Original Article Series, Volume 18, Number 7, pages 69–79
© 1982 March of Dimes Birth Defects Foundation

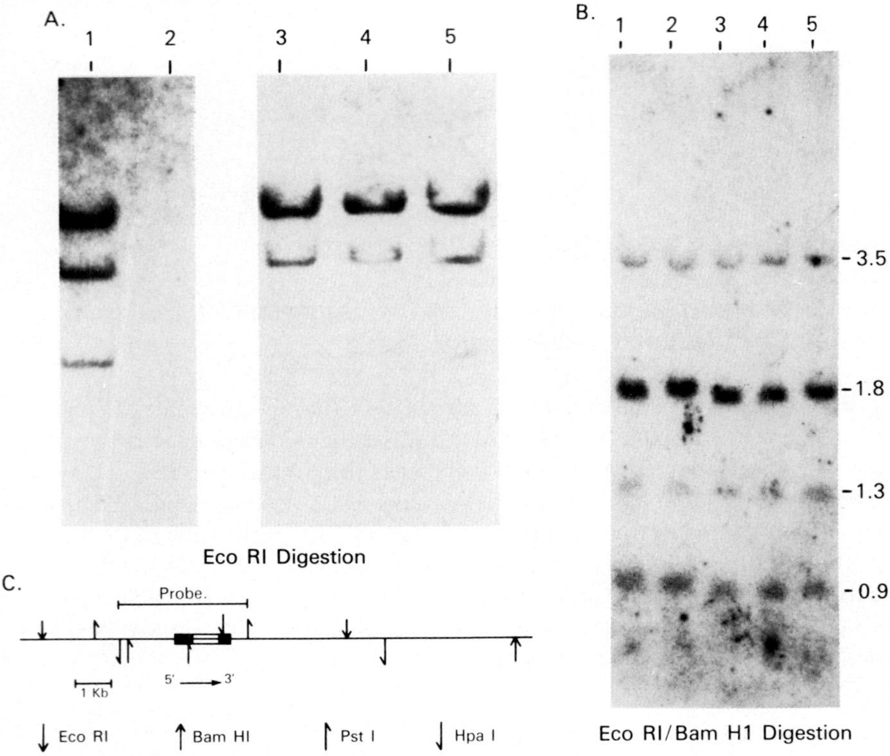

Fig. 1. Southern blot analysis of DNA from thalassemic and normal individuals following restriction endonuclease digestion. Panel A) Digestion was with Eco RI. Lane 1, β^+-thal homozygote; lane 2, homozygous hereditary persistence of fetal hemoglobin; lane 3, normal; and lanes 4 and 5, β^+-thal heterozygotes. Panel B) Digestion was with Eco RI and Bam HI simultaneously. Lane 1, normal; lanes 2-4, β^+-thal homozygotes; and lane 5, β^+-thal heterozygote. Panel C) Shown is the map of several restriction endonuclease sites in the β-globin gene region. The probe used was a cloned DNA fragment which included the entire β-globin gene as shown. (From Tam JWO et al: Analysis of globin gene structure in patients with β-thalassemia by restriction endonuclease mapping. Hemoglobin 5:209, 1981, with permission.)

hundreds of base pairs long to reach the threshold level for detection. Point mutations or small deletions, unless they affected a restriction endonuclease site directly, would not be revealed by the Southern blotting methodology. Clearly, more sensitive techniques were required to define mutations which cause β-thalassemia.

QUANTITATION OF THE β-GLOBIN mRNA PRECURSOR

The focus of efforts in our laboratory has been to study gene function in individual patients by examination of RNA metabolism. We reasoned that by defining the functional consequences of mutations in specific patients, namely by determining their effect on RNA transcription, processing, or stability in bone marrow cells, we would obtain clues as to the nature of mutations which cause thalassemia. Such clues would suggest which genes would be most interesting to study by DNA sequence analysis after molecular cloning using recombinant DNA techniques.

Transcription of a globin gene is thought to begin at a point corresponding to the 5′ end of mature messenger RNA [3]. The gene is copied in its entirety including the 3 coding blocks or exons and the 2 introns or intervening segments of DNA. Termination of transcription may occur somewhere downstream but, early in its metabolism, globin RNA is polyadenylated at a point corresponding to the 3′ end of mature messenger RNA. By measuring the concentration of the RNA precursor which contains the sequences transcribed from introns in thalassemic bone marrow RNA samples, we could distinguish defects affecting transcription from those in which the mutation led to retarded or incomplete removal of intervening sequence RNA. To measure precursor concentration we chose a cloned DNA segment containing the entire large intron (along with small amounts of coding sequence DNA) as a molecular hybridization probe [15]. The rate of annealing of this double-stranded DNA probe in the presence of added bone marrow RNA compared to its rate of self-annealing in the absence of added RNA provided a measure of the concentration of precursor molecules which contain RNA sequences transcribed from the large intron.

Comparison of the results obtained using this method of analysis with bone marrow RNA from a patient with sickle cell anemia and from one with homozygous β-thalassemia is shown in Figure 2. The rate of annealing of the probe in the presence of thalassemic bone marrow RNA is approximately twice that observed with RNA from a patient without a thalassemic mutation. Four thalassemic patients were studied; in each, the RNA sequences homologous to the β-globin gene large intron were present in roughly twice the concentration found in non-thalassemic bone marrow RNA. These data indicated that in a significant percentage of patients with homozygous β-thalassemia, the RNA precursor was normal, or even increased in concentration, suggesting that transcription of the β-globin genes was normal in these patients. Our efforts were, therefore, focused on defining mutations which influenced posttranscriptional RNA metabolism.

RNA METABOLISM IN THALASSEMIC BONE MARROW CELLS

To compare the rate of synthesis of α- and β-globin mRNA sequences, thalassemic bone marrow cells were incubated in [^{3}H] uridine for 20 minutes [15]. The RNA was recovered and the α-and β-sequences were purified by absorption to filters to which either α- or β-cloned cDNA sequences had been bound. The

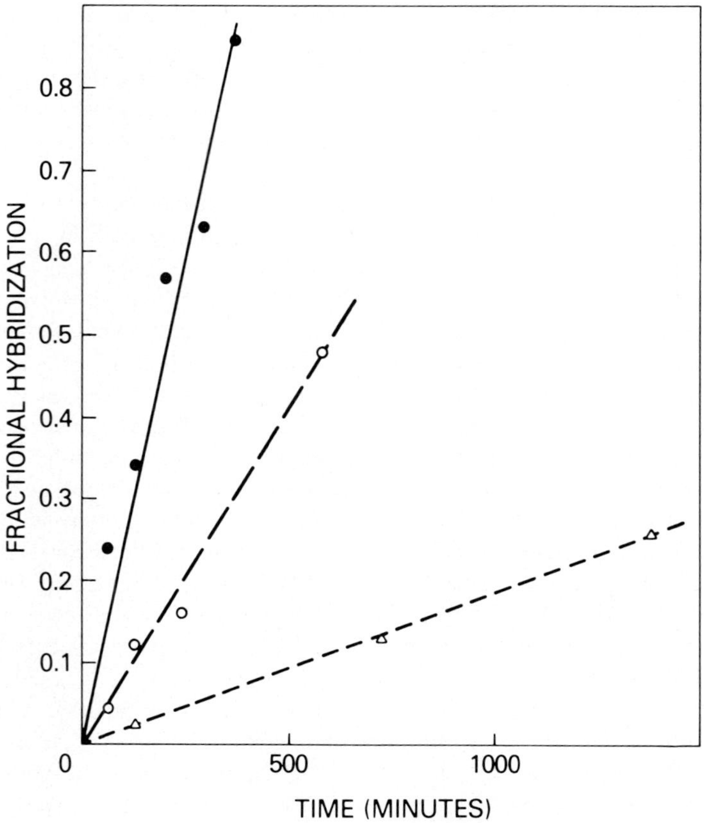

Fig. 2. Quantitation of β-globin mRNA precursor concentration in total cellular RNA from bone marrow [15]. The rate of annealing of the double-stranded intron probe in the presence of 90 μg of RNA from a patient with homozygous β^+-thalassemia (•), in the presence of 80 μg of RNA from a patient with sickle cell anemia (0), or in the presence of 100 μg of *E. coli* RNA (△) were compared. The quantity of reactive RNA species in the 2 experimental reactions was estimated by comparison of their slopes to that of the control reaction. (From Kantor JA et al: Beta thalassemia: Mutations which affect the processing of the β-globin mRNA precursor. Cell 21:149, 1980, with permission of the copyright holder, MIT.)

absorbed α- or β-mRNA sequences were eluted with formamide and the fraction of bound radioactivity which specifically represented mRNA sequences was determined by annealing to a complementary DNA probe. Incubation of bone marrow in the presence of [^{3}H]uridine for 2 hours, followed by removal of the label and incubation of the cells in fresh medium for several additional hours, was performed in order to compare the relative stability of newly synthesized α- and β-mRNA sequences.

TABLE 1. Analysis of Globin mRNA Synthesis and Stability

	2 hr pulse (β/α)	2 hr pulse, 20 hr chase (β/α)
A. Total Cellular		
Controls (3)	1.01	1.03
β^+-thal 1	0.56	0.34
β^+-thal 2	0.76	0.14
B. Nuclear		
Control (1)	1.2	
β^+-thal 1	1.4	—
β^+-thal 2	1.4	—
C. Cytoplasm		
Control (1)	0.71	
β^+-thal 1	0.44	—
β^+-thal 2	0.44	—

The data shown in Table 1 indicate that the ratios of newly synthesized β-and α-mRNA sequences were roughly equivalent in the nuclei from the 2 thalassemic bone marrow samples studied, and were comparable to the ratios in non-thalassemic bone marrow cells. However, the β-mRNA sequences were relatively deficient in the cytoplasm even at 2 hours of incubation. On prolonged incubation (20 hours) the relative proportion of β-mRNA sequences declined precipitously. These data support the interpretation that transcription of the β-globin genes is normal in these thalassemic patients, but that a post-transcriptional defect in RNA metabolism leads to reduced accumulation of β-mRNA sequences.

CHARACTERIZATION OF β-GLOBIN RNA SPECIES PRESENT IN THALASSEMIC BONE MARROW CELLS

Polyadenylated RNA was purified from total cellular RNA using oligo dT cellulose chromatography [15]. Following denaturation with methylmercury, the RNA species present were resolved, based on size, by agarose gel electrophoresis [16]. Transfer of the RNA to diazobenzyloxymethyl-paper was performed using the standard Northern blotting technique. In the experiment shown in Figure 3, the cloned DNA fragment corresponding to the large β-globin gene intron was used as a probe to detect RNA molecules containing homologous sequences.

This probe detects the 16S precursor to β-globin mRNA present at an abundance of roughly 100 mol/erythroid cell. Equivalent amounts of this species were found in nuclear RNA from a patient with sickle cell anemia (Fig. 3, lane

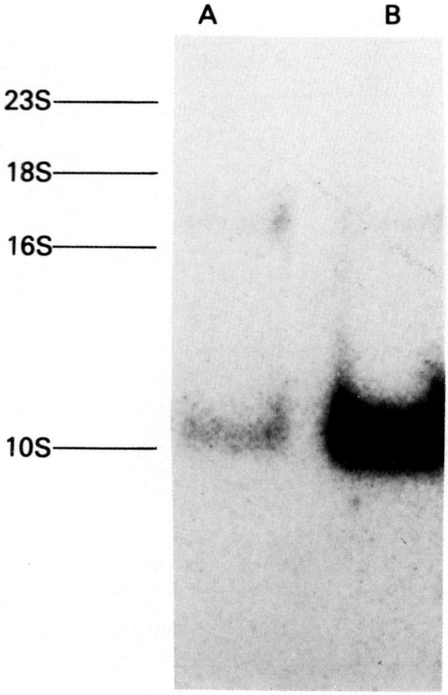

Fig. 3. Electrophoretic resolution of the β-globin RNA species present in 3 μg of nuclear RNA A) from a patient with sickle cell anemia, and B) from a patient with homozygous β-thalassemia. Following electrophoresis, the RNA was transferred to diazobenzyloxymethyl-paper and annealed to the Bam HI-Eco RI genomic DNA fragment derived from the human β-globin gene; this fragment contains the entire large intron and a small portion of coding sequence [15]. The position of ribosomal and messenger RNA species used as size markers is indicated.

1), and in nuclear RNA from a patient with homozygous β-thalassemia (Fig. 3, lane 2). These results provide further evidence that the β-globin mRNA precursor concentration is normal in this thalassemic bone marrow sample. The intron probe also anneals to mature messenger RNA (because it contains a small part of coding sequence). The faintness of this band in non-thalassemic bone marrow RNA (Fig. 3, lane 1) reflects the fact that only a very small part of the probe is complementary to its sequence; its intensity does not give an estimate of the relative abundance of mature mRNA compared to the precursor. Note that the corresponding band in thalassemic RNA is far more intense. Both nuclear RNA samples contain equivalent amounts of mature β-mRNA sequences as shown by a quantitative analysis using β-cDNA as a probe in solution hybridization experiments [15]. The intensity of this band on the Northern blot analysis of this thalassemic RNA indicates the presence of an RNA species which retains at least a portion of the large intervening sequence. This RNA species is roughly the size of mature messenger RNA and was shown in separate experiments to be polyadenylated [15].

S_1 NUCLEASE ANALYSIS OF THALASSEMIC BONE MARROW RNA

Clearly the experiments described above establish the presence and relative frequency of mutations affecting RNA processing in thalassemic patients. However, only limited insight could be obtained into the nature of the precise defects that were present. A refined method of analysis which could pinpoint specific processing errors by providing data as to the types and relative abundance of aberrantly processed RNA molecules was needed. A modification of the method of S_1 nuclease analysis first described by Berk and Sharp [17] was developed in our laboratory for this purpose.

The general strategy of this method of analysis is outlined in Figure 4. Radioactive probes complementary to a portion of the β-globin gene coding sequence, and spanning either the 5′ or 3′ end of messenger RNA or one of the RNA splice junctions, were utilized. We used the M13 cloning system to obtain uniformly labeled single-stranded probes of high specific activity for this purpose. Six segments of the normal β-globin gene were cloned into M13; these allowed specific analysis of each end and splice junction of the messenger RNA molecules [18]. The secreted single-stranded form of each recombinant served as a template for synthesis of a [^{32}P]-labeled probe of high specific activity.

In an individual experiment, 10 μg of total bone marrow RNA was annealed to 20,000 cpm of probe. As illustrated in Figure 4, mRNA protects that portion of the probe complementary to its sequence from subsequent S_1 nuclease analysis. If an RNA species is present from which a portion, but not all, of the intervening sequence has been removed, then a DNA segment corresponding to the length of the coding sequence in the probe plus retained intervening sequence is protected. If the entire intervening sequence is present in the RNA molecule to which the probe anneals, then the entire segment of the probe derived from human DNA will be protected as illustrated in Figure 4.

Shown in Figure 4 are results of an analysis of bone marrow RNA from 3 patients homozygous for β-thalassemia. The probe used spans the 3′ splice junction of intron 1 and extends across the entire intron and a short distance into exon 1. Normally processed β-globin mRNA should protect a 134 nucleotide DNA segment derived from this probe as illustrated in Figure 4. All 3 bone marrow samples protected a portion of the probe which migrated in this position. Two of the thalassemic bone marrow RNA samples also contain an RNA species which retains a portion of the small intervening sequence. This RNA species protects

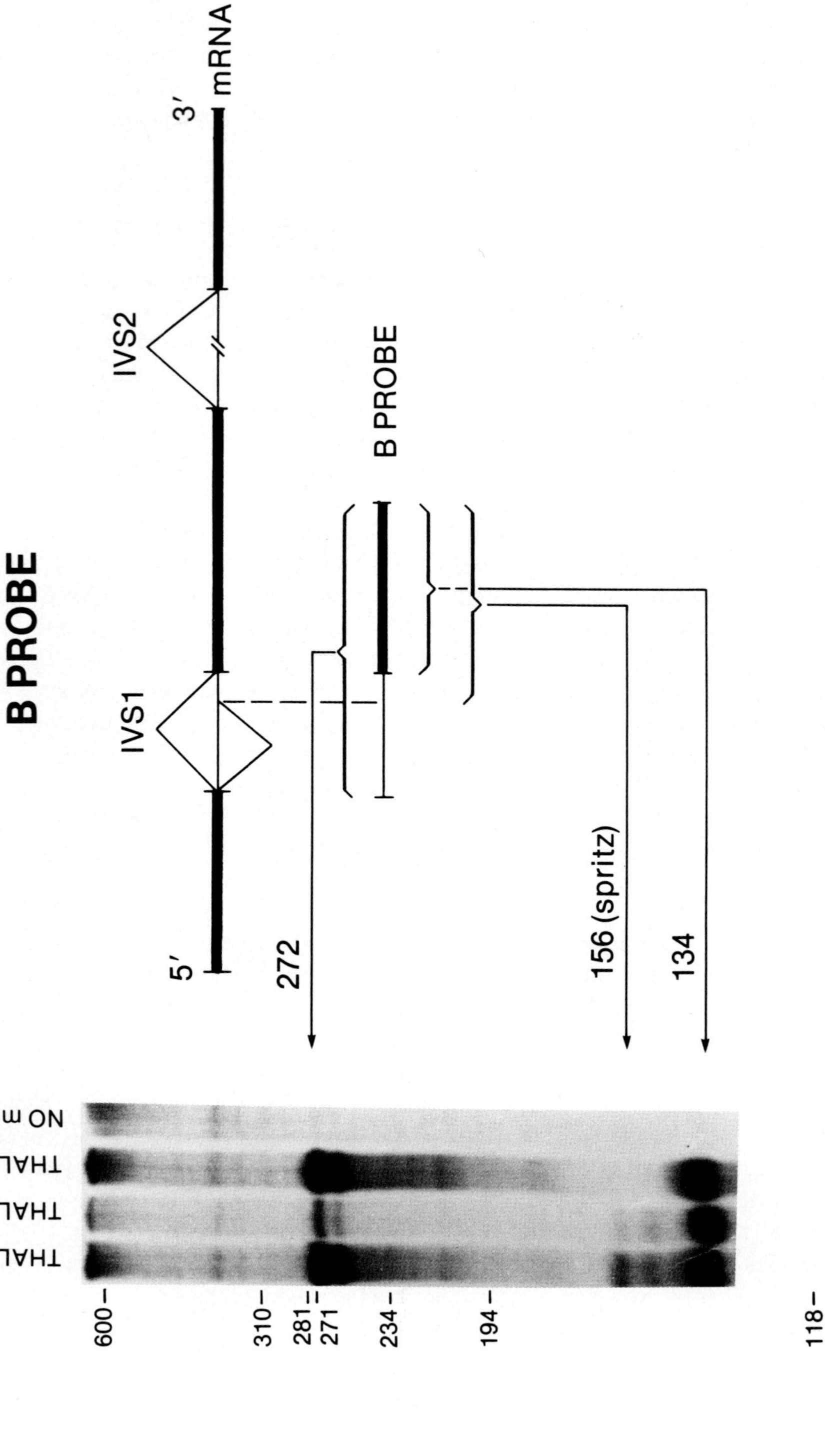
B PROBE
IVS1
IVS2
5′
3′
mRNA
B PROBE
272
156 (spritz)
134
NO mRNA
THAL
THAL
THAL
600
310
281
271
234
194
118

153 nucleotides of the probe yielding the band at this position in the first and third lanes (Fig. 4). One of the thalassemic bone marrow RNA samples (the center of the 3 in Fig. 4) contains a normal amount of precursor which still retains the sequences transcribed from intron 1. A moderately intense DNA band 272 nucleotides long arises because of protection of the entire human segment of the probe by this RNA species. The other 2 thalassemic bone marrow RNA samples contain a markedly increased amount of a precursor species from which the RNA transcribed from intron 1 has not been removed.

The RNA species which retains a portion of the sequences transcribed from intron 1 in 2 patients' bone marrow samples undoubtedly reflects the presence of the mutation described by Spritz et al [19]. By DNA sequence analysis of a cloned thalassemic gene, they discovered a single nucleotide change in the thalassemic gene; an adenosine substituted for a guanosine in intron 1. This substitution perfects an alternative acceptor site within the intron. The RNA species which arises from use of this acceptor site retains 19 nucleotides of IVS1. The presence of an in-phase terminator codon within this aberrantly processed RNA molecule effectively prevents synthesis of β-globin on this RNA template. A quantitative reduction in β-globin production is the consequence.

In experiments now published, Ley and colleagues [18] have analyzed 15 bone marrow samples from individual thalassemic patients by S_1 nuclease analysis using probes specific for the ends and splice junctions of β-mRNA. Several bone marrow RNAs contained a species which reflected the presence of the IVS1 alternative acceptor site mutation [19-21]. Several additional bone marrow RNAs contained increased amounts of an RNA species from which none of the RNA sequences transcribed from intron 1 had been removed. Data from 2 of these are shown in Figure 4. This aberrantly processed molecule presumably represents the presence of a mutation affecting either the donor or acceptor site of

---

Fig. 4. Illustrated on the left is a schematic representation of the technique of S_1 nuclease analysis. In our experiments, uniformly labeled single-stranded DNA probes were generated using templates derived from M13 recombinants. The probe is purified after synthesis by gel electrophoresis. Annealing to total cellular RNA is under standard hybridization conditions [15]. RNA-DNA duplexes which form are exposed to S_1 nuclease digestion; only DNA sequences protected by mRNA survive digestion. Illustrated is the circumstance in which 2 types of mRNA molecules are present, one processed correctly, and one processed using an alternative acceptor splice site 19 bp into intron 1 [19-21]. The data were obtained by analysis of total bone RNA from 3 separate patients homozygous for β-thalassemia. On the left are indicated the migration positions of [^{32}P]-labeled $\phi\chi$ Hae III fragments. The first patient is doubly heterozygous for a mutation which retards removal of RNA transcribed from intron 1 and the 3′ intron 1 alternative acceptor splice site mutation. The second patient is heterozygous for the alternative acceptor site mutation, while the third patient is heterozygous for a mutation leading to increased amounts of precursor from which RNA transcribed from intron 1 has not been removed.

intron 1, thus preventing removal of these sequences from precursor molecules. Analysis of bone marrow RNA from additional patients provided no evidence for aberrantly processed RNA molecules; such patients may have genes which are affected by mutations altering transcriptional rate or polyadenylation efficiency.

SUMMARY

Our studies have shown that globin-gene structure, as revealed by Southern blot analysis, is normal in most patients who are homozygous for β-thalassemia. In many, but not all patients, evidence for mutations which alter the metabolism of β-globin RNA molecules was obtained by several methods of analysis. The most specific and sensitive of these involves the use of single-stranded, highly radioactive probes generated using the M13 cloning system. Such probes allow detection of aberrantly processed RNA molecules by S_1 nuclease analysis, thereby providing clues as to the position and nature of mutations within individual thalassemic globin genes. Of greatest potential interest are those genes which provide no evidence, in bone marrow RNA, of aberrantly processed intermediates. Analysis of these genes by molecular cloning and DNA sequencing may lead to identification of sequences which are important for initiation or termination of RNA transcription.

Mutations which cause β-thalassemia continue to provide a rich source of information about the nature of DNA sequences which are essential for efficient gene expression. By study of thalassemic patients, new insights are obtained into normal mRNA metabolism.

REFERENCES

1. Nienhuis AW, Propper R: The thalassemias: Disorders of hemoglobin synthesis. In Nathan D, Oski F (eds): "Hematology of Infancy and Childhood." Philadelphia: WB Saunders Co, 1981, vol I, p 726.
2. Bank A, Mears JG, Ramirez F: Disorders of human hemoglobin. Science 207:486, 1980.
3. Stamatoyannopoulos G, Nienhuis AW (eds): "Organization and Expression of Globin Genes." New York: Alan R Liss, Inc, 1981.
4. Southern EM: Detection of specific sequences among DNA separated by gel electrophoresis. J Mol Biol 98:503, 1975.
5. Orkin SH, Old JM, Weatherall DJ, Nathan DG: Partial deletion of β-globin genes in certain patients with β^0-thalassemia. Proc Natl Acad Sci USA 76:2400, 1979.
6. Flavell RA, Bernards R, Kooter JM, DeBoer E, Little PFR, Annison G, Williamson R: The structure of the human β-globin gene in β thalassemia. Nucleic Acids Res 25:2749, 1979.
7. Tam JWO, Kaufman RE, Nienhuis AW: Analysis of globin gene structure in patients with β thalassemia by restriction endonuclease mapping. Hemoglobin 5:209, 1981.
8. Mears JG, Ramirez F, Leibowitz D, Bank A: Organization of human δ and β-globin genes in cellular DNA and the presence of intragenic inserts. Cell 15:15, 1978.
9. Flavell RA, Kooter JM, DeBoer E, Little PFR, Williamson R: Analysis of the β-δ-globin gene loci in normal and Hb Lepore DNA: Direct determination of gene linkage and intragene distance. Cell 15:25, 1978.

10. Lawn RM, Fritsch EF, Parker RC, Balke G, Maniatis T: The isolation and characterization of linked δ- and β-globin genes from a cloned library of human DNA. Cell 15:1157, 1978.
11. Fritsch EF, Lawn RM, Maniatis T: Molecular cloning and characterization of the human β-like globin gene cluster. Cell 19:959, 1980.
12. Kaufman RE, Kretschmer PJ, Adams JW, Coon HC, Anderson WF, Nienhuis AW: Cloning and characterization of DNA sequences surrounding the human γ-, δ-, and β-globin genes. Proc Natl Acad Sci USA 77:4229, 1980.
13. Fritsch EF, Lawn RM, Maniatis T: Characterization of deletions which affect the expression of fetal globin genes in man. Nature 279:598, 1979.
14. Bernard R, Flavell RA: Physical mapping of the globin gene deletion in hereditary persistence of fetal hemoglobin (HPFH). Nucleic Acids Res 8:1521, 1980.
15. Kantor JA, Turner PH, Nienhuis AW: Beta thalassemia: Mutations which affect the processing of the β-globin mRNA precursor. Cell 21:149, 1980.
16. Alwine JC, Kemp DJ, Stark GR: Method for detection of specific RNAs in agarose gels by transfer to diazobenzyloxymethyl-paper and hybridization with DNA probes. Proc Natl Acad Sci USA 74:5350, 1977.
17. Berk AJ, Sharp PA: Sizing and mapping of early adenovirus mRNAs by gel electrophoresis of S_1 endonuclease-digested hybrids. Cell 12:721, 1977.
18. Ley T, Anagnou N, Pepe G, Nienhuis AW: RNA processing errors in patients with β-thalassemia. Proc Natl Acad Sci USA 79:1982.
19. Spritz RA, Jagadeeswaran P, Choudary PV, Biro PA, Elder JT, deRiel JK, Manley JL, Gefter ML, Forget BG, Weissman SM: Base substitution in an intervening sequence of a β^+-thalassemic human globin gene. Proc Natl Acad Sci USA 78:2455, 1981.
20. Westaway D, Williamson R: An intron nucleotide sequence variant in a cloned β^+-thalassemia globin gene. Nucleic Acids Res 9:177, 1981.
21. Busslinger M, Moschonas N, Flavell RA: β^+ Thalassemia: Aberrant splicing results from a single point mutation in an intron. Cell 27:289, 1981.

STRUCTURE AND SYNTHESIS OF FETAL HEMOGLOBIN

The Polymorphism of Human Fetal Hemoglobin*

Titus H.J. Huisman, PhD, DSc

INTRODUCTION

The structural heterogeneity of human fetal hemoglobin (Hb F) has been studied extensively ever since it was discovered that position 136 of the γ chain can be occupied by a glycyl or an alanyl residue [1]. Soon it became evident that the $^{A}\gamma$ and $^{G}\gamma$ chains are the products of nonallelic γ structural genes, and recent structural DNA analyses have indicated that duplicated γ genes are located on chromosome #11 [2–4]. Several γ chain variants have been discovered; some are $^{A}\gamma$ chain and others $^{G}\gamma$ chain mutants (a list is provided in HEMOGLOBIN 5:280, 1981). One variant, Hb F-Sardinia or $\alpha_2\gamma_2$ 75(E19)Ile → Thr, was discovered by Griffoni et al [5] in a patient who had β-thalassemia. Ricco et al [6] searched for this variant in additional β-thalassemia patients and observed it in 39 of 42 homozygotes. The relatively high incidence of Hb F-Sardinia in subjects with β-thalassemia who originate from the Mediterranean littoral, has been confirmed by others [7,8]. Structural analyses have indicated that the γ chain of Hb F-Sardinia is a variant of the $^{A}\gamma$ chain [9,10] and is presently designated as the $^{A}\gamma^{T}$ chain (T = threonine) while the $^{A}\gamma^{I}$ (I=isoleucine) symbol is assigned to the most commonly occurring $^{A}\gamma$ chain.

Recently, several micro procedures have been developed which are useful for the separation and quantitation of the $^{A}\gamma^{T}$, $^{A}\gamma^{I}$, and $^{G}\gamma$ chain [for a review, see ref. 11]. Application of these methods greatly facilitates a reevaluation of the γ chain heterogeneity in normal subjects and in persons with pathologic conditions. We have used a high pressure liquid chromatographic (HPLC) procedure to further analyze the γ chain heterogeneity of the Hb F from numerous newborn babies and from patients with β-thalassemia and $\delta\beta$-thalassemia of different racial or ethnic origins. The results of these studies form the basis of this presentation.

*Supported in part by USPHS research grants HLB-05168 and HLB-15158.

Birth Defects: Original Article Series, Volume 18, Number 7, pages 83–99
© 1982 March of Dimes Birth Defects Foundation

TECHNICAL INFORMATION

Subjects

Cord blood samples were obtained from over 430 Black and 200 Chinese newborns. These samples were submitted to the laboratories of the Comprehensive Sickle Cell Center as part of a general testing program or were mailed by a foreign investigator (Dr. Zeng, Shanghai) with whom an official collaborative study was initiated. Blood samples from adult patients with β- or $\delta\beta$-thalassemia (heterozygotes, homozygotes, or subjects with a combination of β- or $\delta\beta$-thalassemia) were obtained locally (Black patients) or were mailed to the author by collaborators in foreign countries (Dr. G. D. Efremov, Yugoslavia; Dr. A. Gurgey, Turkey; Dr. B. Ibarra, Mexico). These samples were mailed by air as washed red cells or as isolated Hb F; diagnoses were established locally and confirmed in the authors' laboratories when possible.

Methods

Each sample was studied by starch gel electrophoresis [12]. The level of Hb F in adult red cell lysates was determined by alkali denaturization [13] and the % Hb A_2 by DEAE-cellulose chromatography [14]. The same chromatographic procedure was used to isolate Hb F for structural analyses. All isolated hemoglobin samples contained at least 40% Hb F as judged by visual inspection of a starch gel. Cord blood red cell lysates were analyzed without prior purification. The ${}^A\gamma^T$, ${}^A\gamma^I$, and ${}^G\gamma$ chains were separated and quantitated by the HPL chromatographic method which has been described in detail elsewhere [11, 15–18]. The method requires less than 100 mg Hb F and one analysis is completed in 3 to 4 hours. Quantitation of the chains is reproducible with a SD not exceeding 2%; values of ${}^A\gamma^T$ and ${}^A\gamma^I$ chains below 2% are considered unreliable. The references quoted above present numerous examples of chromatograms that can be obtained; Figure 1 shows the separation of heme, α and β^A and β^C chains, and the ${}^A\gamma^T$, ${}^G\gamma$, and ${}^A\gamma^I$ chains in the red cell lysate of a newborn Hb C heterozygote who had an additional ${}^A\gamma^T$ heterozygosity. Experience has taught that samples should be analyzed as quickly as possible, preferably within 2 weeks after the preparation of the lysates or the isolation of the Hb F.

RESULTS AND DISCUSSION

Newborn Babies

The presence of the ${}^A\gamma^T$ *chain.* Table 1 summarizes the data describing the occurrence of the ${}^A\gamma^T$ chain in Black babies with and without the Hb S abnormality, and in normal Chinese babies. Results for newborn and adult patients with sickle cell anemia are also included [these data are from ref. 19]. Both ${}^A\gamma^T$ heterozygotes and homozygotes were observed. The ${}^A\gamma^T$ gene frequencies among Black and Chinese babies were significantly different and considerably less than that

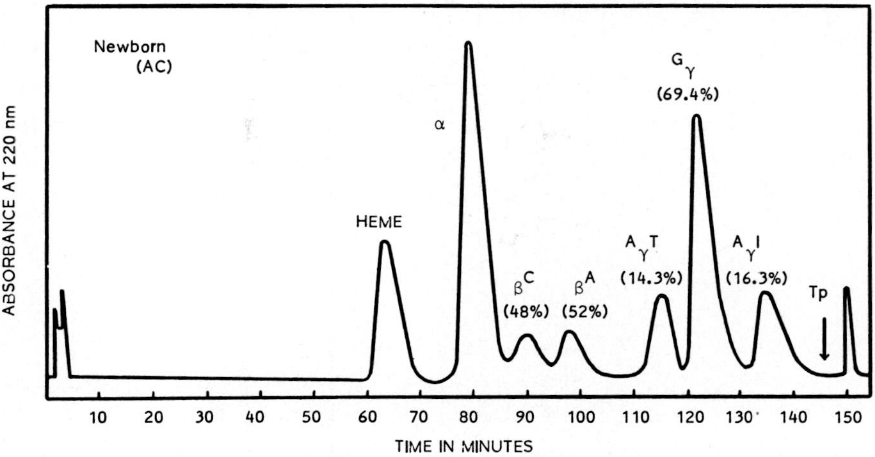

Fig. 1. Separation of the $^{A}\gamma^{T}$, $^{G}\gamma$, and $^{A}\gamma^{I}$ chains by HPL chromatography. About 100 μg Hb from a cord blood cell lysate of a baby with the Hb C heterozygosity is mixed with 25 μl phosphate solution, pH 2.86, and applied to a C_{18} Waters μBondapak column equipped with a guard column. A Perkin Elmer Series 3 Microprocessor with LC-55B Digital Spectrophotometer and Microcell, Model 23, recorder with AUFS at 0.02 range is used. The solvents consist of mixtures of acetonitrile and methanol (UV High Purity Solvent grade), and a solution of 49 mM KH_2PO_4 and 5.4 mM H_3PO_4 per liter at pH 2.86. T_p is time of purging the column. Flow rate: 1.5 ml/min. For further details, see references [11, 15–18]. Quantitation of the 2 β chains and of the 3 γ chains is based on the relative areas under the peaks which can be determined by weighing.

calculated from data for Italian newborns [6]. The low $^{A}\gamma^{T}$ frequency (0.036) in the SS population adequately explains the lower percentage of $^{A}\gamma^{T}$ heterozygotes among Black AS newborns. Apparently, the genotype with the $^{A}\gamma^{T}$ *in trans* to the β^{S} mutant occurs about 3 times more frequently than that in which the $^{A}\gamma^{T}$ mutant is *in cis* to the β^{S} mutation.

These results suggest that the $^{G}\gamma$, $^{A}\gamma^{T}$, δ, β genotype was likely introduced in the Black and Chinese populations through admixture of genes from the Mediterranean littoral where the $^{A}\gamma^{T}$ mutation presumably originated. Thus, most persons with a heterozygosity for Hb S or Hb C (and probably also other β chain variants) will have the $^{A}\gamma^{T}$ gene *in trans* of the β determinant although a rather frequently occurring crossing-over within the $^{G}\gamma$, $^{A}\gamma$, δ, β gene region may explain the observation that about 25% of AS heterozygotes with the additional $^{A}\gamma^{T}$ heterozygosity have this $^{A}\gamma^{T}$ gene *in cis* to the β^{S} mutation [19].

The percentages of $^{A}\gamma^{T}$ chain in heterozygous and homozygous babies. Table 2 lists the average percentages of the two types of $^{A}\gamma$ chain in heterozygotes. No differences have been observed between Black and Chinese babies. The relative amount of the $^{A}\gamma^{T}$ chain is slightly less than that of the $^{A}\gamma^{I}$ chain (45% vs 55%).

TABLE 1. The Occurrence of the $^{A}\gamma^{T}$ Gene in Different Populations

Population	N	$^{A}\gamma^{T}$ Heterozygote		$^{A}\gamma^{T}$ Homozygote		Gene Frequency	
		N	(%)	N	(%)	$^{A}\gamma^{T}$	$^{A}\gamma^{I}$
Black AA newborn	285	51	(17.9)	4	(1.4)	0.104	0.897
Black AS newborn	144	19	(13.2)*	1	(0.7)	—	—
Black SS newborn and adults	138	8	(5.8)	1	(0.7)	0.036	0.964
Chinese AA newborn	201	29	(14.4)	1	(0.5)	0.077	0.923

*It is estimated that 5 cases have the $^{A}\gamma^{T}$ gene *in cis* and 14 cases have the $^{A}\gamma^{T}$ gene *in trans* to the β^{S} variant [19].

TABLE 2. The Average Percentages of $^{A}\gamma^{T}$ and $^{A}\gamma^{I}$ Chains in the Hb F of Newborn Babies With an $^{A}\gamma^{T}$ Heterozygosity

	$^{A}\gamma^{T}$		$^{A}\gamma^{I}$		
Origin	%	SD	%	SD	$^{A}\gamma^{T} \cdot 100/[^{A}\gamma^{T}+^{A}\gamma^{I}]$
Black AA (N = 52)	12.6 ±	3.0	15.3 ±	3.1	45.2
Black AS (N = 19)	13.0 ±	1.8	16.3 ±	2.3	44.4
Chinese AA (N = 29)	14.2 ±	1.8	17.0 ±	2.5	45.5

TABLE 3. The Average Percentages of the $^{G}\gamma$ Chain in the Hb F of Newborn Babies of Different Ethnic Origins Divided in Subgroups I, II, and III

	Group I*			Group II*			Group III*		
Origin	N	%	SD	N	%	SD	N	%	SD
Black AA (N = 285)	2	40.0	± 5.0	272	70.4	± 3.0	11	82.8	± 2.4
Black AS (N = 144)	0	—		137	71.2	± 3.1	7	82.7	± 2.4
Chinese (N = 201)	6	41.5	± 1.8	188	68.8	± 2.9	7	80.3	± 1.3

*See Figure 2.

The average % $^{A}\gamma^{T}$ chain in the 6 $^{A}\gamma^{T}$ homozygous newborns [25.3% ± 1.8% (SD)] was slightly less than that in the numerous $^{A}\gamma^{I}$ homozygous Black newborns [29.6% ± 1.9 (SD)] or $^{A}\gamma^{I}$ homozygous Chinese newborns [31.2% ± 1.3 (SD)].

The percentages of $^{G}\gamma$ chain. Figure 2 illustrates the distribution of the $^{G}\gamma$ chain values among Black AA, AS, and SS babies and normal Chinese babies (some of this information has been presented in ref. 18, while detailed data on the Chinese studies will be published elsewhere) and Table 3 lists average percentages. Most babies have $^{G}\gamma$ values of about 70% (group II) confirming previously published data [1, 20, 21]. Two additional subgroups have been observed.

Group I. This subgroup consists of 2 healthy Black newborn and 6 healthy Chinese babies with an average $^{G}\gamma$ chain level of about 40%. The 2 Black babies, who are first cousins, have been followed for nearly one year. The data on Figure 3 [from ref. 18 where these studies are described in great detail] indicate persistently low $^{G}\gamma$ chain levels in these infants—about 10% at the age of nearly one year. (The relatively low $^{G}\gamma$ level in baby A.W. who suffered from a vitamin-E deficiency-related hemolytic anemia was corrected after appropriate treatment). The mothers, who are sisters, also had low $^{G}\gamma$ levels in their Hb F, similar to the percentages observed in their babies (Fig. 4). The follow-up of the Chinese babies with the low $^{G}\gamma$ chain values has been limited thus far; however, again low $^{G}\gamma$ chain values were seen in samples collected at the age of 3 months.

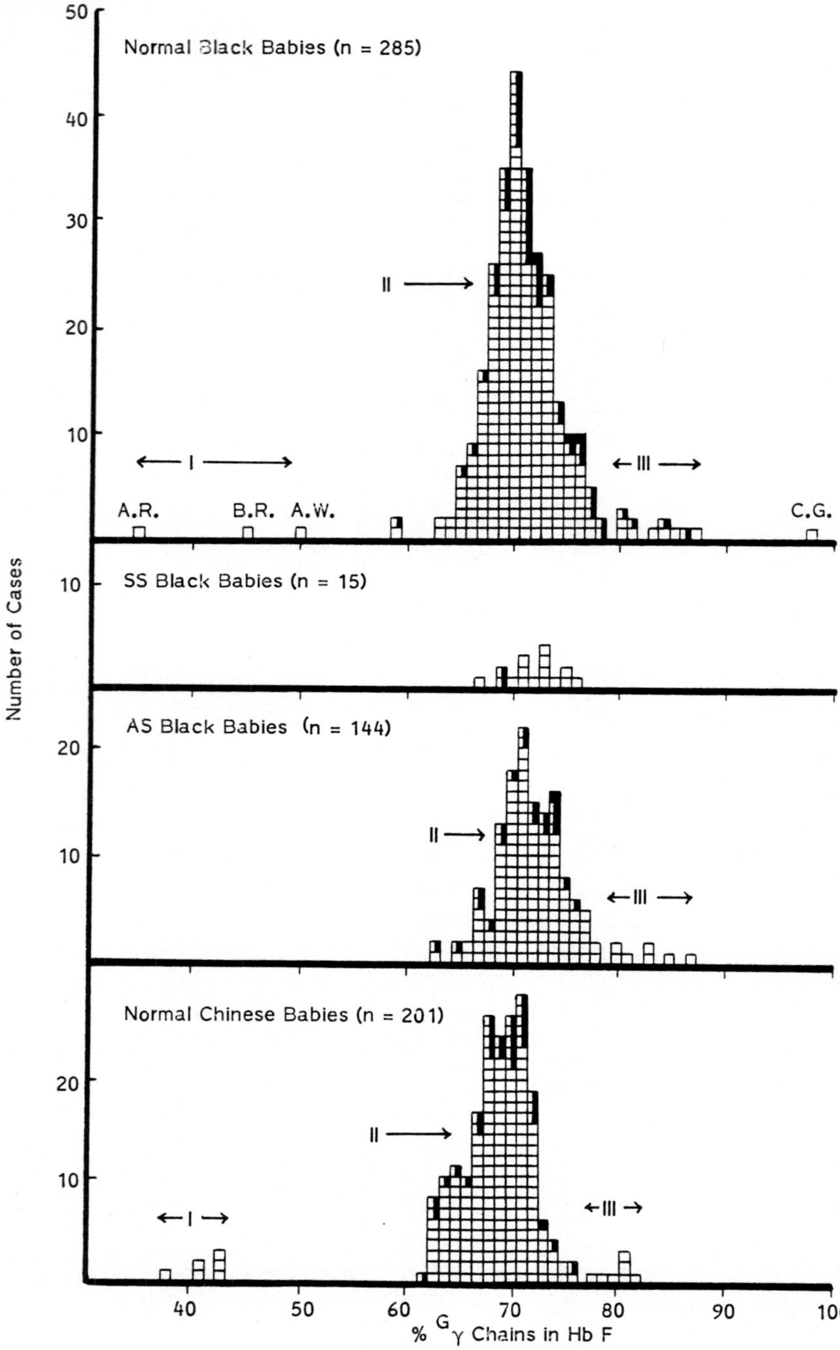

Fig. 2. The levels of $^{G}\gamma$ chain in the Hb F of newborns with normal Hb patterns (Black AA and Chinese AA) and with a Hb S trait (Black AS) or sickle cell anemia (Black SS). □ $^{A}\gamma^{T}$ negative; ◧ $^{A}\gamma^{T}$ heterozygote; ■ $^{A}\gamma^{T}$ homozygote.

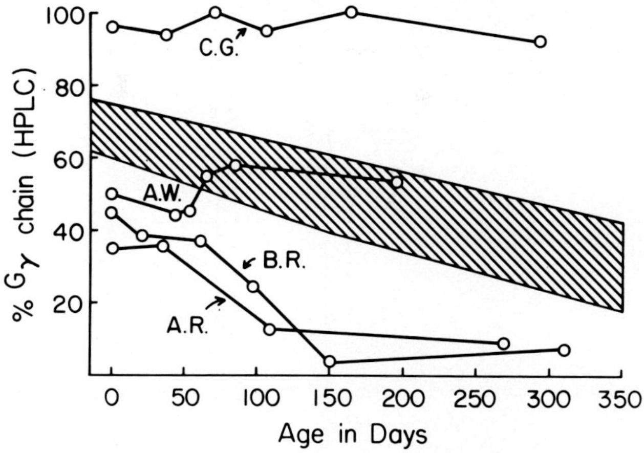

Fig. 3. The levels of $^{G}\gamma$ chain in 4 newborns with high or low $^{G}\gamma$ levels, determined at various time intervals during the first year of life [from ref. 18].

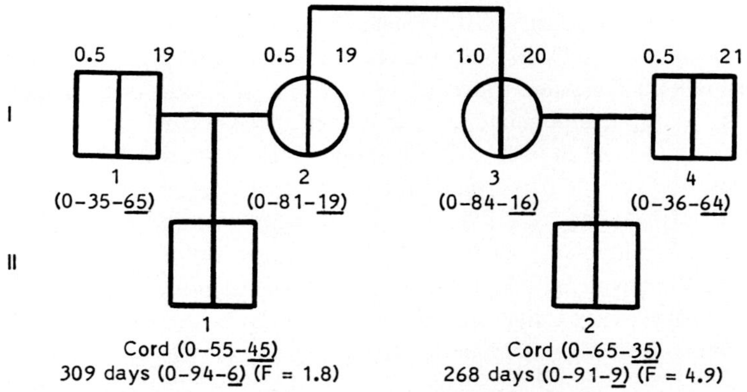

Fig. 4. *Family R* from Georgia with unusually low levels of $^{G}\gamma$ chain in the Hb F of 2 newborns. The % F_{AD} is listed at the upper left hand corner and the age at the upper right hand corner; (30-30-40) indicate percentages of the $^{A}\gamma^{T}$, $^{A}\gamma^{I}$, and $^{G}\gamma$ chains.

The clinical condition and normal hematologic values seen in these babies nearly exclude the possible presence of a $^{G}\gamma$ chain deficiency (ie a $^{G}\gamma$-thalassemia trait). It appears more likely that the infants carry 3 $^{A}\gamma$ chain genes and 1 $^{G}\gamma$ chain gene either through a mechanism of unequal crossing-over or because they belong to a small group of persons in whom the Ala → Gly mutation is absent in 1 of the 2 γ chain genes because a Gly → Ala back- mutation had occurred.

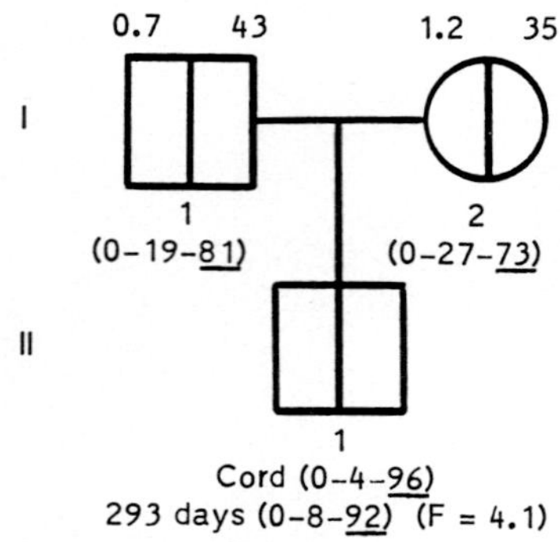

Fig. 5. *Family G* from Georgia with a newborn having a homozygous $^{A}\gamma^{+}$-thalassemia with extremely low $^{A}\gamma$ levels. The % F_{AD} is listed at the upper left hand corner, and the age at the upper right hand corner; (30-30-40) indicate percentages of $^{A}\gamma^{T}$, $^{A}\gamma^{I}$, and $^{G}\gamma$ chains.

Group III. Previous studies [21] have indicated that some babies have $^{G}\gamma$ values which are slightly higher than the normal level of 70%. This was again observed in both Black and Chinese babies (Fig. 2 and Table 3; the incidence of this condition in the 2 populations is about 4%). One normal newborn (C.G. of Fig. 2) had a $^{G}\gamma$ level of 96% which remained high in several samples collected during his first year of life (Fig. 3; the Hb F level at the age of 309 days was 1.8% with a Hb A_2 level of 2.3%). It is of interest to note that the normal parents of this infant had low levels of Hb F (0.7% and 1.2%) with a $^{G}\gamma$ chain percentage (73 and 81%) considerably higher than usually seen in normal persons (Fig. 5).

These results suggest that the babies with $^{G}\gamma$ chain levels of about 80% are heterozygous for a regulatory deficiency which affects the synthesis of the $^{A}\gamma$ chain. Baby C.G., who produced over 90% $^{G}\gamma$ chains but a detectable percentage of $^{A}\gamma$ chains, is likely homozygous for this condition. The suppression of the $^{A}\gamma$ chain synthesis appears incomplete and, thus, this anomaly can be considered a form of $^{A}\gamma^{+}$-thalassemia. This deficiency seems not to influence the clinical or hematologic condition of the affected newborn mainly because of the high production rates by the $^{G}\gamma$ chain genes.

β-Thalassemia

The presence of the $^{A}\gamma^{T}$ chain. Limited data, published previously [17], suggest that 1 of 5 Black β-thal heterozygotes has a $^{A}\gamma^{T}$ heterozygosity. Similar data are shown in Figure 6 which lists information on 103 Black normal adults, 121 Black β-thal traits, and 52 β-thal traits from the Mediterranean area. Results on members of a few families are included; however, it appears that 23.5% of the

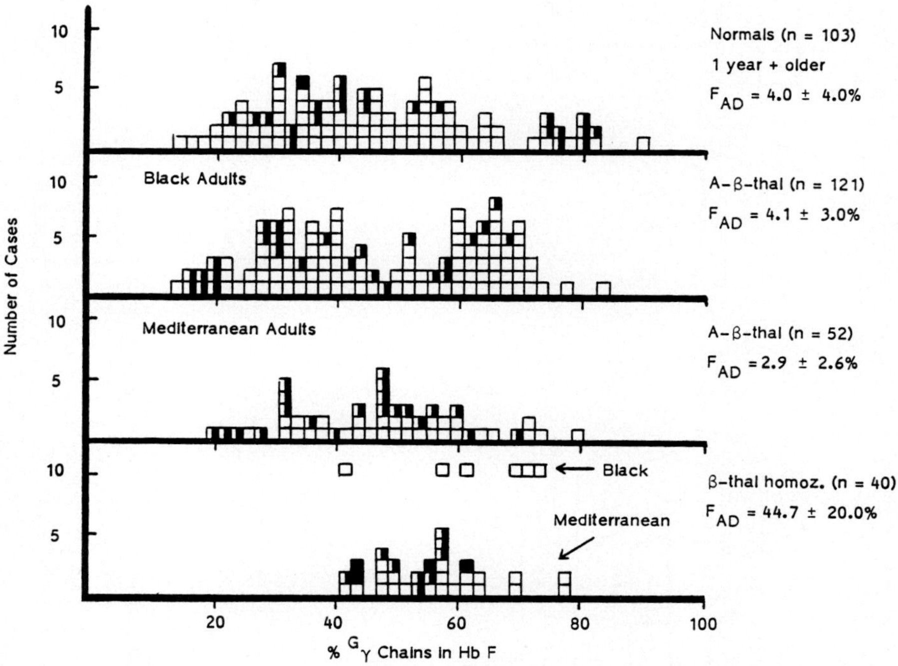

Fig. 6. The levels of ${}^G\gamma$ chain in the Hb F of normal adults, and adults with a heterozygosity or homozygosity for β-thalassemia. □ ${}^A\gamma^T$ negative; ◧ ${}^A\gamma^T$ heterozygote; ■ ${}^A\gamma^T$ homozygote.

Black normal adults are ${}^A\gamma^T$ positive (one person is a homozygote), 20.5% of the Black β-thal trait are ${}^A\gamma^T$ heterozygotes, and 38% of the non-Black β-thal traits carry the ${}^A\gamma^T$ heterozygosity, corresponding to gene frequencies of 0.12, 0, 10, and 0.20, respectively.

The percentages of ${}^G\gamma$ chain in normal adults and β-thal traits. The results illustrated in Figure 6 indicate a large variation which is ill-understood. Normal adult data seem to fall in 2 groups; a major group has ${}^G\gamma$ values between 14 and 66%, and a minor group has values between 72 and 88%. It may well be that the latter values are characteristic for a ${}^A\gamma^+$ thalassemia trait (see above).

A similar large variation is observed for Black β-thal heterozygotes. However, 2 distinct groups are observed with low ("adult") ${}^G\gamma$ values and high ("newborn") ${}^G\gamma$ values, confirming data reported earlier [22,23]. Surprisingly,

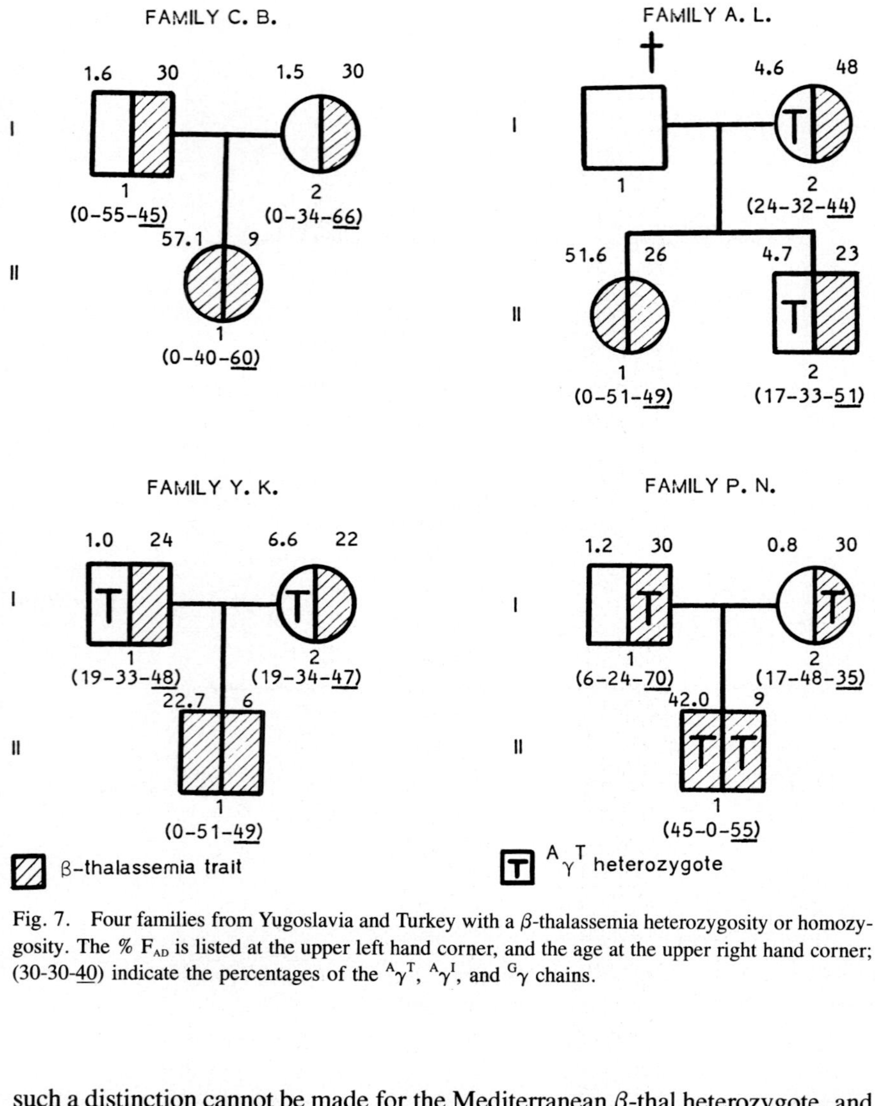

Fig. 7. Four families from Yugoslavia and Turkey with a β-thalassemia heterozygosity or homozygosity. The % F_{AD} is listed at the upper left hand corner, and the age at the upper right hand corner; (30-30-40) indicate the percentages of the $^{A}\gamma^{T}$, $^{A}\gamma^{I}$, and $^{G}\gamma$ chains.

such a distinction cannot be made for the Mediterranean β-thal heterozygote, and the $^{G}\gamma$ chain values for this group of 52 individuals vary as much as is seen for the normal adults. The large variation of these data is puzzling and only partly influenced by technical problems encountered in these analyses; high $^{G}\gamma$ and low $^{G}\gamma$ values are reproducible in duplicate analyses and for duplicate blood samples.

The percent $^{A}\gamma^{T}$ chain in β-thalassemia heterozygotes. The % $^{A}\gamma^{T}$ chain (as % of total $^{A}\gamma$ chain) varied from 6 to 94% and was to some extent dependent on the location of the $^{A}\gamma^{T}$ mutation, ie either *in cis* or *in trans* to the β-thal determinant.

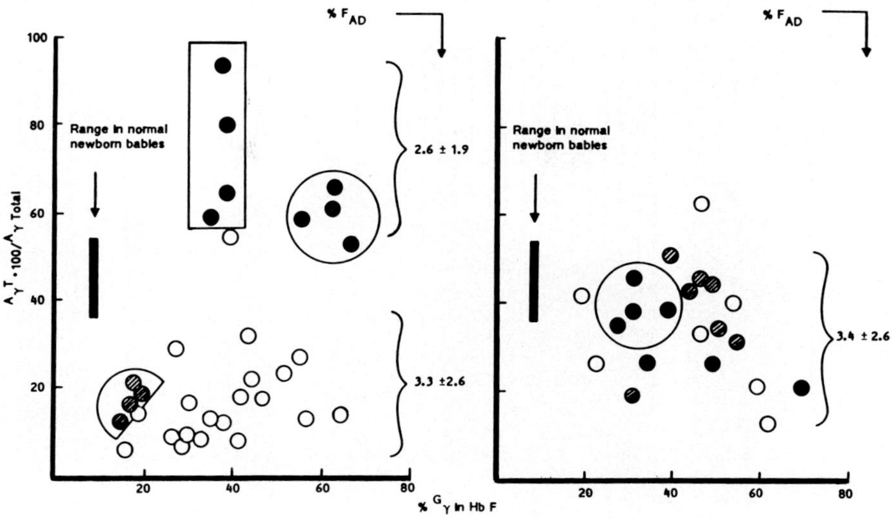

Fig. 8. The percent $^{A}\gamma^{T}$ chain (as % of total $^{A}\gamma$ chain) plotted against the percent $^{G}\gamma$ chain in β-thalassemia heterozygotes of Black (left panel) and Mediterranean (right panel) origin. ● $^{A}\gamma^{T}$ *in cis;* ◍ $^{A}\gamma^{T}$ *in trans;* ○ relation of $^{A}\gamma^{T}$ to β-thal is undetermined. Boxed in values are from families.

Determination of the *in cis* or *in trans* position was made by family studies as shown for Black families in ref. 17 and for Caucasian families in Figure 7. The 4 examples of families, ie parents with a child homozygous for β-thalassemia with or without a $^{A}\gamma^{T}$ anomaly, demonstrate the method used to designate the genotype in the heterozygote (the possibility of cross-over was not considered). Figure 8 lists the $^{A}\gamma^{T}$ percentages in relation to the $^{G}\gamma$ chain levels for both Black and Mediterranean β-thalassemia heterozygotes. Cases with the $^{A}\gamma^{T}$ anomaly *in cis* or *in trans* to the β-thal determinant are clearly identified in this figure, while data on family members can also be readily recognized. The average percentages of $^{A}\gamma^{T}$ chain (as % of total $^{A}\gamma$ chain) in Black β-thal traits are 16.4 ± 7.3 % (SD) when the $^{A}\gamma^{T}$ chain gene is *in trans,* and 65.7 ± 12.6% (SD) when this gene is *in cis* to the β-thal determinant. This information indicates that at least two-thirds of the γ chain production in Black β-thal traits originates by the γ chain genes *in cis* to the β-thal abnormality. This appears to be different for the Mediterranean β-thal heterozygotes because no distinction could be made between the subjects with either an *in cis* or *in trans* location of the $^{A}\gamma^{T}$ gene. The average percentage of $^{A}\gamma^{T}$ chain [34.6 ± 11.1 (SD)] suggests that the contribution to the γ chain production by γ chain genes *in cis* and *in trans* to the β-thal determinant is about the same.

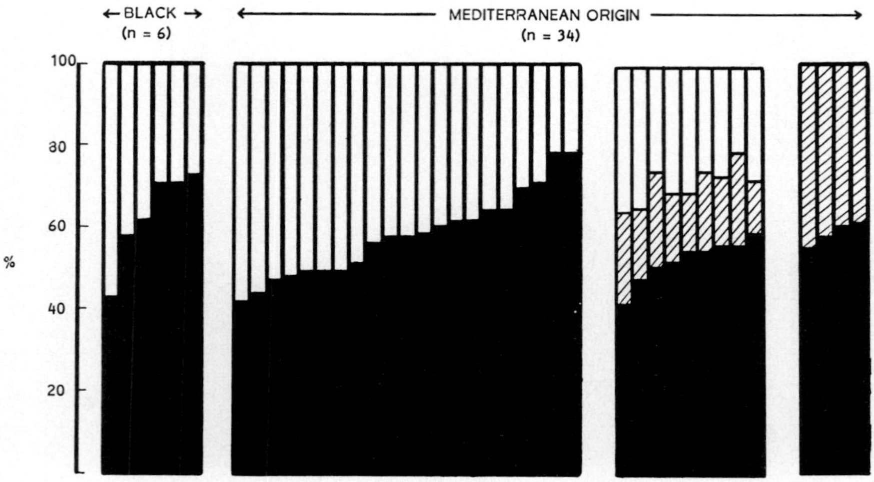

Fig. 9. The relative amounts of the $^{G}\gamma$ (■), $^{A}\gamma^{T}$ (▨), and $^{A}\gamma^{I}$ (□) chain in the Hb F of 40 β-thalassemia homozygotes. The $^{A}\gamma^{T}$ 100/total $^{A}\gamma$ ratio in the 9 $^{A}\gamma^{T}$ heterozygotes averaged 39%.

The percentages of $^{G}\gamma$ *and* $^{A}\gamma^{T}$ *chains in β-thalassemia homozygotes.* Figure 9 shows data for 6 Black and 34 Mediterranean homozygotes (identity of the types of β thal in the Mediterranean patients, is $\beta^{+}\beta^{+}$, $\beta^{+}\beta^{0}$, $\beta^{0}\beta^{0}$, was not made mainly because of transfusion requirements; the 6 Black homozygotes were of the β^{+} β^{+} sub-class). None of the Black patients had the $^{A}\gamma^{T}$ chain and of the Mediterranean patients only 9 (including 2 brothers) were $^{A}\gamma^{T}$ heterozygotes, 4 (including 1 brother and sister) were homozygotes, and 21 (including 1 brother and sister) were $^{A}\gamma^{T}$ negative. The gene frequency (0.22 which is similar to that calculated for the Mediterranean β-thal heterozygotes) is low mainly because of a strikingly lower occurrence of the $^{A}\gamma^{T}$ chain anomaly in the Turkish patients. The average $^{A}\gamma^{T}$ value (as % of the total $^{A}\gamma$-chain) was 39% which is comparable to the 45% observed in newborn heterozygotes (Table 2).

The $^{G}\gamma$ chain levels varied from 42 to 78% which are comparable to values reported previously [17, 22, 23].

δβ-Thalassemia

Two types of this condition have been studied; they are characterized by different types of deletions [2, 24]. Data for the Black $^{G}\gamma$-δβ-thalassemia traits have been reported before [17] and are again summarized in Table 4. About 10% Hb F

TABLE 4. The Levels of Hb F and the Three Types of γ Chain in $\delta\beta$-Thalassemia Heterozygotes

Type of Condition	N	% F_{AD} (SD)	% $^{G}\gamma$ (SD)	% $^{A}\gamma^{T}$ (SD)	% $^{A}\gamma^{I}$ (SD)
Black $^{G}\gamma$-$\delta\beta$-Thal $^{A}\gamma^{T}$ negative	15	11.2 ± 4.8	94.6 ± 2.8	0	5.2 ± 1.1
Mediterranean $^{A}\gamma^{G}\gamma$-$\delta\beta$-thal $^{A}\gamma^{T}$ negative	1	14.1	39.7	0	60.3
Mediterranean $^{A}\gamma^{G}\gamma$-$\delta\beta$-thal $^{A}\gamma^{T}$ positive (*in cis*)	9	10.5 ± 3.1	38.8 ± 4.7	58.1 ± 4.2	3.1 ± 2.3
Mediterranean $^{A}\gamma^{G}\gamma$-$\delta\beta$-thal $^{A}\gamma^{T}$ positive (*in trans*)	1	7.1	29.9	11.8	58.3

is present. Only 5% of this Hb F is of the $^{A}\gamma$ type suggesting a major contribution by the $^{G}\gamma$ chain gene *in cis* to this type of $\delta\beta$-determinant. An $^{A}\gamma^{T}$ positive $^{G}\gamma$-$\delta\beta$-thalassemia heterozygote has not yet been observed.

Ten of the 11 Mediterranean $^{A}\gamma^{G}\gamma$-$\delta\beta$-thal heterozygotes [see also ref. 25, 26] were positive for the $^{A}\gamma^{T}$ chain; 8 of these belonged to 2 relatively large families (Fig. 10). Four members of the Mexican families (top section of Fig. 10) were β-thal traits with the $^{A}\gamma^{T}$ chain *in cis* because the normal mother (*I-1*) of 2 β-thal traits was $^{A}\gamma^{T}$ negative. The 3 children of one $^{A}\gamma^{T}$ positive β-thal heterozygote and an $^{A}\gamma^{T}$ positive $\delta\beta$-thal heterozygote were $^{A}\gamma^{T}$ positive; the 2 youngest children had the β-$\delta\beta$ thal condition with an $^{A}\gamma^{T}$ homozygosity. Thus, the $\delta\beta$-thal traits *I-4* and *II-3* carry the $^{A}\gamma^{T}$ chain anomaly *in cis* to the $\delta\beta$-thal determinant. A similar conclusion can be drawn from the data obtained for the 6 $\delta\beta$-thal heterozygotes of *Family D* from Yugoslavia (bottom section of Fig. 10; see also ref. 8). It is noteworthy that the 10-year-old β-$\delta\beta$-thal patient in this family is a $^{A}\gamma^{T}$ heterozygote but her condition is otherwise not different from that of patients *II-4* and *II-5* of *Family 0* who have an $^{A}\gamma^{T}$ chain homozygosity.

Table 4 summarizes the results for all $\delta\beta$-thalassemia traits. The high percentage of the $^{A}\gamma^{T}$ chain (as % of total $^{A}\gamma$ chain) in the $^{A}\gamma^{G}\gamma$-$\delta\beta$-thal heterozygotes indicates that at least 95% of the relatively high level of Hb F is due to an increased production by the γ chain genes *in cis* to the $\delta\beta$-thal determinant. In this respect the $^{G}\gamma$-$\delta\beta$- and $^{A}\gamma^{G}\gamma$-$\delta\beta$-thal condition are comparable.

Figure 11 shows the pedigree of a family with $^{G}\gamma^{A}\gamma$-$\delta\beta$-thal and β-thalassemia. This family study indicates that the $^{A}\gamma^{T}$ anomaly is *in trans* to the $\delta\beta$-thal determinant; the $^{A}\gamma^{I}$ chain is present in an amount far exceeding that of the $^{A}\gamma^{T}$ chain (see also Table 4).

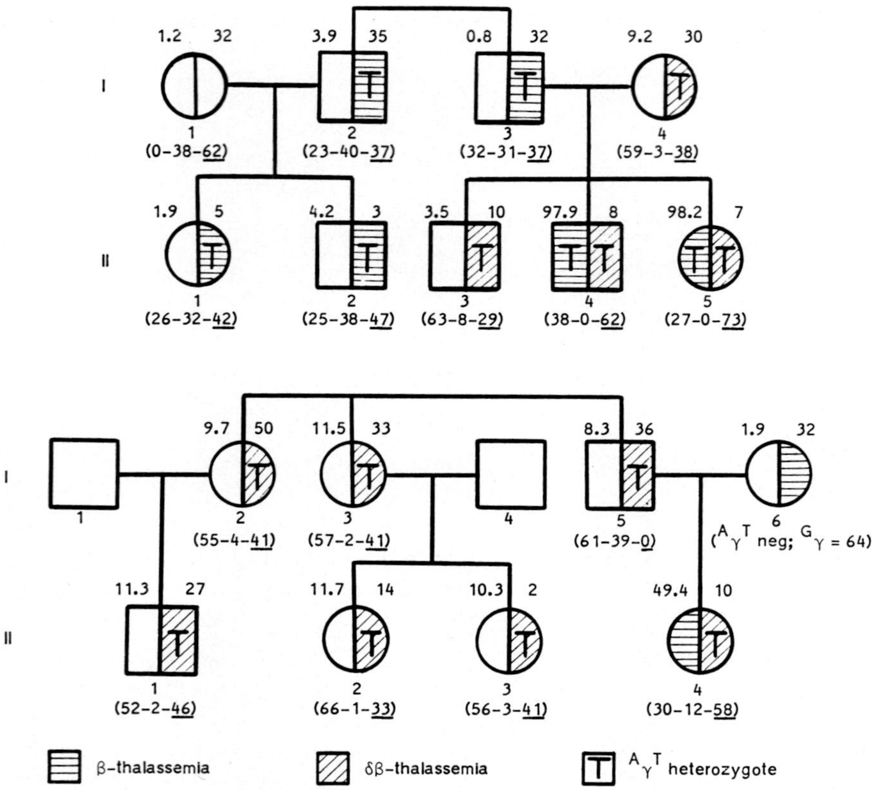

Fig. 10. Two families with the $^{A}\gamma^{G}$ -$\delta\beta$-thalassemia having the $^{A}\gamma^{T}$ chain gene *in cis* to the $\delta\beta$-thalassemia determinant. The % F_{AD} is listed at the upper left hand corner and the age at the upper right hand corner; (30-30-40) indicate the percentages of the $^{A}\gamma^{T}$, $^{A}\gamma^{I}$, and $^{G}\gamma$ chains. Pedigree at the top: *Family O* from Mexico [see also ref. 25]. Pedigree at the bottom: *Family D* from Yugoslavia [see also ref. 8].

CONCLUSIONS

Application of simplified methodology to the study of the γ-chain heterogeneity has facilitated the quantitation of the 3 most commonly occurring chains. This report contains a large body of data obtained by a newly developed high pressure liquid chromatographic method. The results concern numerous newborns, and adults with a β- or $\delta\beta$-thalassemia heterozygosity or homozygosity.

Evidence has been presented for the existence of a $^{A}\gamma^{+}$ type of thalassemia which is readily detectable in a newborn and which has no clinical consequences. No definite indication exists as yet for a $^{G}\gamma$ thalassemia, although some newborn

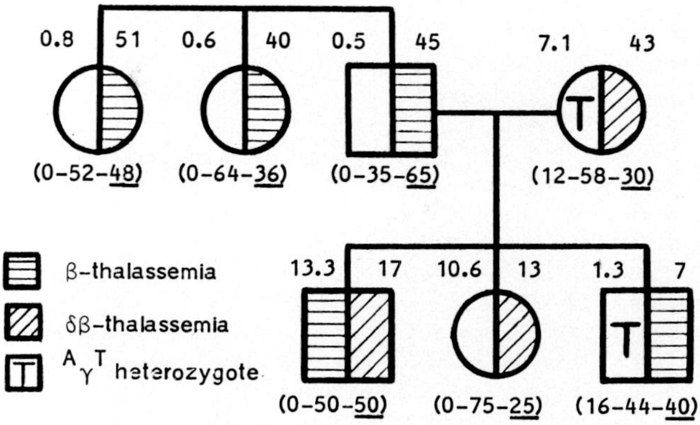

Fig. 11. *Family M* with a $^{A}\gamma^{G}\gamma$-$\delta\beta$-thalassemia heterozygote with a $^{A}\gamma^{T}$ heterozygosity *in trans* to the $\delta\beta$-thal determinant. The % F_{AD} is listed at the upper left hand corner, and the age at the upper right hand corner; (30-30-40) indicate the percentages of $^{A}\gamma^{T}$, $^{A}\gamma^{I}$, and $^{G}\gamma$ chains.

babies exhibit unusually low levels of $^{G}\gamma$ chains. The presence of an $^{A}\gamma^{T}$ chain heterozygosity was useful in evaluating some of these conditions.

Although most data presented for the patients with β-thalassemia or $\delta\beta$-thalassemia are not different from those reported in earlier publications the simultaneous quantitation of the $^{A}\gamma^{T}$, $^{A}\gamma^{I}$, and $^{G}\gamma$ chains offered data useful for an evaluation of the contribution by the γ-chain genes *in cis* or *in trans* to thalassemia determinant(s). Subtle differences might exist in this respect between Black and Mediterranean β-thalassemia heterozygotes. There seems little doubt that over 90% of the Hb F in the $\delta\beta$-thalassemia heterozygotes originated through an increased activity of the γ-chain gene(s) *in cis* to these thal determinants.

The newly developed HPLC procedure is useful for the determination of the $^{A}\gamma^{T}$ frequencies in various populations.

ACKNOWLEDGMENTS

The author is greatly indebted to his colleagues overseas who provided the samples from newborn babies (Dr. Zeng, Shanghai) and patients with β- or $\delta\beta$-thalassemia (Dr. G.D. Efremov, Yugoslavia, Dr. A. Gurgey, Turkey, Dr. B. Ibarra, Mexico); to his many collaborators who assisted in the data collection: M.B. Gardener, M.E. Gravely, K. Okonjo, A. Reese, A. Reynolds, H. Rocha, B. Webber; and to his friends who helped in the sample collection in the USA (B.L. Abraham, B. Joseph, H.F. Harris, L. Walker).

REFERENCES

1. Schroeder WA, Huisman THJ, Shelton JR, Shelton JB, Kleihauer EF, Dozy AM, Robberson B: Evidence for multiple structural genes for the γ chain of human fetal hemoglobin. Proc Natl Acad Sci USA 60:537, 1968.
2. Fritsch EF, Lawn RM, Maniatis T: Characterization of deletions which affect the expression of fetal globin genes in man. Nature 279:598, 1979.
3. Bernards R, Little PFR, Annison G, Williamson R, Flavell RA: Structure of the human $^{G}\gamma$-$^{A}\gamma$-δ-β globin gene locus. Proc Natl Acad Sci USA 76:4827, 1979.
4. Maniatis T, Fritsch EF, Lauer J, Lawn RM: The molecular genetics of human hemoglobins. Annu Rev Genet 14:145, 1980.
5. Griffoni V, Kamuzora H, Lehmann H, Charlesworth D: A new Hb variant: Hb F- Sardinia γ75 (E19) Isoleucine → Threonine, found in a family with Hb G-Philadelphia, β-chain deficiency and a Lepore-like haemoglobin indistinguishable from Hb A_2. Acta Haematol 53:347, 1975.
6. Ricco G, Mazza U, Turi RM, Pich PG, Camaschella C, Saglio G, Bernini LF: Significance of a new type of human fetal hemoglobin carrying a replacement Isoleucine → Threonine at position 75 (E19) of the γ chain. Hum Genet 32:305, 1976.
7. Huisman THJ, Schroeder WA, Reese A, Wilson JB, Lam H, Shelton JR, Shelton JB, Baker S: The $^{T}\gamma$ chain of human fetal hemoglobin at birth and in several abnormal hematological conditions. Pediatr Res 11:1102, 1977.
8. Schroeder WA, Huisman THJ, Efremov GD, Shelton JR, Shelton JB, Phillips P, Reese A, Gravely M, Harrison JM, Lam H: Further studies of the frequency and significance of the $^{T}\gamma$ chain of human fetal hemoglobin. J Clin Invest 63:268, 1979.
9. Efremov GD, Wilson JB, Huisman THJ: The chemical heterogeneity of human hemoglobin F: Direct evidence for the existence of three types of γ chains, the $^{IG}\gamma$, $^{IA}\gamma$, and $^{TA}\gamma$ chains. Biochim Biophys Acta 579:421, 1979.
10. Saglio G, Ricco G, Mazza U, Camaschella C, Pich PG, Gianni AM, Gianazza E, Righetti PG, Giglioni B, Comi P, Gusmeroli M, Ottolenghi S: Human $^{T}\gamma$ globin chain is a variant of $^{A}\gamma$ chain ($^{A}\gamma$ Sardinia). Proc Natl Acad Sci USA 76:3420, 1979.
11. Huisman THJ, Wilson JB: Recent advances in the quantitation of human fetal hemoglobins with different gamma chains. Am J Hematol 9:225, 1980.
12. Huisman THJ, Jonxis JHP: "The Hemoglobinopathies: Techniques of Identification." New York: Marcel Dekker, 1977.
13. Betke K, Marti H, Schlicht I: Estimation of small percentages of foetal haemoglobin. Nature 184:1877, 1959.
14. Abraham EC, Reese A, Stallings M, Huisman THJ: Separation of human hemoglobins by DEAE-cellulose chromatography using glycine-KCN-NaCl developers. Hemoglobin 1:27, 1976.
15. Huisman THJ, Webber B, Okonjo K, Reese AL, Wilson JB: The separation of human hemoglobin chains by high pressure liquid chromatography. In Hanash SM, Brewer GJ (eds): "Advances in Hemoglobin Analysis." New York: Alan R Liss, 1981, pp 23–38.
16. Huisman THJ, Altay CA, Webber B, Reese AL, Gravely ME, Okonjo K, Wilson JB: Quantitation of three types of γ chain of Hb F by high pressure liquid chromatography; application of this method to the Hb F of patients with sickle cell anemia or the S-HPFH condition. Blood 57:75, 1981.
17. Huisman THJ, Gravely ME, Webber B, Okonjo K, Henson J, Reese AL: The gamma chain heterogeneity of fetal hemoglobin in Black β-thalassemia and HPFH heterozygotes. Blood 58:62–70, 1981.
18. Huisman THJ, Altay C: The chemical heterogeneity of the fetal hemoglobin of Black newborn babies and adults; a reevaluation. Blood (In press)

19. Huisman THJ, Webber B: The frequency of the $^{A}\gamma^{T}$ gene in the presence and absence of the β^{S} or β^{C} gene in the Black population of the Southeastern USA. Hemoglobin 5:441–451, 1981.
20. Schroeder WA, Shelton JR, Shelton JB, Apell G, Huisman THJ, Bouver NG: Worldwide occurrence of nonallelic genes for the γ-chain of human foetal haemoglobin in newborns. Nature 240:273, 1972.
21. Huisman THJ, Schroeder WA, Felice A, Powars D, Ringelhann B: An anomaly in the γ chain heterogeneity of the newborn. Nature 265:63, 1977.
22. Schroeder WA, Huisman THJ, Shelton JR, Shelton JB, Apell G, Bouver N: Heterogeneity of fetal hemoglobin in β-thalassemia of the Negro. Am J Hum Genet 22:505, 1970.
23. Huisman THJ, Schroeder WA, Efremov GD, Duma H, Mladenovski B, Hyman CB, Rachmilewitz EA, Bouver N, Miller A, Brodie AR, Shelton JR, Shelton JB, Apell G: The present status of the heterogeneity of fetal hemoglobin in β-thalassemia: An attempt to unify some observations in thalassemia and related conditions. Ann NY Acad Sci 232:107, 1974.
24. Orkin H, Alter P, Altay C: Deletion of the $^{A}\gamma$-globin gene in $^{G}\gamma$- $\delta\beta$-thalassemia. J Clin Invest 64:866, 1979.
25. Cantu JB, Ibarra B, Vaca G, Ramirez ML, Sanchez-Corona J: Partial mispairing and crossing-over between β^{0} and δ genes as the origin of the $\delta\beta^{0}$ thalassemia gene. Hum Genet 49:191, 1979.
26. Stamatoyannopoulos G, Schroeder WA, Huisman THJ, Shelton JR, Shelton JB, Apell G, Bouver N: Nature of foetal haemoglobin in F-thalassemia. Br J Haematol 21:633, 1971.

MODEL SYSTEM FOR REGULATION OF GLOBIN GENE EXPRESSION: ANIMALS AND CELL CULTURE

Hemoglobin Switching in Sheep: Analysis Following Transplantation of Fetal Cells to Adult Animals

W.G. Wood, PhD, **and C. Bunch,** MB, ChB, MCRP

INTRODUCTION

In primates and ruminants, a developmentally related change in the pattern of hemoglobin production occurs in the perinatal period whereby the production of mainly fetal hemoglobin (Hb F) switches to the production of almost exclusively adult hemoglobin [1]. This switch provides an excellent system for examining developmentally regulated gene expression; but as yet has yielded little information about the control of this process [2]. Several mechanisms have been proposed [reviewed in ref. 3] including 1) developmental changes in the proliferation of two, or more, separate populations of cells producing different major hemoglobin types; 2) production at a specific time in development of an inductive factor which alters the subsequent pattern of hemoglobin production; 3) changes in extracellular signals produced by the "environment" in which the hemopoietic cells develop; and 4) a biologic clock built into the hemopoietic cells controlling the developmental changes. None of these processes can be excluded on the available data, although there is considerable circumstantial evidence that the production of adult hemoglobin is unlikely to be the result of the proliferation of a new or previously dormant hemopoietic cell lineage.

A critical experiment which should help to resolve this question is to determine the type of hemoglobin synthesized by the progeny of fetal hemopoietic cells which have undergone differentiation in an adult "environment" [1-4]. Continued production of Hb F by the transplanted fetal cells would be consistent with control by a time-restricted inducer, the period of induction being bypassed by the transplantation procedure. If continuous "environmental" signals were responsible for controlling hemoglobin type, the fetal cells should switch fairly rapidly to adult hemoglobin production after transplantation, irrespective of their gestational age (Fig. 1). Conversely, if the fetal cells contain an internal program regulating switching, they should begin producing adult hemoglobin after transplantation at a time which would be inversely related to their gestational age (Fig. 2).

Birth Defects: Original Article Series, Volume 18, Number 7, pages 103–110
© 1982 March of Dimes Birth Defects Foundation

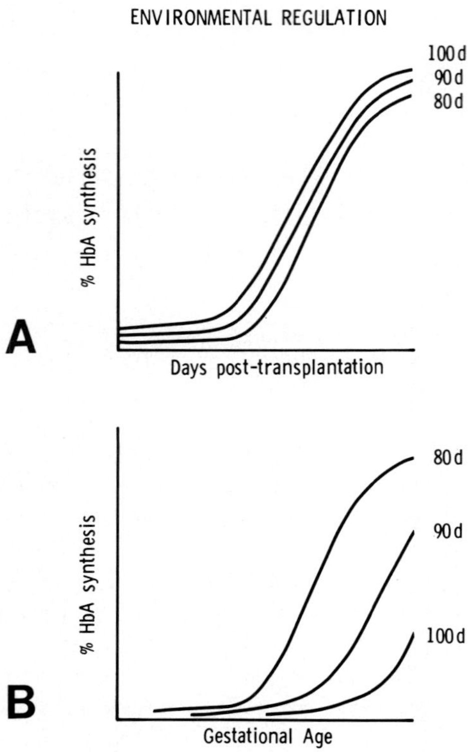

Fig. 1. A) Diagrammatic representation of the pattern of hemoglobin synthesis by fetal cells in an adult environment assuming that the environment is responsible for the induction of adult hemoglobin production. Increasing adult hemoglobin production is correlated with time posttransplantation; B) and not the gestational age of the fetus donating the cells.

We have undertaken a program of fetal to adult hemopoietic cell transplants in sheep to determine the conditions for successful transplantation of this type, hoping ultimately to be able to answer this question [5]. The sheep is a suitable animal model since the overall pattern of developmental changes in hemoglobin is similar to that in man [6,7]. Furthermore, sheep are polymorphic at the β-chain locus, with 2 common alleles, β^A and β^B. Thus, it is possible to select donor and recipient animals to be of different adult hemoglobin types, and hence, have a marker to monitor the origin of any adult hemoglobin produced.

EXPERIMENTAL DESIGN AND METHODS

Donor fetuses, homozygous for the β^A- or β^B-allele, were obtained at 85-100 days gestation (term ~ 145 days) and a suspension of bone marrow and fetal

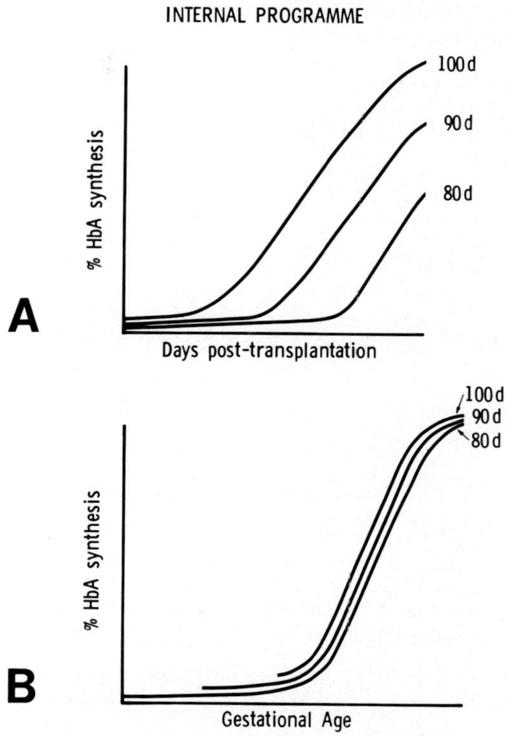

Fig. 2. B) Diagrammatic representation of the pattern of hemoglobin synthesis by fetal cells in an adult environment assuming that the process of switching is inherently programmed into the hemopoietic cells. Increasing adult hemoglobin production is correlated with the gestational age; A) and not with time posttransplantation.

liver hemopoietic cells prepared. These cells were infused (via a previously implanted jugular vein catheter) into recipient lambs of opposite Hb type which had received 10-12 Gy total body irradiation (1 Gy = 100 rad) a few hours earlier. Following transplantation, the recipients received appropriate supportive care with intravenous fluid replacement, parenteral feeding, antibiotics, and platelet transfusions. Bone marrow samples were monitored regularly for evidence of engraftment by assessing cellularity, determining the pattern of globin-chain synthesis and, when donor and fetus were of opposite sex, by chromosomal analysis. Full details of these techniques have been published previously [5].

RESULTS

The results of the initial experiments in this series have been reported in detail previously [5]; included here are 2 successfully engrafted animals (10 and 11)

TABLE 1. Details of Donor Fetuses and Recipient Lambs and the Outcome of 7 Experiments Involving the Transplantation of Fetal Hemopoietic Cells to Irradiated, Postswitched Lambs

	Donor			Recipient				
Expt.	Gestational Age (Days)	Hb	Sex	Age (Months)	Hb	Sex	Survival (Days)	Outcome
10	94	BB	M	2	AA	F	24	Successful engraftment
11	96	BB	F	2	AA	F	26	Successful engraftment
12	85	BB	M	6	AA	F	12	Successful engraftment
13	88	BB	M+F	8	AA	M	14	Successful engraftment
14	85	BB	F+F	9	AA	M	16	Transient engraftment
15	99	AA	M	5	BB	F	5	Unevaluated
16	95	BB	F	10	AA	M	16	Transient engraftment

from the earlier series together with results of 5 subsequent attempts (animals 12-16) (Table 1).

Transplantation

While in initial experiments a radiation dose of 10 Gy was used to prepare the recipient, successful engraftment has been achieved only with a radiation dose of 12 Gy. However, gastrointestinal problems have been severe at this dose and were responsible for the deaths of animals 12 and 13 following perforation of the bowel and peritonitis. At attempt at a compromise level of 11 Gy in animal 14 did not result in prolonged engraftment.

In animals 10-13, there was good evidence for engraftment. Bone marrow cellularity increased from day 7 onwards and by day 14 their marrows were extremely cellular, in marked contrast to marrows from animals without successful engraftment. In the latter, a transient appearance of a few hemopoietic cells was observed between days 7 and 10, but the degree of cellularity was much less than in the successfully engrafted animals; the hemopoietic cells disappeared by day 14. Chromosomal evidence of engraftment was obtained in animals 10 and 13 where 98% and >89% of the mitoses were of donor karyotype. It is interesting that in animal 13, a male infused with hemopoietic cells from twin fetuses of opposite sexes, the karyotypes were nearly all female, suggesting that one of the fetuses had contributed to the engraftment to a much greater extent than the other.

Hemoglobin Synthesis

The pattern of hemoglobin synthesis in bone marrow samples was examined serially at various times after transplantation. In all cases the predominant non-α-globin chain produced was the γ-chain of Hb F. Although we had no marker to demonstrate that this was of donor origin, a series of control experiments involving irradiated but untransplanted animals, autologous transplants, or allogeneic lamb to lamb marrow transplants demonstrated that little, if any, reactivation of γ-chain synthesis occurs in such animals [5]. A small amount of globin-chain synthesis of recipient origin (ie β^A-chains and β^C-chains, the latter being produced by animals with Hb A when subjected to erythroid stress) was observed in the fetal to lamb transplants but rarely exceeded 15%. Since these chains are separated from the γ- and β^B-chains of donor origin, the latter can be quantitated separately, and the proportion of β^B-chain synthesis expressed as a percentage of the donor non-α-chain synthesis (Fig. 3A). The results show that in 3 instances, a rise in donor β-chain synthesis occurred 7-10 days posttransplantation, while in the other 3 cases no such increase had occurred by the time the animal died. These results are plotted against the postconceptional age of the donor cells in Figure 3B.

DISCUSSION

The theoretic basis of these experiments, as discussed above, should allow us to distinguish between three possible mechanisms of the control of hemoglobin switching, a time-restricted inducer, continuous "environmental" regulation and an internally programmed hemopoietic cell. Despite advances in bone marrow transplantation in other species, these experiments have been difficult to perform in practice and, as yet, only partial success has been achieved in a small proportion of attempts. A number of factors may be responsible. Experience with marrow transplantation in sheep is limited and many variables have to be examined. The major histocompatibility system of the sheep has not been as well studied as that in human or other species used for transplant research; but recent studies suggest that tissue typing is unlikely to be of much assistance since there is considerable allelic variation in the major histocompatibility loci in sheep [8]. While an inbreeding program could produce matched donor and recipient, it would be a long and costly process, particularly to maintain both the β^A-and β^B-globin gene alleles in the population. A further potential difficulty in the studies described here is that the number of donor cells transplanted is limited by the small size of the fetus, yet cell dose is known to be a very important factor in successful allogeneic transplantation [9]. For this reason young lambs were chosen as recipients. That successful engraftment (if not survival) was obtained in lambs transplanted from fetuses of 86-95 days' gestation suggests that cell dose may not be limiting unless earlier fetuses are required. Finally, it is clear that conditioning with 12 rather than 10 Gy total body irradiation may be necessary to prevent graft rejection, but this dose is not well tolerated by the ruminant digestive system and affects survival even when marrow engraftment is successful.

The results of hemoglobin synthesis measurements in the partially successful

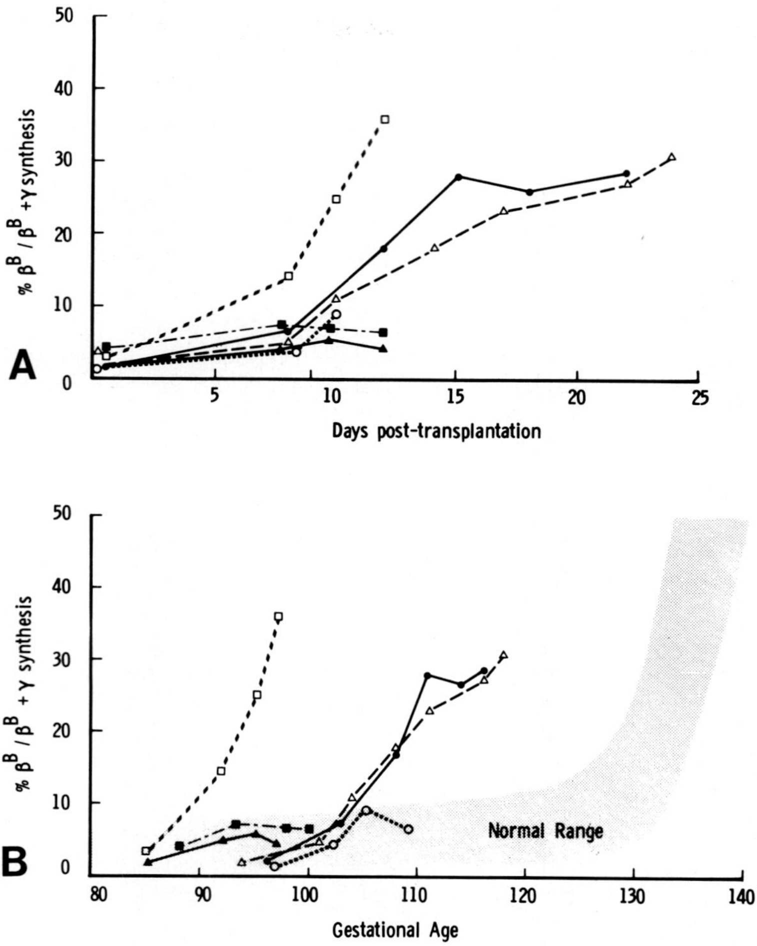

Fig. 3. A) β-chain synthesis of donor cell origin (expressed as a percentage of total donor non-α-chain synthesis) in bone marrow samples of 6 irradiated lambs at various times after transplantation with fetal hemopoietic cells. B) The same results plotted according to the postconceptional age of the fetal cells. ● expt. no. 10; △ 11; ▲ 12; ■ 13; □ 14; ○ 16.

transplants demonstrate unequivocally that for the first 3-4 weeks after transplantation, the fetal cells continue to synthesize predominantly fetal hemoglobin. This is in contrast to the result of the only previously successful experiment of this type [10] in which the rapid appearance of donor type adult hemoglobin in the recipient was interpreted as evidence for a rapid switch to adult hemoglobin synthesis in the adult environment. There were several differences between that experiment and those described here, including the method of hemoglobin analysis, the fact that the donor fetuses were slightly older (100 days) than any we have used, and that the recipient was an adult sheep rather than a lamb. It is not possible at present to account for the apparently contradictory results.

In our experiments, an increase in the proportion of donor β-chains was seen in 3 out of the 6 evaluated cases. This would appear to exclude a switch control mechanism which relied on the production of an inducer immediately prior to the switch to convert the program of hemoglobin synthesis from fetal to adult; since, if this were the case, an increase in β-chain production should not have occurred. The results in these cases are also not consistent with an *immediate* inductive effect of the adult "environment" converting the cells to adult hemoglobin production or with a *strictly* controlled internal program. However, they do not exclude the reasonable possibility that an environmentally induced event acts gradually, or that an "internal program" may have been modified by the process of the experiment itself, for instance by increased stem-cell proliferation in a rapidly regenerating bone marrow. In those animals which showed increased β-chain synthesis, this occurred at an earlier time than if the cells had remained in the fetus in utero; also it appeared to be better correlated with the time post-translation than with the gestational age. However, in 3 other animals no such increase was observed at 10–12 days posttransplantation.

Clearly, it would be premature to place too much emphasis on these results from experiments which were only partially successful. When we succeed in obtaining transplants which survive long enough for the switch to go to completion (assuming it does), the pattern in the first few weeks, before the cells have settled into something approaching a steady state, may be seen to be unstable and relatively uninformative. Nevertheless, we believe that these experiments have demonstrated the potential of this system and future results will be of importance in determining the direction of subsequent research into developmental changes in hemoglobin production.

REFERENCES

1. Wood WG, Clegg JB, Weatherall DJ: Developmental biology of human hemoglobins. In Brown EB (ed): "Progress in Hematology." New York: Grune & Stratton, 1977, vol X, pp 43–90.
2. Wood WG, Jones RW: Erythropoiesis and hemoglobin production: A unifying model involving sequential gene activation. In Stamatoyannopoulos G, Nienhuis AW (eds): "Hemoglobins in Development and Differentiation." New York: Alan R Liss, 1981.
3. Wood WG: Haemoglobin production during development. In Hollan SR, Gardos G, Sarkardi B (eds): "Advances in Physiological Sciences." New York: Pergamon Press, 1981, vol 6.
4. Weatherall DJ, Clegg JB, Wood WG: A model for the persistence or reactivation of fetal haemoglobin production. Lancet 2:660–663, 1976.

5. Bunch C, Wood WG, Weatherall DJ, Robinson JS, Corp MJ: Haemoglobin synthesis by fetal erythroid cells in an adult environment. Br J Haematol 49:325–336, 1981.
6. Bard H, Battaglia FC, Makowski EL, Meschia G: The synthesis of fetal and adult hemoglobin in sheep during the perinatal period. Proc Soc Exp Biol Med 139:1148–1150, 1972.
7. Wood WG, Pearce K, Clegg JB, Weatherall DJ, Robinson JS, Thorburn GD, Dawes GS: The switch from fetal to adult haemoglobin synthesis in normal and hypophysectomised sheep. Nature 264:799–801, 1976.
8. Cullen PR, Bunch C, Brownlie J, Morris PJ: The major histocompatibility complex of the sheep. I: A preliminary study of sheep leucocyte antigens. (Submitted for publication)
9. Storb R, Prentice RL, Thomas ED: Marrow analysis of factors associated with graft rejection. N Engl J Med 296:61–66, 1977.
10. Zanjani ED, McGlave PB, Bhakthavathsalan A, Stamatoyannopoulos G: Sheep fetal haematopoietic cells produce adult haemoglobin when transplanted in adult animal. Nature 280:495–496, 1979.

A Cellular Model for Hemoglobin Switching*

Blanche P. Alter, MD, and David G. Nathan, MD

The switch from Hb F to A which occurs during ontogeny in primates is incomplete in the adult. In addition, Hb F may reappear during erythroid stress. Colonies derived in vitro from erythroid progenitors also produce both Hbs F and A. At each stage of normal ontogeny, the relation between the proportion of F synthesized in the colonies derived from progenitors in vitro and in the reticulocytes or erythroblasts (precursors) which developed in vivo is not immediately apparent. Data from our previously published studies of rhesus monkeys [1] are summarized in Figure 1.

There are several possible models to explain the phenomenon of the ontogenic switch. These have been described elsewhere by others [2].

1) Cellular: One population of stem cells, with a specific Hb potentiality (eg for high F) is replaced by one or more other population(s), with different and decreasing Hb potential (eg for low F).

2) Environment: The fetal environment contains "factors" (cellular or humoral) which direct F synthesis by the progenitor and its progeny, while the adult environment directs A synthesis.

3) Biologic clock: With time, erythroid stem cells undergo continual, inexorable, and irreversible modification of their F potential, with ever decreasing F synthesis in the progeny. Reappearance of F occurs because the F loss is asynchronous, and some earlier progenitors remain, not yet fully modulated.

4) Cell–cycle related: F progenitors are not normally in cycle in adults, but they are in cycle in fetuses, or in adult erythroid stress.

Features of Hb analysis which may complicate analyses but are not contradictory to any of the above models are the influence on Hb F of colony maturity, time of burst development, plating efficiency, and burst size.

Any model for Hb switching must be compatible with the available data. In particular, we must explain why the synthesis of Hb F in colonies derived from

*Supported by NIH grants HD 11471, HL 26132, HL 27395, National Cancer Institute grant 2P3006516, and an Irma T. Hirschl Career Scientist Award (to Dr. Alter).

Birth Defects: Original Article Series, Volume 18, Number 7, pages 111–116
© 1982 March of Dimes Birth Defects Foundation

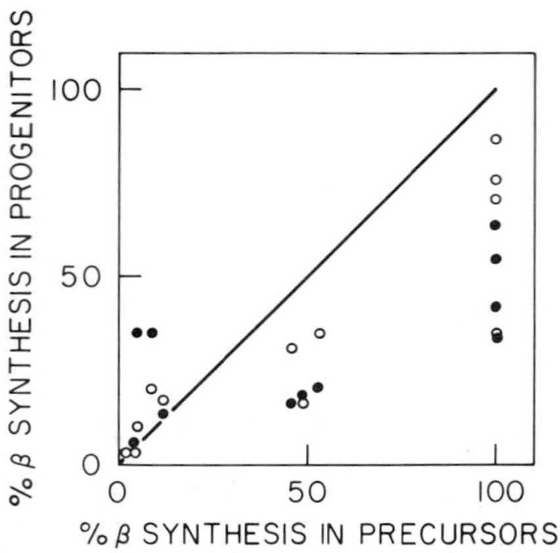

Fig. 1. Percent β-globin synthesis in erythroid progenitor-derived colonies compared with differentiated precursors, in rhesus monkeys. The solid line is the hypothetic line of identity if progenitor-derived colonies produced the same percent β-globin as simultaneously acquired marrow erythroid precursors. ○ = CFU-E-derived colonies. ● = BFU-E-derived colonies. (From Alter BP, Jackson BT, Lipton JM, Piasecki GJ, Jackson PL, Kudisch M, Nathan DG: Control of the simian fetal hemoglobin switch at the progenitor cell level. J Clin Invest 67:458–466, 1981, with permission.)

progenitors is less than in precursors in the early switch period, and yet colony F synthesis exceeds that of precursors in the mid– and post–switch periods.

One possible explanation for this apparently anomalous result is that there are at least 2 different types of progenitors, which change their relative quantities during ontogeny. The first of these, a truly "fetal" progenitor, gives rise to progeny which produce essentially only Hb F. The relative number of these fetal progenitors, and of each type (BFU-E, CFU-E, and erythroblasts) of fetal-differentiated progeny, decreases with ontogeny. A new type of adult progenitor and progeny emerges. This new type is "fetal-like," but distinct from the truly fetal progenitor, in that these new progenitors do have the possibility of losing Hb F synthesis.

The loss of F synthesis may occur on a stochastic basis in the fetal-like cell line. Thus, a series of events may occur (possibly but not necessarily cell divisions), which result in a reduction in the Hb F synthetic potential by a specific amount at each event. The simplest assumptions required for consideration of this 2-cell (fetal and fetal-like) model include:

1) The F potential in the pluripotent stem cell is 100%, even in the fetal-like stem cell.

2) The decrease in F potential occurs with a fixed probability. (The probability may change, but this adds unnecessary complications.) P is defined as the probability for retention of F.

3) The loss of F potential occurs at specific stochastic events (? cell divisions).

4) There are ~6 stochastic events during the differentiation and maturation series in vivo. If these are cell divisions, it means one stem cell produces 64 mature erythroblasts. There is one stochastic event before the BFU-E stage, and one more to the CFU-E stage.

5) The number of stochastic events does not change significantly during ontogeny (although there could be 1 or 2 less in fetuses without affecting the results).

6) In vitro cultures result in erythroid colonies which reflect the Hb potential program of the progenitor (an "arrested development") at that point in time, not its potential if left in vivo; ie "P" does not operate in vitro.

The rhesus monkey data previously published [1] will be used to demonstrate the applicability of the 2-cell model. Table 1 summarizes the data on the percent of Hb F synthesis by colonies derived from BFU-E or CFU-E, or by precursors, at each switch period. In the pre-switch, essentially all Hb produced in vivo is F. In the early switch, ~ 10% Hb A synthesis occurs, and in the mid switch, ~ half is F and half A. The adult rhesus monkey produces no detectable F in vivo.

Using the assumptions listed above, the pre-switch period appears to be associated with only truly fetal progenitor cells. The probability for retention of F is thus ~ 1.0 (it could be 0.99 and still result in ≥ 94% F after 4–6 stochastic events, ie $0.99^6 = 0.94$). Thus, the findings in the pre-switch period can be explained.

For the adult, the P value is clearly < 1.0. If we assume that one stochastic event occurred up to the BFU-E stage, P appears to be ~ 0.5. One more stochastic event to the CFU-E stage still fits with P ~ 0.5 (expect F synthesis to be 0.5^2 or 0.25, find 0.28). Three or 4 more events (total of 5 or 6, ie 0.5^5 or 0.5^6) with P = 0.5 would lead to F synthesis of 3.13 or 1.56%, or ~ 2% or less, as found.

TABLE 1. Percent Hb F Synthesized During Ontogeny*

Switch period	% Hb F synthesis		
	BFU-E	CFU-E	Precursors
Pre	>95	>95	>95
Early	72 ± 13	85 ± 6	91 ± 4
Mid	79 ± 4	73 ± 5	51 ± 4
Adult	48 ± 13	28 ± 17	<2

*Mean ± SD of 3 separate studies at each time point.

The results in the early and mid-switch periods could thus be explained by mixtures of the fetal (P = 1.0) and fetal-like (P = 0.5) cells. The actual proportion of each cell type can be determined mathematically:

$$x(a) + (1-x)(b) = c \qquad x = \frac{b-c}{b-a}$$

x = proportion of fetal-like (adult) cells, where P = 0.5
a = % Hb F if only fetal-like cells were present
b = % Hb F if only truly fetal cells were present (ie 100% HbF)
c = % Hb F measured in early or mid-switch colonies or precursors

For example, using data in Table 1: Mid-switch erythroblasts, where a = $(0.5)^6 \leq 2$, b = 100, and c = 51%;

$$x = \frac{100-51}{100-2} = \frac{49}{98} = 0.5$$

Thus, this population could consist of 50% fetal and 50% fetal-like derived cells.

Another example, for early switch CFU-E:

$$a = 28,\ b = 100,\ c = 85;$$

$$x = \frac{100-85}{100-28} = \frac{15}{72} = 0.21$$

The formula shown above was used for each data point in Table 1 to determine the proportion of fetal-like (adult) progenitors which were in the mixture. For each calculation, a = 48% at the BFU-E stage, 28% at CFU-E, and 2% in the precursors; b = 100% at each point; and c varied and was the actual % F measured in early or mid switch BFU-E, CFU-E, or precursors. Table 2 shows the results of these calculations in each switch period and for each type of colony or precursor. The same results are depicted graphically in Figure 2.

The findings in the pre-switch and adult periods are readily explained by the presence of only fetal or only adult (fetal-like) progenitors and their progeny in the respective states. The early switch period is heralded by the appearance in the BFU-E compartment of up to 50% fetal-like (adult) BFU-E. Since CFU-E develop from BFU-E, the proportion of the CFU-E compartment which is fetal-

TABLE 2. Proportion of Adult (Fetal-Like) Cells During Ontogeny

Switch period	Proportion of fetal-like cells		
	BFU-E	CFU-E	Precursors
Pre	0	0	0
Early	54*	21	9
Mid	40*	38*	50
Adult	100	100	100

*Because of errors in measurement, these numbers are not significantly different from 50.

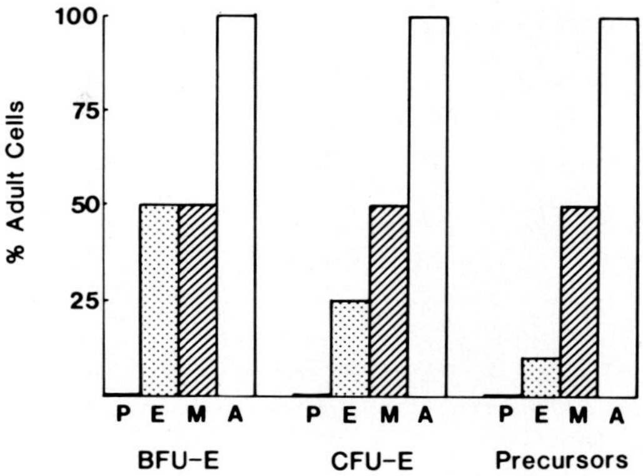

Fig. 2. Model for hemoglobin regulation during ontogeny. The percent adult (fetal-like) cells in colonies derived from BFU-E or CFU-E, or in marrow precursors at each ontogenic stage was calculated in Table 2. P = Pre-switch; E = Early switch; M = Mid switch; A = Adult (post switch).

like is < 50% (~ 20%). Erythroblasts, which develop from further differentiation of CFU-E, are still of predominantly fetal origin. In the mid switch, the proportion of BFU-E which are of adult fetal-like derivation may still be half. However, the rate of differentiation to CFU-E from BFU-E is identical for fetal or fetal-like progenitors, so the 50% fetal-like progenitors in the BFU-E have now had time to penetrate into the CFU-E compartment. Finally, the erythroblasts in the mid switch also reflect the 50:50 status of the earlier compartments. Of course, by the time of the adult switch period, the fetal progenitors have disappeared, leaving only the population with P = 0.5.

While this 2-cell model is by no means proven by the data, it is compatible with the results. It is also testable. BFU-E-derived colonies can be grown at the early or mid-switch period, and examined individually for F synthesis. If P for the fetal-like cells is ~ 0.5, and P for the fetal cells ~ 1.0, two groups of colonies should be readily distinguishable. One group would have a mean F of close to 100%, while the other group should be normally distributed around a mean of ~ 50% F.

There is an additional possible ally in the quest to distinguish fetal from fetal-like cells. We found that the rhesus monkey has 2 γ globin chains, similar to the $^{G}\gamma/^{A}\gamma$ heterogeneity in man. In the rhesus, the electrophoretically fast $\gamma(\gamma_2)$ comprised > 70% of the total. In adult colonies, γ_2 was < 70%. Thus the bimodality of % F predicted for individual colonies during the switch may be paralleled at the level of % γ_2.

Further experiments will test the oversimplified model proposed here. If incorrect, attention can then be directed to the other types of switching models, which are more difficult to approach experimentally.

ACKNOWLEDGMENTS

We are very grateful to Dr. Arthur Axelrad for his permission to include his stochastic theory of hemoglobin regulation in the adult. We acknowledge the expert contributions of Drs. Jeffrey Lipton, Michele Kudisch, and Roger Macklis.

REFERENCES

1. Alter BP, Jackson BT, Lipton JM, Piasecki GJ, Jackson PL, Kudisch M, Nathan DG: Control of the simian fetal hemoglobin switch at the progenitor cell level. J Clin Invest 67:458–466, 1981.
2. Nienhuis A: This volume.

Hemoglobin Expression in Clones of K-562 Cell Line*

Ugo Testa, MD, William Vainchenker, MD, Yves Beuzard, Philippe Rouyer-Fessard, Monique Titeux, Jacqueline Bouguet, Janine Breton-Gorius, and Jean Rosa

INTRODUCTION

The human K-562 cell line is a Philadelphia chromosome-positive cell line [1] which possesses erythroid features [2–13]. In particular, Rutherford et al [6, 7, 10] and Benz et al [8] have rigorously shown that embryonic Hbs (Hb Portland and Hb Gower), as well as small quantities of fetal Hb (Hb F), are produced by the K-562 cells after exposure to hemin. Thus, this cell line provides a new tool to study erythroid differentiation and the switch between embryonic and fetal hemoglobins.

Human development is characterized by the sequential appearance of embryonic, fetal, and adult hemoglobins [14]. The 3 embryonic hemoglobins are formed by the combination of 4 types of globin chains: Hb Gower 1 ($\zeta_2\epsilon_2$), Hb Portland ($\zeta_2\gamma_2$), and Hb Gower 2 ($\alpha_2\epsilon_2$) [15, 16]. These hemoglobins are replaced by fetal hemoglobin ($\alpha_2\gamma_2$) during development. In addition, adult hemoglobin ($\alpha_2\beta_2$) synthesis has been detected as early as the 9th week of development; at this time, embryonic and fetal hemoglobins are also evident [14]. The mechanisms of the embryonic to fetal hemoglobin switch remain unknown.

Cloning appears to be a crucial step in the study of the globin gene expression in K-562 cell line since evidence has been provided that its cellular composition could be heterogeneous [17–19]. A minority of cells exhibits a cytochemical marker (platelet peroxidase) characteristic of the megakaryocytic cell lineage, while other markers of megakaryocytes were absent [19]. The initial cloning of the K-562 cell line has shown a heterogeneity in the Hb content of the different clones [19, 20]. The aim of the present study was to analyze the Hb expression in primary and secondary clones of K-562 cell line and to investigate the subse-

*Supported by a grant from INSERM (ATP 78/88 and 36 76 68).

Birth Defects: Original Article Series, Volume 18, Number 7, pages 117–130
© 1982 March of Dimes Birth Defects Foundation

quent effect of hemin on the expression of embryonic, fetal, and adult globin genes.

MATERIAL AND METHODS

For cloning we used a subline of the K-562 cell line provided by Dr. Turcz (Villejuif, France).

Culture

The K-562 cell line was grown in suspension culture in a modified RPMI 1640 medium containing 10% heat inactivated fetal or newborn calf serum in a humidified atmosphere with 5% CO_2 [7]. Karyotypic analysis showed a single Ph^1 chromosome in all metaphases studied.

Sodium-butyrate (1 mM) or hemin (0.1 mM) were added in culture for a long period of time (4 days) to study the induction of hemoglobin expression. Viable cells were counted with a hemocytometer using the trypan blue exclusion test. Morphology (May Grunwald Giemsa), and peroxidase activity of hemoglobin were determined on cytocentrifuged cell preparations.

Cloning of K-562 Cell Line

The K-562 cell suspension was diluted to a concentration of 10 cells/ml by serial dilution. Aliquots (0.1 ml) of this suspension were placed in individual microwells. Cells which proliferate and give rise to cellular colonies after 8–14 days were picked off, and subsequently grown in a large amount of medium. The number of clones observed corresponded to 30% of the number expected if all the cells were proliferating. This technique permitted us to study more than 100 primary clones. Three such primary clones exhibiting different features were subsequently cloned by the technique described.

Hemoglobin Studies

Hemoglobins were analyzed by 2 methods: electrophoresis on cellulose acetate strips at 4°C [21], and isoelectric focusing (IEF) (using LKB ampholines with a pH 6–9 gradient) [22]. At the end of electrophoresis, benzidine staining was performed to detect the peroxidase activity of hemoglobin. The hemoglobin nature of the bands positively stained by benzidine was proved by their displacement after addition of haptoglobin, which specifically binds to hemoglobin, prior to the electrophoresis of a duplicate sample [23]. Haptoglobin formed a complex with all the embryonic hemoglobins (unpublished results).

For studies of Hb synthesis, 100 μl of cells were incubated for 2 hours in NCTC 109 leucine-free medium (Eurobio, Paris, France) to which 100 μCi ^3H leucine was added. Cells were then harvested, washed 3 times in saline solution and lysed. The radioactivity incorporated into globin chains was evaluated by electrophoresis of globin chains in polyacrylamide gel containing urea [24], followed by fluorography in 8 M urea [25]. Prior to electrophoresis or chromatography, Hbs were completely or partially purified from the non-heme proteins by affinity chromatography on Sepharose-haptoglobin [26].

RESULTS

Hemoglobin Expression in the K-562 Cell Line and in the Different Clones

The combination of isoelectric focusing and of cellulose acetate electrophoresis allowed us to identify all the Hb fractions. The Hb synthesis represented less than 3% of the total synthesis of soluble proteins as shown by the purification of hemoglobin by affinity chromatography on Sepharose-haptoglobin.

A dilution technique produced 110 primary clones, and their Hb production was investigated. Great differences in the amount of Hb and in the Hb pattern were observed from one clone to another (Table 1). The clones were subsequently classified into 3 groups according to their Hb phenotype (Table 1). Group I included the 17.3% of the clones (19 clones) which did not contain detectable amounts of Hb.

Group II corresponded to the 66.3% of the clones (73 clones) which exhibited Hb Portland. Group III included the 16.4% of the clones (18 clones) which expressed Hb Gower 1 in addition to Hb Portland. Hb Gower 1 was never present alone. Hb Barts ($\gamma 4$) often could be detected in clones of groups II and III.

Three primary clones (Nos. 48, 201, and 209) were recloned by dilution. The Hb phenotype was heterogeneous in these secondary clones but much less than in the primary clones (Fig. 1). The repartition of the secondary clones in the 3 groups was clearly dependent upon the Hb phenotype of the primary clone. The primary clone, which did not express Hb (group I), did not give rise to secondary clones of group III. Conversely, the primary clone of group III gave rise to a tiny proportion of group I secondary clones.

The Hb synthesis was investigated after Hb purification by gel electrophoresis and chromatography of globin chains. The results, summarized in Table 2, show different patterns of globin synthesis from one clone to another. No globin chain

TABLE 1. Hemoglobin Pattern in 110 Primary Clones of the K-562 Cell Line Grown Without Inducer

Hb Undetectable	Hb Portland	Hb Portland + Hb Gower 1
19 (17.3%)	73 (66.3%)	18 (16.4%)

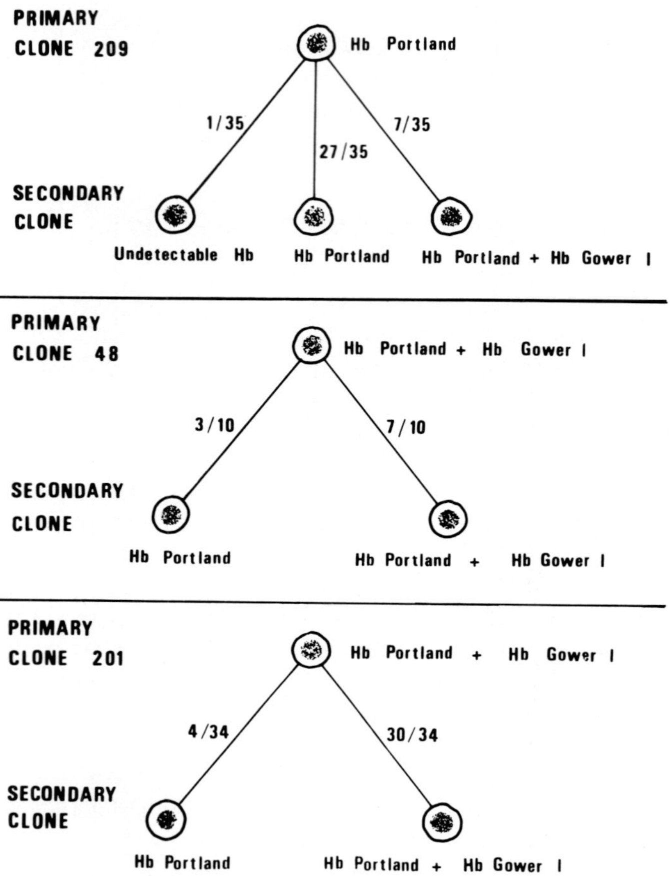

Fig. 1. Hemoglobin expression in secondary clones derived from 3 primary clones of the K-562 cell line. A) in the absence, or B) in the presence of 1×10^{-4}M hemin.

synthesis was detected in clones of group I confirming the absence of Hb in these clones. The γ chains and the ζ chains were always simultaneously synthesized by clones II and III. The presence of ϵ chain was characteristic of group III clones (Fig. 3). In all cases, the results obtained by the study of the Hb and by the electrophoresis of newly synthesized Hb chains were in agreement.

The γ-chain synthesis varied from 17.4% to 90% of the total globin synthesis. The two γ-genes, $^G\gamma$ and $^A\gamma$ were always expressed, but in various proportions. The $^G\gamma/^G\gamma + {}^A\gamma$ ratio, which decreases during development from 0.7 in fetus to 0.4 in adult [27], changed dramatically in clones of the K-562 cell line from 0.45 to 0.81 (Table 2). This ratio was not dependent upon the proportion of the total

TABLE 2. Globin Chain Synthesis in Total K-562 Cell Line and in Some Primary Clones Grown in the Presence or in the Absence of Hemin.

		Proportion Globin Chain Synthesis					Ratios of Globin Chain Synthesis		
Sample	Hemin	$^{G}\gamma$	$^{A}\gamma$	ζ	ϵ	α	$^{G}\gamma/^{G}\gamma + {}^{A}\gamma$	$\alpha + \zeta/\gamma + \epsilon$	$\epsilon/\epsilon + {}^{G}\gamma + {}^{A}\gamma$
K-562	−	59	28.5	7.5	5	0.2	0.67	0.07	0.05
Cell line	+	19.5	9.9	40	29	1.6	0.66	0.70	0.50
39	−	59.6	13.9	26.5	—	—	0.81	0.36	0
	+	18.8	22.7	12.5	46	—	0.59	0.14	0.52
48	−	7.9	9.5	32.6	50	—	0.45	0.51	0.74
	+	5.5	15.9	14	57.8	6.8	0.26	0.26	0.67
63	−	32.9	15.1	22	30	—	0.68	0.28	0.42
	+	20.4	11.5	26	40	2.5	0.68	0.40	0.54
68	−	45	40	10.1	4	0.9	0.53	0.12	0.04
	+	33.9	23.9	16	24.6	1.6	0.59	0.21	0.29
213	−	27.3	14.8	57.8	—	—	0.65	1.38	0
	+	28	10.5	46.1	—	15.4	0.73	0.84	0
229	−	37.6	16	30.9	15.4	—	0.70	0.45	0.26
	+	25.3	16.2	39	19.5	0.5	0.61	0.65	0.32

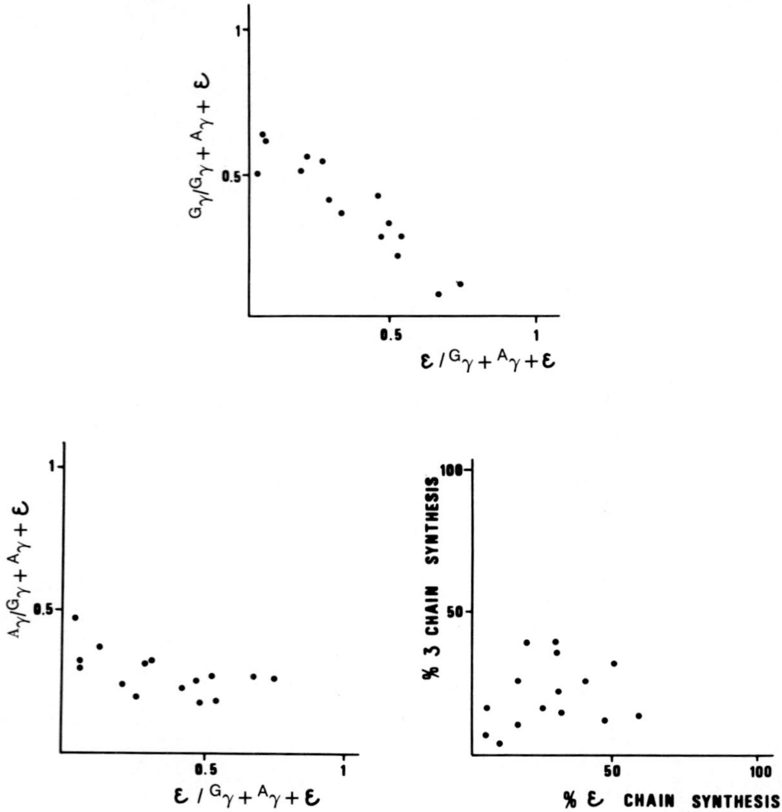

Fig. 2. Relationship between the proportion of different globin chain synthesis in different primary clones of the K-562 cell line.

TABLE 3. Hemoglobin Phenotype in 35 Primary Clones of the K-562 Cell Line Classified in Three Groups According to Their Hb Pattern.

Group	Before hemin induction	After hemin induction
I	Undetectable Hb (10)	Undetectable Hb (1) Hb Portland (9)
II	Hb Portland (17)	Hb Portland (8) Hb Portland + Hb Gower 1 (9)
III	Hb Portland+Hb Gower 1 (8)	Hb Portland + Hb Gower 1 (8)

γ-chain synthesis. The α-chain synthesis was occasionally present in minute amounts in clones of groups II and III. In all clones, the α- and non-α-like globin syntheses were unbalanced (Table 2).

Effect of Hemin

In clones which exhibited Hb before induction, hemin (1×10^{-4}M) added in the culture medium a few days later (2–5 days), induced an increase in the Hb synthesis from 2 to 10 times without affecting the total protein synthesis. Furthermore, hemin was able to induce Hb accumulation in most of the clones (9/10) which did not contain detectable Hb before induction (Table 3).

Another effect of hemin was to modify the phenotype of Hb expression of the different clones. Hemin induced the expression of Hb Gower 1 in more than 50% of the group II (Table 3) clones which only contained Hb Portland before induction. Hb Barts, minute amounts of Hb F as well as the Hb X fraction were more frequently detected after hemin addition than in the absence of the inducer.

In addition, the effect of hemin was studied in secondary clones derived from clones 48, 201, and 209. The results summarized in Figure 3 and Table 4 showed

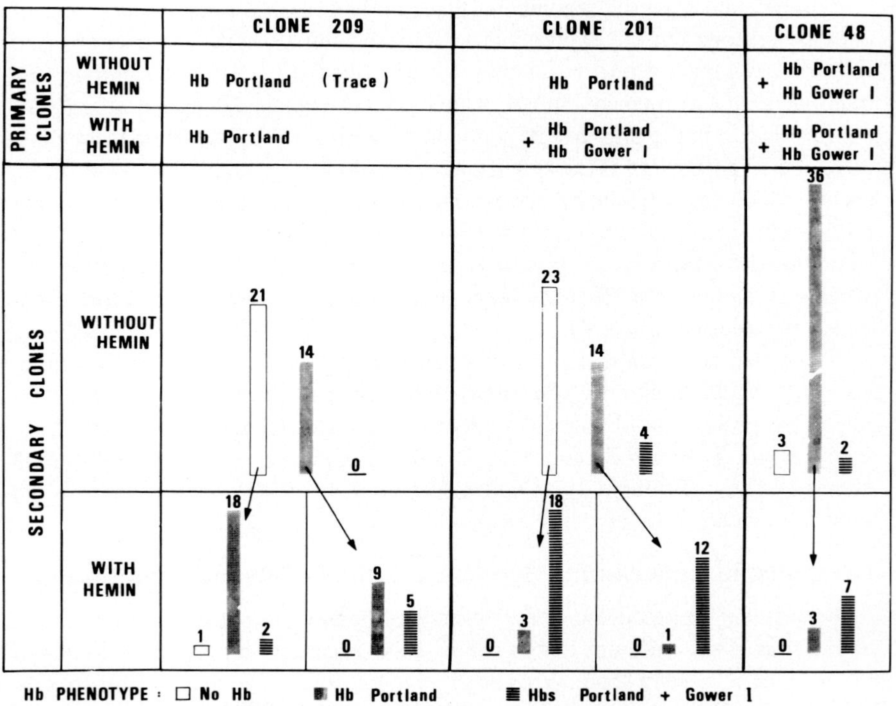

Fig. 3. Hemoglobin expression in secondary clones derived from 3 primary clones.

TABLE 4. Hemoglobin Phenotype in Secondary Clones Derived From 3 Primary Clones. All the Clones Were Grown in the Presence of 1 × 1⁻⁴M Hemin.

Clone Number	Primary clones	Secondary clones
209	Hb Portland	Undetectable hemoglobin (1/35) Hb Portland (27/35) Hb Portland + Hb Gower 1 (7/35)
48	Hb Portland + Hb Gower 1	Undetectable Hb (0) Hb Portland (3/10) Hb Portland + Hb Gower 1 (7/10)
201	Hb Portland + Hb Gower 1	Undetectable Hb (0) Hb Portland (4/34) Hb Portland + Hb Gower 1 (30/34)

that hemin induced a shift in the Hb pattern in comparison to that of the uninduced state.

The Hb pattern of the secondary clones in the presence of hemin was dependent as well on their Hb expression before induction as on the Hb phenotype of the primary clones from which they were derived (Fig. 1). For example, the majority of the secondary clones, which did not contain Hb in the absence of hemin, shifted in the presence of hemin to group II for those deriving from clone 209, and to group III for those deriving from clone 201. Similarly, most of the secondary clones which exhibited Hb Portland in the absence of hemin were not modified by hemin addition for those deriving from clone 209, while they shifted to group III for those deriving from clone 201. Thus, after hemin induction, the secondary clones were 70–85% homogeneous in comparison to the clone from which they derive (Table 4).

The effect of hemin was also investigated at the level of globin-chain synthesis. The results summarized in Table 2 showed that, in most cases, hemin reduced the proportion of γ-chain synthesis, induced the synthesis of ϵ-chains in many clones of group II, and enhanced the proportion of ϵ-chain synthesis in clones of group III (Table 2). In addition, hemin enhanced α-chain synthesis but to a low extent.

Relationship Between the Synthesis of the Different Globin Chains

Both in the presence and in the absence of hemin, the pattern and the rate of expression of the different globin chains was variable in the different clones of the K-562 cell line. In spite of this heterogeneity, some general characteristics do exist:

1) The ${}^{A}\gamma$-, and ${}^{G}\gamma$-, and ζ-globin chains were present in all the clones exhibiting Hb, but in various proportions.
2) The synthesis of ${}^{G}\gamma$-chain was inversely correlated to that of the ϵ-chain, as shown in Figure 2A. The 2 genes are neighbors on chromosome 11 [28].
3) In contrast, the synthesis of ${}^{A}\gamma$-chain was not proportional to that of the ${}^{G}\gamma$-chain and was less correlated to the ϵ-chain synthesis (Fig. 2B). The ${}^{G}\gamma/{}^{G}\gamma + {}^{A}\gamma$ ratio was variable from one clone to another and often changed after hemin induction (Table 2).
4) The synthesis of ζ- and ϵ-chains was not correlated (Fig. 2C).
5) The expression of the two globin-gene clusters, the non-α-genes on chromosome 11, and the α-globin genes on chromosome 16, was not balanced even after hemin induction (Table 2).

Effect of Sodium Butyrate

Sodium butyrate per se did not change significantly the total amount of hemoglobin or of globin chains. However, it modified the proportion of hemoglobins or globin chains increasing the proportion of Hb Gower 1 and of ϵ-globin chain, as shown in Figure 4. The pattern of non-heme proteins was not significantly modified by the inducers as shown in the upper part of Figure 4.

DISCUSSION

The present results confirm previous studies, which showed that synthesis of embryonic and fetal hemoglobin is a peculiar and constant characteristic of the K-562 cell line [6–8, 10, 11, 13, 29]. Analysis of Hb production in primary clones, before and after induction by hemin, revealed a sequential pattern of globin gene expression. Three groups of clones were observed according to the types of Hb production: first, clones with no Hb accumulation; second, clones with mainly synthesis of Hb Portland; and third, clones with production of both Hbs Gower 1 and Portland. The induction by hemin modified the distribution towards the second and third group; for instance, hemin induced the synthesis of Hb Portland in clones of the first group. Analysis of hemoglobin chain synthesis confirmed these results which showed the existence of a sequential program of Hb expression: no Hb → Hb Portland → Hb Portland + Hb Gower 1.

Hemin affected the K-562 cell line in 2 ways. It increased the synthesis of Hb (2–10 times), and it modified the pattern of globin gene expression. In addition, hemin determined a significant increase of α-chains which were either absent or present at a very low level before induction. Previous studies on Friend erythroleukemia cells have shown that hemin is able to exert specific effects on globin gene expression at the pretranslational, as well as the translational, level [30–35], without triggering commitment to the terminal differentiation program

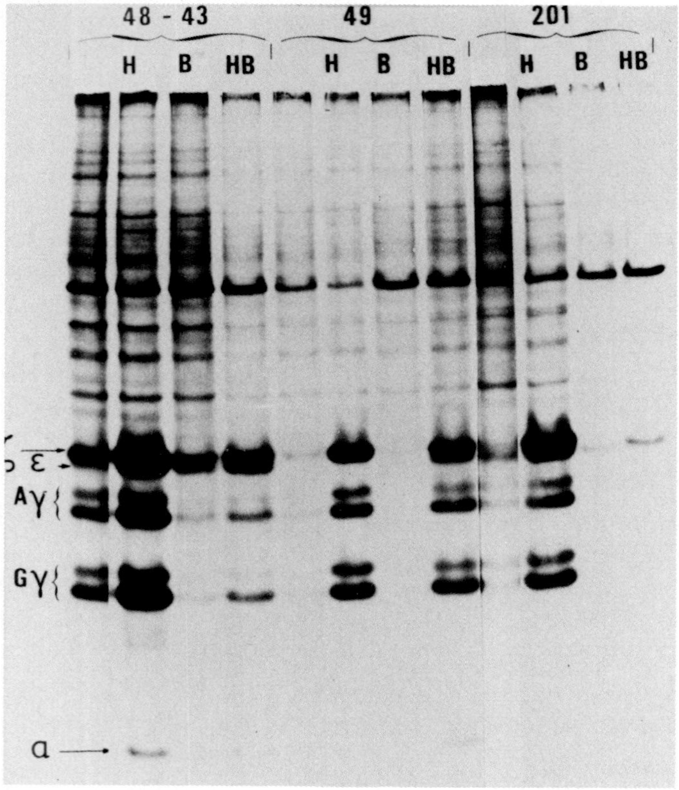

Fig. 4. Hemoglobin chain synthesis in subclones of the K-562 cell line in the absence of inducer and in the presence of hemin (H), sodium butyrate (B), or both (B + H) analyzed by isoelectric focusing. Hemoglobin was only partially purified by affinity chromatography on Sepharose-haptoglobin to compare the synthesis of globin chains with respect to other proteins which are present in the upper part of the figure.

[36–38]. RNA studies have shown that hemin increased by two- to threefold the level of globin mRNA expression in K-562 cells [8, 11]. This result, as well as the induction of specific globin gene expression reported here, suggests that hemin acts on K-562 cells at the pretranslational level.

In contrast, sodium butyrate did not significantly modify the degree of hemoglobinization; other markers, however, were significantly modified by butyrate without triggering K-562 cells into a terminal erythroid differentiation (Testa et al in preparation).

Analysis of globin-chain synthesis suggests that 2 switches of globin genes (one on chromosome 11 and the other on chromosome 16) occur in the K-562 cell line.

The switch on chromosome 11 occurs from the "fetal" $^{G}\gamma$-gene to the "embryonic" ϵ-gene. This hypothesis is supported by the sequence of the hemoglobin expression in the different clones, and also upon hemin addition. The sequence of the Hb expression was from Hb Portland ($\zeta_2\gamma_2$) to Hb Gower ($\zeta_2\epsilon_2$), and never the reverse. In addition, at the level of the hemoglobin-chain synthesis, an inverse correlation between the $^{G}\gamma$- and the ϵ-chains was constantly observed in clones which exhibited γ- and ϵ-chains.

The switch on chromosome 16 occurred in the direction from ζ- to α-gene expression. However, a low ζ-chain output is incompletely compensated by the expression of α-chains, resulting in an α-thalassemia phenotype as previously reported [29]. The switches occurring in the 2 gene clusters are in the opposite direction to that occurring during normal human development, and are not fully coordinated in the K-562 cell line.

These results indicated that the differences in Hb production are an intrinsic characteristic of the cells proliferating in each clone. However, the origin of the clonal heterogeneity remains speculative. Papayannopoulou et al and other investigators have provided some evidence that in different ontogenic stages (fetal, neonatal, and adult) globin gene expression is related to the differentiation of the erythroid progenitors [39–43], and to the late maturation process of erythroid cells [44, 45]. Taking into account this model, one can assume that the differential expression of globin genes is related to the differentiation of stem cells, and thus represents a marker of differentiation. Following this assumption, 2 hypotheses could explain the different phenotypes observed in K-562 clones.

First, each clone arises from the proliferation of stem cells corresponding to different levels of differentiation. In agreement with this hypothesis, a heterogeneity in the cellular commitment was observed [19]. Second, the heterogeneity is the reflection of different blocks occurring during the differentiation of a stem cell. In this case, these blocks represent the direct consequence of the leukemic process and can be partially bypassed by the inducer. A similar hypothesis was previously proposed by Sachs et al to understand the heterogeneity in the phenotype of different clones isolated from a murine myeloid cell line [46]. Whatever the mechanism determining this heterogeneity, the K-562 cell line represents a unique tool for molecular biology to investigate the sequential expression and the regulation of embryonic and fetal globin genes.

ACKNOWLEDGMENTS

We are indebted to Drs. B. Forget and Turcz for providing two different sources of K-562 cells.

Our thanks are also extended to M. Segear and A.M. Dulac for preparing the manuscript, and to Ph. Reboul for photographic assistance.

REFERENCES

1. Lozzio CB, Lozzio BB: Human chronic myelogeneous leukemia cell line with positive Philadelphia chromosome. Blood 45:321–334, 1975.
2. Andersson LC, Jokinen M, Gahmberg CG: Induction of erythroid differentiation in the human leukaemia cell line K 562. Nature 278:364–365, 1979.
3. Jokinen M, Gahmberg CG, Andersson LC: Biosynthesis of the major human red cell sialoglycoprotein, glycophorin A, in a continuous cell line. Nature 279:604–607, 1979.
4. Andersson LC, Nilsson K, Gahmberg CG: Expression of the major sialoglycoprotein (glycophorin A) in human leukemic cells. Int J Cancer 23:143–147, 1979.
5. Gahmberg CG, Jokinen M, Andersson LC: Expression of the major red cell sialoglycoprotein, glycophorin A, in the human leukemic cell line K 562. J Biol Chem 254:7442–7448, 1979.
6. Rutherford T, Clegg JB, Higgs DR, Jones RJ, Weatherall DJ: The pattern of haemoglobin synthesis in the human leukaemic cell line K 562. In Rossi GB (ed): "In Vivo and In Vitro Erythropoiesis: The Friend System." New York: Elsevier/North Holland, 1980, pp 467–475.
7. Rutherford TR, Clegg JB, Weatherall DJ: K-562 human leukaemic cells synthesize embryonic haemoglobin in response to haemin. Nature 280:164–165, 1979.
8. Benz EJ, Murnane MJ, Tonkonow BL, Berman BW, Mazar EM, Cavallesco C, Jenko T, Snyder EL, Forget BG, Hoffman R: Embryonic-fetal erythroid characteristics of a human leukemic cell line. Proc Natl Acad Sci USA 77:3509–3513, 1980.
9. Hoffman R, Ibrahim N, Murnane MJ, Diamond A, Forget B, Levere RD: Heme control of heme biosynthesis and catabolism in a human leukemia cell line. Blood 56:567–570, 1980.
10. Rutherford T, Clegg JB, Higgs DR, Jones RJ, Thompson J, Weatherall DJ: Embryonic erythroid differentiation in the human leukemic cell line K-562. Proc Natl Acad Sci USA 78:348–352, 1981.
11. Cioe L, McNab A, Hubbell HR, Meo P, Curtis P, Rovera G: Differential expression of the globin genes in human leukemia (K 562) cells induced to differentiate by hemin or butyric acid. Cancer Res 41:237–243, 1981.
12. Hoffman R, Murnane MJ, Benz EJ, Prohaska R, Floyd V, Dainiak N, Forget BG, Furthmayr H: Induction of erythropoietic colonies in a human chronic myelogeneous leukemia cell line. Blood 54:1182–1187, 1979.
13. Guerrasio A, Vainchenker W, Breton-Gorius J, Testa U, Rosa R, Thomopoulous P, Titeux M, Guichard J: Embryonic and fetal hemoglobin synthesis in K 562 cell line. Blood Cells 7:165–176, 1981.
14. Wood WG, Clegg JB, Weatherall DJ: Developmental biology of human hemoglobins. In Brown B (ed): "Progress in Hematology." New York: Grune & Stratton, 1977, vol X, pp 43–90.
15. Pataryas HA, Stamatoyannopoulos G: Hemoglobins in human fetuses: Evidence for adult hemoglobin production after the 11th gestational week. Blood 39:688–696, 1972.
16. Gale RE, Clegg JB, Huehns ER: Human embryonic haemoglobins Gower I and Gower II. Nature 280:162–164, 1979.
17. Lozzio BB, Lozzio CB, Bamberger EG, Feliu AS: A multipotential leukemia cell line (K 562) of human origin. Proc Soc Exp Biol Med 166:546–550, 1981.
18. Lozzio CB, Lozzio BB, Feliu AS, Bamberger EG: Letter to the Editor. Blood 57:979–980, 1981.
19. Vainchenker W, Testa U, Guichard J, Titeux M, Breton-Gorius J: Heterogeneity in the cellular commitment of a human leukemic cell line: K 562. Blood Cells 7:357–375, 1981.
20. Vainchenker W, Guerrasio A, Testa U, Titeux M, Guichard J, Beuzard Y, Rosa J, Breton-Gorius J: Multipotential capacities of differentiation and hemoglobin pattern of K-562 cell line. In Stamatoyannopoulos G, Nienhuis AW (eds): "Hemoglobins in Development and Differentiation." New York: Alan R Liss, 1981, pp 507–518.
21. Beuzard Y, Varet B, Lejeune JA, Bouguerra M, Gaillardon J, Rosa J: Etude d'une hemoglobine

Lepore: Hypothèse de regulation de la synthèse, des chaînes Lepore et anti-Lepore. Nouv Rev Fr Hématol 12:595–608, 1972.
22. Basset P, Beuzard Y, Garel MC, Rosa J: Isoelectric focusing of human hemoglobin. Its application to screening, to the characterization of 70 variants and to the study of modified fractions of normal hemoglobins. Blood 51:971–982, 1978.
23. Testa U, Beuzard Y, Vainchenker W, Goossens M, Dubart A, Monplaisir N, Brizard CP, Papayannopoulou Th, Rosa J: Elevated Hb F associated with an unstable hemoglobin, Hb Saint-Etienne: Hb synthesis in blood BFU-E in culture. Blood 54:334–343, 1979.
24. Alter BP, Goff SC, Efremov GD, Gravely ME, Huisman THJ: Globin chain electrophoresis: A new approach to the determination of the Gγ/Aγ ratio in fetal haemoglobin and to studies of globin synthesis. Br J Haematol 44:527–534, 1980.
25. Clegg JB, Naughton WA, Weatherall DJ: Abnormal human hemoglobin-separation and characterization of the alpha and beta chains by chromatography, and the determination of two new variants, Hb Chesapeake and Hb J Bangkok. J Mol Biol 19:91–108, 1966.
26. Tsapis A, Hinard N, Testa U, Dubart A, Vainchenker W, Rouyer-Fessard Ph, Beuzard Y, Rosa J: Globin chain affinity chromatography on Sepharose-haptoglobin: A new method of study of hemoglobin synthesis in reticulocytes, in bone marrow and in colonies of erythroid precursors. Eur J Biochem 112:513–519, 1980.
27. Alter B, Goff SC: Variable globin chain synthesis in mouse erythroleukemia cells. Blood 52:1047–1057, 1978.
28. Fritsch EF, Lawn RM, Maniatis T: Molecular cloning and characterization of the human β-like globin gene cluster. Cell 19:959–972, 1980.
29. Alter BP, Goff SC: Electrophoretic separation of human embryonic globin demonstrates "α-thalassemia" in human leukemia cell line K 562. Biochem Biophys Res Commun 94:843–848, 1980.
30. Ross J, Sautner D: Induction of globin mRNA by hemin cultured erythroleukemia cells. Cell 8:513–520, 1976.
31. Dabney BJ, Beaudet AL: Increase in globin chains and globin mRNA in erythroleukemia cells in response to hemin. Arch Biochem Biophys 179:106–112, 1977.
32. Rovera G, Surrey S: Use of resistant or hypersensitive variant clones of Friend cells in analysis of mode factors of inducers. Cancer Res 38:3737–3744, 1978.
33. Lowenhaupt K, Lingrel JB: Synthesis and turnover of globin mRNA in murine erythroleukemia cell induced with hemin. Proc Natl Acad Sci USA 76:5173–5177, 1979.
34. Rutherford TR, Weatherall DJ: Deficient heme synthesis as the cause of non-inducibility of hemoglobin synthesis in a Friend erythroleukemia cell line. Cell 16:415–423, 1979.
35. Hoffman LM, Ross J: The role of heme in the maturation of erythroblasts: The effect of inhibition of pyridoxine metabolism. Blood 55:762–771, 1980.
36. Mager D, Bernstein A: The role of heme in the regulation of the late program of Friend cell erythroid differentiation. J Cell Physiol 100:467–480, 1979.
37. Gusella JF, Weil SC, Tsiftsoglou AS, Vollach V, Newmann JR, Keys C, Housman DE: Hemin does not cause commitment of murine erythroleukemia (MEL) cells to terminal differentiation. Blood 56:481–487, 1980.
38. Lo SC, Aft R, Mueller GC: Role of non-hemoglobin heme accumulation in the terminal differentiation of Friend erythroleukemia cells. Cancer Res 41:864–870, 1981.
39. Papayannopoulou Th, Brice M, Stamatoyannopoulos G: Hemoglobin F synthesis in vitro: Evidence for control at the level of primitive erythroid stem cells. Proc Natl Acad Sci USA 74:2923–2927, 1977.
40. Vainchenker W, Testa U, Hinard N, Beuzard Y, Dubart A, Tsapis A, Monplaisir N, Rouyer-Fessard Ph, Rosa J: Hemoglobin synthesis in 7-day and 14-day old erythroid colonies from the bone marrow of normal individuals. Hemoglobin 4:53–67, 1980.
41. Stamatoyannopoulos G, Rosenblum BB, Papayannopoulou Th, Brice M, Nakamoto B, Shepart

Th: Hb F and Hb A production in erythroid cultures from human fetuses and neonates. Blood 54:440–450, 1979.

42. Beuzard Y, Vainchenker W, Testa U, Dubart A, Monplaisir N, Breton-Gorius J, Rosa J: Fetal to adult hemoglobin switch in cultures of early erythroid precursors from human fetuses and neonates. Am J Hematol 7:207–218, 1979.
43. Rowley PT, Ohlsson-Wilhelm B, Farley BA, Kosciolek B: Hemoglobin synthesis in cultures of hepatic erythroid cells from the human fetus. Proc Natl Acad Sci USA 76:1477–1480, 1979.
44. Papayannopoulou Th, Kalmantis T, Stamatoyannopoulos G: Cellular regulation of hemoglobin switching: Evidence for inverse relationship between fetal hemoglobin synthesis and degree of maturity of human erythroid cells. Proc Natl Acad Sci USA 76:6420–6424, 1979.
45. Chui DHK, Wong SC, Enkim MW, Patterson M, Ives RA: Proportion of fetal hemoglobin synthesis decreases during erythroid cell maturation. Proc Natl Acad Sci USA 77:2757–2761, 1980.
46. Sachs L: Constitutive uncoupling of pathways of gene expression that control growth and differentiation in myeloid leukemia: A model for the origin and progression of malignancy. Proc Natl Acad Sci USA 77:6152–6156, 1980.

In Vitro Regulation of Hb Synthesis: Studies in Normal Subjects and Thalassemic Patients*

Cesare Peschle, MD, Anna Rita Migliaccio, PhD, Giovanni Migliaccio, PhD, Gianfranco Mastroberardino, MD, Alessandro Massimo Gianni, MD, Paola Comi, PhD, Sergio Ottolenghi, MD, and Barbara Giglioni, PhD

Recent studies from our laboratories have been focused on the Hb switch in ontogenic development and erythroblastic differentiation [1-5]. The technical approach involved evaluation of synthesis of α-, ϵ-, β-, $^{G}\gamma$-, $^{A}\gamma$-globin chains in single bursts, and pooled CFU-E clusters, by means of analytic IEF. The Hb synthesis program of the progenitors was thereby evaluated on the basis of the globin-chain synthesis in their clonal progeny.

Our observations are compatible with a monoclonal model for the Hb switch (Fig. 1), which includes a single population of BFU-E. These progenitors are programmed for Hb F + some A synthesis in the fetal age. They are gradually reprogrammed in the perinatal phase, thus leading to an adult pool prevailingly committed to Hb A (+ A_2) synthesis. It is emphasized, however, that all adult BFU-E maintain the potential for some Hb F synthesis.

The time-programmed mechanism underlying the perinatal Hb switch has not been unveiled yet. Different mechanisms may be postulated, of either ''extrinsic'' (humoral factor(s), cell-cell interaction) or ''intrinsic'' (critical number of mitosis) type [6-8]. The evidence supporting these various hypotheses, however, is unsatisfactory at best.

*Supported by grants from: Volkswagen Foundation, Hannover (CP); EURATOM, Bruxelles (No. BIO-C-353-I) (CP); CNR, Rome (Progetto Finalizzato ''Controllo della crescita Neoplastica'' No. 80.01615.96 (CP), 81.01437.96 (CP), and 80.01943.96 (AMG); Progetto Finalizzato ''Medicina Preventiva'' No. 80.01133.83 (SO).

Glossary and Abbreviations: Hb F ($\alpha_2\gamma_2$); Hb A ($\alpha_2\beta_2$), A_2 ($\alpha_2\delta_2$). Isoelectric focusing, IEF, Burst-forming unit, erythroid, BFU-E; primitive BFU-E, P-BFU-E; intermediate or mature BFU-E, M-BFU-E. Colony-forming unit, erythroid, CFU-E. Burst-promoting activity, BPA. Fetal calf serum, FCS. Bromodeoxyuridine, BrdU. Thymidine, dT. Hereditary persistence of Hb F, HPFH.

Birth Defects: Original Article Series, Volume 18, Number 7, pages 131–138
© 1982 March of Dimes Birth Defects Foundation

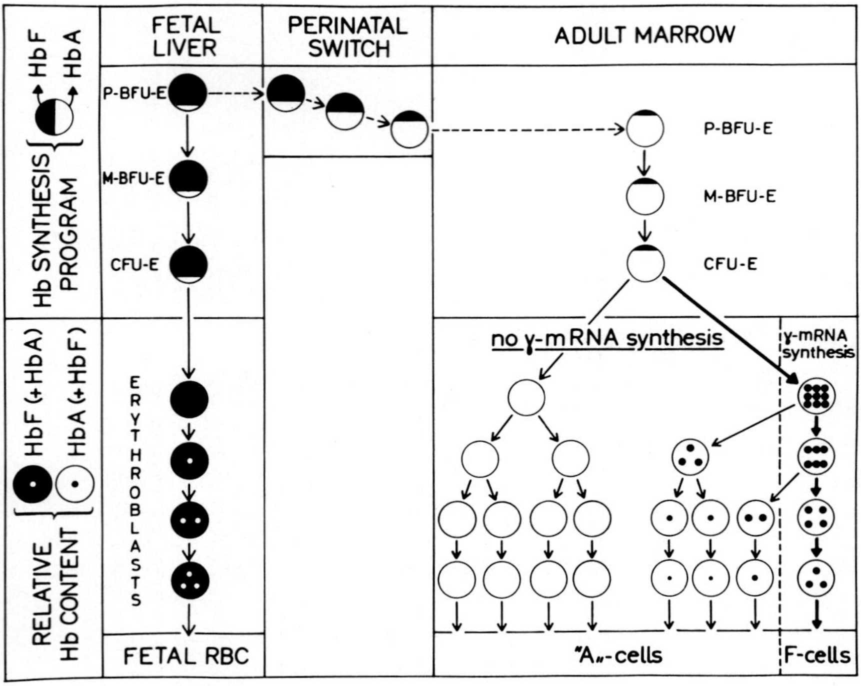

Fig. 1. A model for the regulation of Hb synthesis in ontogenic development and erythropoietic differentiation.

Theoretically, the Hb synthesis program may or may not be modulated in the differentiation pathway of erythroid progenitors. In this regard, Stamatoyannopoulos and co-workers [9,10] suggested that PBFU-E → M-BFU-E → CFU-E differentiation is linked with gradual obliteration of the program for Hb F synthesis. This concept was largely based on immunofluorescence studies on adult bursts. Some colonies were HbF^+, while others seemed F^-. More important, F^+ bursts apparently contained both F^+ and F^- subcolonies. These results, however, may be related to the asynchronous hemoglobinization of different bursts in a single plate, as well as of the various subcolonies in a single burst. Conceivably, bursts and subcolonies scored as F^- by immunofluorescence may have been composed essentially of immature erythroblasts. These would contain a very low level of Hb, thus rendering the minor Hb F aliquot undetectable by the employed assay. This bias may be circumvented, if analysis of globin-chain synthesis in erythroid colonies is performed by means of the sensitive IEF method. This approach has indeed demonstrated that some Hb F is produced in *all* adult bursts and subcolonies [3,11]. On the other hand, if the Hb F synthesis program is gradually obliterated in the course of P-BFU-E → M-BFU-E → CFU-E differentiation, it follows that the 3 different types of colonies generated by these 3 classes of progenitors should show a progressive decrease of Hb F production. This corollary was verified in strictly standardized cultures of normal adult marrow [1,5]. The 3 types of colonies were picked out and labeled at a corresponding hemoglobinization stage, in order to avoid the maturation bias (see below). These studies did not show a gradual decrease of Hb F synthesis in the clonal progeny of P-BFU-E, M-BFU-E and CFU-E. This suggests, that *under strictly homogeneous in vitro conditions,* the Hb synthesis program remains substantially unmodified in the differentiation of erythroid progenitors. On the other hand, if culture conditions are heterogeneous, the program might still be modulated. In this regard BFU-E kinetics are largely controlled by BPA [12]. It has been claimed that in vitro addition of BPA induces an enhanced γ-chain synthesis in adult bursts [13]. These studies, however, are inconclusive, since the analysis was not carried out on colonies of corresponding hemoglobinization stage (see below). In a retrospective analysis of our studies, it is apparent that adult bursts were grown in cultures supplemented by different FCS batches, either rich or poor BPA. Single well-hemoglobinized bursts grown in BPA-rich cultures showed a higher level of relative γ-synthesis (~5-15%) (Fig. 2A) than those in BPA-poor plates (~1-3%) (Fig. 2B). More important, the latter values are distinctly closer to those normally observed in vivo. These results are compatible with the concept that the in vivo BPA levels in the adult age may at least contribute in modulating the level of γ-synthesis, via mechanisms operating at the erythroblastic level (see below). Further studies are obviously required to elucidate these crucial aspects.

Expression of the Hb synthesis program is asynchronous, in that γ-chain synthesis peaks earlier than β-chain production in the erythroblastic maturation. The asynchrony has been documented in both fetal, neonatal, and adult erythroid colonies [1,4,14,15], as well as in vivo [16]. Thus, the $\gamma \rightarrow \beta$ switch occurs not only in ontogeny but also in cytogeny. This "maturation phenomenon" may represent a key mechanism underlying modulation of Hb F synthesis in adult life. Particularly, it may explain emergence of a majority of F- vs a minority of A-cells [17,18], as well as enhanced Hb F synthesis in various conditions associated with stress erythropoiesis [19,20]. As previously suggested [1] (Fig. 1), the γ-phase might be heterogeneously modulated in various erythropoietic clones. Accordingly, F-cells would derive from erythroblasts with an amplified γ-phase, in terms of duration and/or intensity of synthetic activity. On the other hand, erythropoietic clones endowed with a less-pronounced γ-phase would give rise to A-cells. This concept predicts that a very small (so far unmeasurable) amount of Hb F is present even in A-cells. Some evidence, however, suggests that at least a majority of A-cells is strictly F^-, in that the Hb F content in RBC may be accounted for solely by the amount of Hb F in F-cells. If most A-cells are strictly

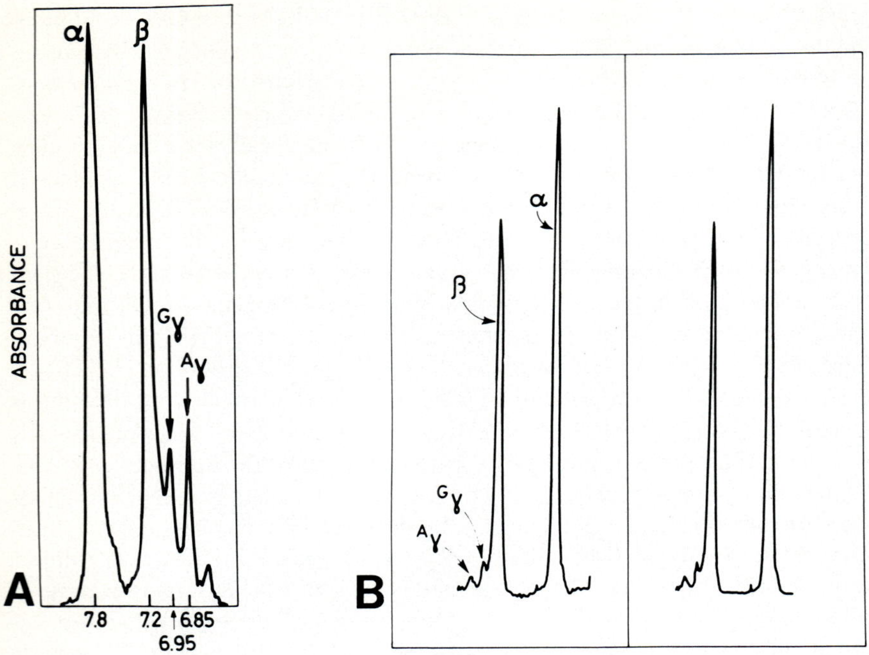

Fig. 2. Densitometric tracing of the radioactive globin pattern from single well-hemoglobinized normal adult blood bursts grown in A) BPA-rich FCS, or B) BPA-poor FCS.

F⁻, production of a few F- vs a majority of A-cells may be explained in terms of a model including: a) heterogeneous modulation of early γ- and late β-synthesis, and b) a series of asymmetric divisions in the early erythroblastic maturation pathway (Fig. 1). Each one of these divisions would generate two cell lineages, respectively endowed or not with the capacity to synthesize some γ-mRNA. The former may give rise to a progeny with sustained γ-synthesis, the relative amount of which would gradually decline in the face of rapidly increasing β-production. This lineage may thereby generate F-cells (Fig. 1). The latter would give rise to a progeny characterized by two different patterns: 1) no γ-mRNA synthesis, if the asymmetric division occurs at very early stages of erythroblastic differentiation. This line would generate strictly F^- A-cells (Fig. 1). 2) Early synthesis of some γ-mRNA, which is then markedly diluted via cell mitosis and catabolism. The dilution would cause a dramatic decrease of absolute, and even more of relative, γ-chain production. This lineage might generate "A"-cells with miniscule, unmeasurable amounts of Hb F (Fig. 1).

An additional mechanism underlying elevation of Hb F in adult RBC may be represented by skipping of terminal divisions, as typically observed in stress erythropoiesis [17]. This would clearly dampen the impact of the late β-synthetic phase.

In an attempt to further explore the asynchrony of globin-chain synthesis in erythroblastic maturation, BrdU (ie a dT analog) has been added at sequential times during adult burst formation. In this regard, BrdU treatment of chick embryos inhibits the initiation of Hb synthesis [21]. Butyric acid-induced differentiation of Friend leukemia cells is also inhibited by BrdU addition [22]: the effect is correlated with the amount of the analog incorporated into nuclear DNA [22]. In our preliminary studies, this agent was supplemented on day 6, 8, and 10 of culture (1 μg/dish). The cloning efficiency in BrdU-treated plates was >70% of control values. Bursts were picked out and labeled on day 11-13, at either early or late stages of hemoglobinization. Interestingly, "red" colonies treated with BrdU on day 6-8 show a significant elevation of the relative γ-synthesis over control levels, while addition on day 10 is ineffective (Fig. 3). No striking difference has been observed between pale colonies, either treated or untreated with BrdU (data not shown). It is suggested that, on day 6 and 8 of culture, the transcription of γ-genes is fully activated, while that of β-genes has not yet reached maximal levels (see the model in [23]). Thus, BrdU addition in this phase inhibits peak β-gene expression, hypothetically via substitution of dT in DNA loci mediating peak transcription of the β-gene. Addition of BrdU on day 10 of culture is ineffective, presumably because full β-gene activation has already occurred. Studies with agents inhibiting DNA methylation are currently in progress in an attempt to gain further insight into these aspects.

The non-α-gene cluster is $5'$-ϵ-$^{G}\gamma$-$^{A}\gamma$-δ-β-$3'$ on chromosome 11 [24]. The $^{G}\gamma/^{A}\gamma$ synthetic quotient is more elevated in the fetal age (~2:1) than in the adult period (~2:3) [25]. In erythroid bursts, γ/β and $^{G}\gamma/^{A}\gamma$ ratios are directly correlated [1-3,26]. This phenomenon is best expressed in cord blood colonies: γ/β quotients are spread over a wide continuous spectrum, ranging from "fetal" to "adult" values, and further correlated with the $^{G}\gamma/^{A}\gamma$ ratios [2,26]. This suggests that a single mechanism may modulate the non-α-gene cluster during ontogenic development.

A correlation between γ/β and $^{G}\gamma/^{A}\gamma$ synthetic ratios also may be observed in adult erythroblastic maturation, particularly in peripheral blood cultures, if very immature bursts are compared with markedly "red" colonies [1]. This suggests that erythropoietic differentiation in the adult is associated with a transcriptional wave progressing along the non-α-gene cluster. The early maturation phase, characterized by peak γ-gene expression, is thus associated with a more elevated $^{G}\gamma/^{A}\gamma$ synthetic ratio. This correlation is also observed in "red" colonies from day 6-8 BrdU-treated plates: these bursts show elevation of both γ-synthesis and $^{G}\gamma/^{A}\gamma$ ratio over control levels (Fig. 3).

We have recently analyzed globin-chain production in erythroid colonies from patients with various disorders of Hb synthesis. Preliminary results on HPFH of

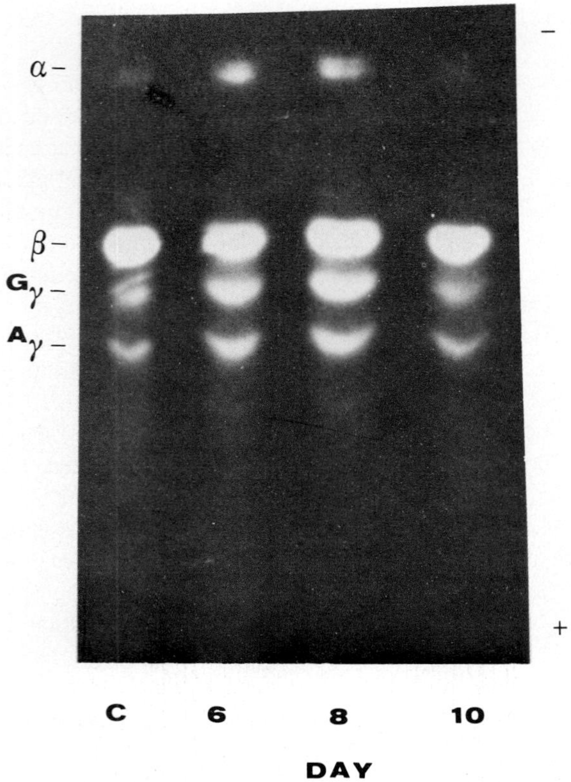

Fig. 3. Fluorogram of the IEF pattern of globins synthesized in well-hemoglobinized normal adult blood bursts, which were grown in either control plates (C) or dishes supplemented with BrdU on day 6, 8, or 10.

hetero- or pancellular type have been presented elsewhere [1]. We wish to discuss here some representative data on a homozygous $\delta°\beta°$-thalassemic patient. As expected, peripheral blood bursts apparently showed no β-chain synthesis (Fig. 4). However, the $^G\gamma/^A\gamma$ production ratio was more elevated in red (grade 3) than in pale-white (grade 1) colonies (Fig. 4). This pattern is clearly the opposite of normal [1]. We suggest that this paradoxic phenomenon may be due to in vitro selection of erythropoietic clones endowed with a more elevated capacity for γ-synthesis, a higher $^G\gamma/^A\gamma$ ratio, and a more balanced α/non-α-synthetic quotient. A paradoxic maturation phenomenon has been similarly observed in the cultures of other patients with thalassemic syndromes (data not shown). In vivo studies are currently in progress in an attempt to strengthen this selection hypothesis.

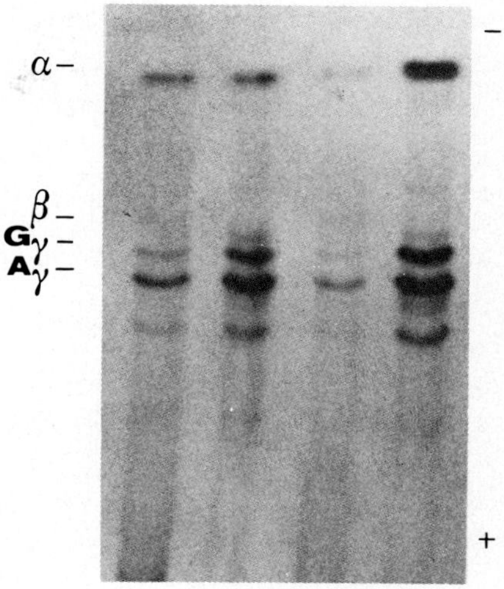

Fig. 4. Fluorogram of the IEF pattern of globins synthesized in blood bursts from a $\delta°\beta°$-thalassemic patient, which were picked out and labeled at either an early (grade 1) or late (grade 3) stage of hemoglobinization.

REFERENCES

1. Peschle C, Migliaccio AR, Migliaccio G, Lettieri F, Maguire YP, Condorelli M, Gianni AM, Ottolenghi S, Giglioni B, Pozzoli ML, Comi P: Regulation of Hb synthesis in ontogenesis and erythropoietic differentiation: In vivo studies on fetal liver, cord blood, normal adult blood or marrow, and blood from HPFH patients. In Stamatoyannopoulos G, Nienhuis A (eds): ''Hemoglobins in Development and Differentiation.'' New York: Alan R. Liss, 1981.
2. Comi P, Giglioni B, Ottolenghi S, Gianni AM, Polli E, Barba P, Covelli A, Migliaccio G, Condorelli M, Peschle C: Globin chain synthesis in single erythroid bursts from cord blood: Studies on γ-β and ${}^{G}\gamma$-${}^{A}\gamma$ switches. Proc Natl Acad Sci USA 77:362–365, 1980.
3. Peschle C, Migliaccio G, Covelli A, Lettieri F, Migliaccio AR, Condorelli M, Comi P, Pozzoli ML, Giglioni B, Ottolenghi S, Cappellini MD, Polli E, Gianni AM: Hemoglobin synthesis in individual bursts from normal adult blood: All bursts and subcolonies synthesize ${}^{G}\gamma$- and ${}^{A}\gamma$-globin chains. Blood 56:218–226, 1980.
4. Gianni AM, Comi P, Giglioni B, Ottolenghi S, Migliaccio AR, Lettieri F, Maguire YP, Peschle C: Biosynthesis of Hb in individual fetal liver bursts: γ-chain production peaks earlier than β-chain in the erythropoietic pathway. Exp Cell Res 130:345–352, 1980.
5. Comi P, Giglioni B, Pozzoli ML, Ottolenghi S, Gianni AM, Migliaccio AR, Migliaccio G, Lettieri F, Peschle C: Biosynthesis of globin chains in fetal liver and adult marrow cultures. Comparative analysis of individual colonies derived from early, intermediate or late erythroid progenitors. Exp Cell Res 133:347–356, 1981.
6. Vainchenker W, Testa U, Dubart A, Beuzard Y, Breton-Gorius J, Rosa J: Acceleration of the

hemoglobin switch in cultures of neonate erythroid precursors by adult cells. Blood 56:541–548, 1980.

7. Zanjani ED, McGlave PB, Bhakthavathsalan A, Stamatoyannopoulos G: Sheep fetal haematopoietic cells produce adult hemoglobin when transplanted in the adult animal. Nature 280:495–496, 1981.
8. Wood WG, Bunch C: Hemoglobin switching in sheep: Analysis following transplantation of fetal cells to adult animals. This volume.
9. Papayannopoulou T, Brice M, Stamatoyannopoulos G: Hemoglobin F synthesis in vitro: Evidence for control at the level of primitive erythroid stem cell. Proc Natl Acad Sci USA 77:2923–2927, 1977.
10. Stamatoyannopoulos G, Papayannopoulou T: Fetal hemoglobin and the erythroid stem cell differentiation process. In Stamatoyannopoulos G, Nienhuis A (eds): "Cellular and Molecular Regulation of Hemoglobin Switching." New York: Grune & Stratton, 1979, pp 323–349.
11. Kidoguchi K, Ogawa M, Karam JD: Hemoglobin biosynthesis in individual erythropoietic bursts in culture. J Clin Invest 63:804–806, 1979.
12. Peschle C: Hemopoietic stem and progenitor cells: Recent advances of physiopathologic relevance. In Willoughby MLN, Siegel SE (eds): "Butterworths International Medical Reviews." Vol 1 Haematology-Oncology. London: Butterworths. (In press)
13. Teresawa T, Ogawa M, Porter PN, Golde DW, Goldwasser E: Effect of burst promoting activity (BPA) and erythropoietin on hemoglobin biosynthesis in culture. Blood 56:1106–1110, 1980.
14. Papayannopoulou T, Kalamantis T, Stamatoyannopoulos G: Cellular regulation of hemoglobin switching: Evidence for inverse relationship between fetal hemoglobin synthesis and degree of maturity of human erythroid cells. Proc Natl Acad Sci USA 76:6420–6424, 1979.
15. Papayannopoulou T, Kurachi S, Brice M, Nakamoto B, Stamatoyannopoulos G: Asynchronous synthesis of HbF and HbA during erythroblast maturation. II. Studies of $^{G}\gamma$, $^{A}\gamma$ and β chain synthesis in individual erythroid clones from neonatal and adult BFU-E cultures. Blood 57:531–536, 1981.
16. Dover GJ, Boyer SH: Quantitation of hemoglobins in individual red cells: Asynchronous biosynthesis of fetal and adult hemoglobin during erythroid maturation in normal subjects. Blood 56:1082–1090, 1980.
17. Boyer SH, Belding K, Margolet L, Noyes N: Fetal hemoglobin restriction to a few erythrocytes (F cells) in normal human adults. Science 188:361–363, 1975.
18. Boyer SH, Dover GJ: The in vivo biology of F cells in man. Supra #10, pp 47–71.
19. Alter BP: Fetal erythropoiesis in bone marrow failure syndromes. Supra #10, pp 87–106.
20. De Simone J, Heller P, Biel SI: Stimulation of fetal hemoglobin synthesis following stress erythropoiesis. Supra #10, pp 139–152.
21. Weintraub H, Campbell G Lem, Holtzer H: Differentiation in the presence of bromodeoxyuridine is "all-or-none". Nature (New Biol) 244:140–142, 1973.
22. Ashman CH, Davidson RL: Inhibition of Friend erythroleukemic cell differentiation by bromodeoxyuridine: Correlation with the amount of bromodeoxyuridine in DNA. J Cell Physiol 102:45–50, 1980.
23. Ottolenghi S, Peschle C, Comi P, Giglioni B, Pozzoli ML, Cappellini N, Migliaccio AR, Lettieri F, Migliaccio G, Barba P, Covelli A, Gianni AM: Hemoglobin synthesis in single erythroid colonies from cord and adult blood. In Rossi GB (ed): "In Vivo and In Vitro Erythropoiesis: The Friend System." Amsterdam: Elsevier, 1980, pp 41–47.
24. Fritsch EF, Lawn RM, Maniatis T: Molecular cloning and characterization of the human β-like globin gene cluster. Cell 19:959–972, 1980.
25. Huisman THJ, Schroeder WA, Efremov GD, Duma H, Mladenovski B, Hyman CB, Rachmilewitz EA, Bouver NG, Miller A, Brodie AR, Shelton JR, Apel G: The present status of the heterogeneity of fetal hemoglobin in β-thalassemia: An attempt to unify some observations in thalassemia and related conditions. Ann NY Acad Sci 232:107–124, 1974.
26. Teresawa T, Ogawa M: Hemoglobin biosynthesis in individual bursts from human adult peripheral and umbilical cord blood: Analysis of the relative rates of synthesis of $^{G}\gamma$ and $^{A}\gamma$ globin chains. J Cell Physiol 105:483–488, 1980.

THALASSEMIA TYPES IN ITALY

Thalassemia Types in Latium

**Ida Bianco, MD, Bruno Graziani, MD, Maria Lerone, BS,
Pietro Congedo, BS, Maria Valente, MD, and Donatella Ponzini, BS**

Every year since October 1975, the Center for the study of microcythemia in Rome carries out a screening of the microcythemias* among the students of the lower secondary school in the whole region of Latium [1,2]. Thus, detailed knowledge of the various forms of thalassemia present in this region and accurate estimates of their frequencies are being obtained.

The study of microcythemics is performed through a whole set of diagnostic tests adopted in this Center [4]. The procedure consists of a number of consecutive steps (Fig. 1) which are applied to progressively smaller groups of specimens. In the first phase, red cell osmotic fragility [5] and morphology are studied. Every sample with even a minimal alteration is passed on to the 2nd phase. All the others (about 60–70% on the average) are classified as normal with no further investigations. In the 2nd phase, specimens' hematologic parameters are determined by an automatic counter. From these findings, both normal and possibly microcythemic samples are subjected to studies of hemoglobin (3rd phase). All classic and slight cases of β-thalassemia, of $\delta\beta$-thalassemia with high Hb F, and the Lepore thalassemias are thus identified. Moreover, at least some of the so-called "isolated high Hb A_2 carriers" [6] are also discovered (dashed line of Fig. 1) through some slight alteration of their red cell morphology.

Those cases which showed thalassemic hematologic features but normal Hbs A_2 and F levels are assayed for serum iron (4th phase). Iron-deficient anemic subjects are thus recognized; remaining samples are further examined by family and globin synthesis studies (5th step) in order to identify the α-thalassemia carriers.

*The term "microcythemia, synonymous with "thalassemia," stands for the healthy heterozygous carrier of a thalassemic gene. It was introduced in 1946 by Silvestroni and Bianco [3] to specify the hereditary hematologic abnormality they found in a number of healthy subjects examined for different purposes. It is meant to stress the most prominent and specific feature of their erythrocytes, namely true microcytosis.

Birth Defects: Original Article Series, Volume 18, Number 7, pages 141–145
© 1982 March of Dimes Birth Defects Foundation

Ample experience has shown [4,7] that this procedure reveals about 99% of the non-α-microcythemias and all the evident α-microcythemias (or α_1- or α^{o}-microcythemias).

The pooled results (Table 1) of the first 5 screenings showed that 4,630 thalassemia carriers were found among a total of 192,147 students examined. This corresponds to an overall incidence of 2.41% in the Latium region. However, considerable fluctuations around this mean incidence are apparent (Table 1, Fig. 2). In fact, one finds an incidence as low as 1.25% in the Rieti province and 2.80% in the Latina province, which is significantly higher than the mean incidence in the rest of the region ($\chi^2_{1df} = 15.50$; $p \ll 0.001$). This finding is in line with well-known north-south cline of the thalassemia gene frequency which is relatively low in northern Italy, intermediate in central Italy, and attains its

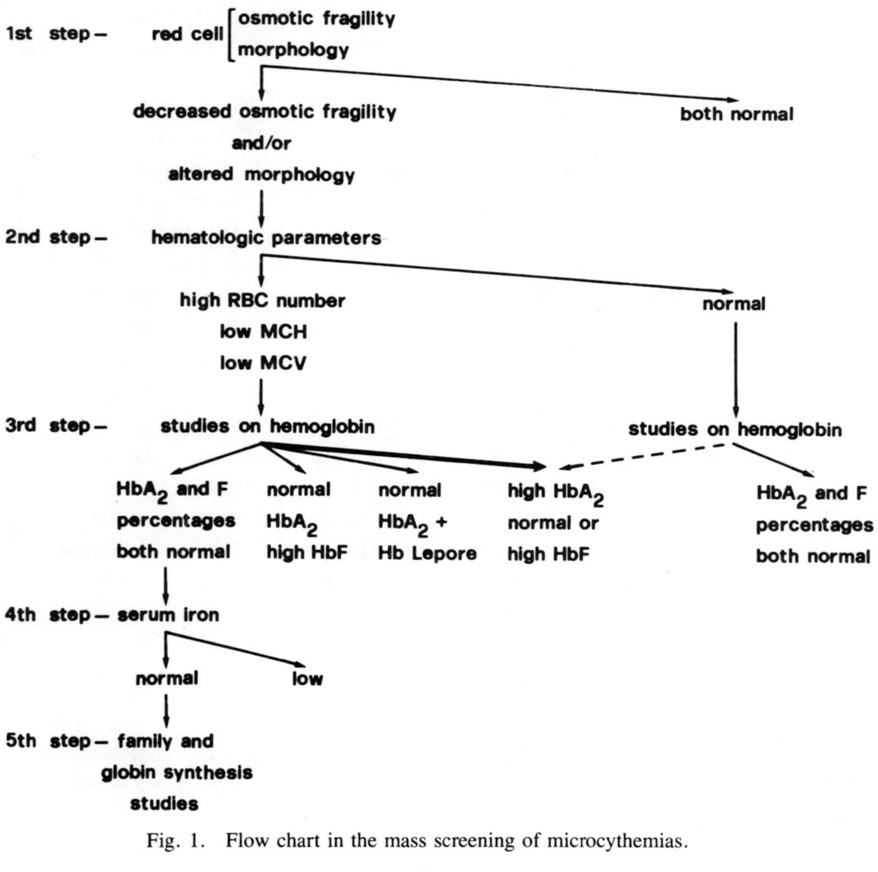

Fig. 1. Flow chart in the mass screening of microcythemias.

highest values in southern and insular Italy, especially in the coastal areas. β-microcythemia represents the most frequent variety found in all Latium provinces. This form alone accounts for about 85–91% of all thalassemias (Table 2).

TABLE 1. Results of 5 Screenings for Thalassemias in Intermediate Schools of Latium

Place	No. Tested	No. Thalassemia	% Thalassemia
Rome	115,581	2,852	2.467 ± 0.046
Province of Rome	28,770	646	2.245 ± 0.091
Prov. of Viterbo	10,605	233	2.197 ± 0.142
Prov. of Latina	21,171	593	2.801 ± 0.113
Prov. Frosinone	13,299	272	2.045 ± 0.123
Prov. of Rieti	2,721	34	1.249 ± 0.213
Total	192,147	4,630	2.410 ± 0.035

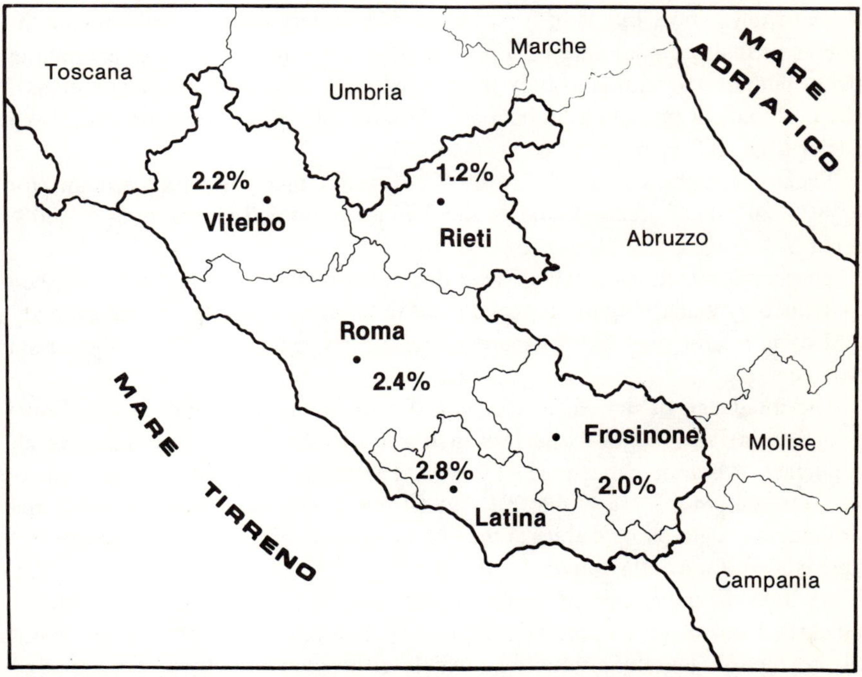

Fig. 2. Frequencies of thalassemias in the 5 provinces of Latium: pooled data of 5 screening campaigns.

TABLE 2. Frequency of α; β and $\delta\beta$ Thalassemias in 4 Provinces of Latium: Pooled Data of 5 Screening Campaigns.

	Types of Thalassemia			
Provinces	β	α	F	Lepore
Rome	3,048 (87.0%)	396 (11.3%)	19 (0.6%)	39 (1.1%)
Latina	501 (85.0%)	77 (13.1%)	—	11 (1.9%)
Viterbo	202 (86.7%)	28 (12.0%)	1 (0.4%)	2 (0.9%)
Frosinone	248 (91.1%)	23 (8.5%)	—	1 (0.4%)

The study of hemoglobin and of its synthesis in a group of patients with Cooley anemia or with thalassemia intermedia, all autochthonous of the Latium region, who were treated in this Center, provided an estimate of the relative frequencies of the β^{o}- and β^{+}-thalassemias. Among 10 Cooley patients, 7 were $\beta^{\text{thal o}}$ homozygotes, while 3 who produced a small quantity of Hb A had at least one $\beta^{\text{thal+}}$ gene; 2 out of 3 patients with thalassemia intermedia showed a high percentage of Hb A and showed that one of their parents was a carrier of a very slight variety of β-microcythemia, that is, $\beta^{\text{thal++}}$. This variety is very common only among the parents of thalassemia intermedia patients [8]. It is particularly frequent among blacks but not uncommon in Italy (mainly in Sicily and other southern regions). The third patient turned out to be a $\beta^{\text{thal o}}$ homozygote who, however, was also a carrier of an α^{thal} gene.

These data show that $\beta^{\text{thal+}}$ and $\beta^{\text{thal++}}$ genes taken together account for 20–40% of all β^{thal} genes found in the Latium region, the remaining 60–80% being $\beta^{\text{thal o}}$ genes.

The α-microcythemia, which was first identified by routine tests and then confirmed by examining the proband's entire family, makes up, on the average, 11% of all microcythemias. Its share seems slightly higher (13.1%) in the Latina province.

The incidence of the carriers of $\delta\beta$-microcythemia with high Hb F (F-microcythemia) was found to be less than 1% of all thalassemias. The overall frequency of Lepore carriers was 1% on the average except in the Latina province where it was 1.9% (Table 2). Almost every Lepore subject found in this province was native to the areas at the border of Campania, the region where this gene is very frequently found.

As far as the prevention of Cooley disease is concerned, the scholastic screening turned out to be extremely useful in spreading correct information about microcythemia, thereby promoting a widely diffused and timely acquaintance of the various routes available for this purpose. The screening has been willingly accepted by this population, and it alone was enough to prompt a further spontaneous mass screening among married or engaged young couples, as well as among pregnant women. This second screening now amounts to about 15,000 subjects examined per year.

REFERENCES

1. Silvestroni E, Bianco I, Graziani B, Carboni C, D'Arca SU: First premarital screening of thalassaemia carriers in intermediate schools in Latium. J Med Genet 15:202, 1978.
2. Silvestroni E, Bianco I, Graziani B, Carboni C, Valente M, Lerone M, D'Arca SU: Screening of thalassaemia in intermediate schools in Latium. J Med Genet 17:161, 1980.
3. Silvestroni E, Bianco I: Una particolare anomalia ematologica: La "microcitemia." Minerva Med II:202, 1946.
4. Graziani B, Bianco I, Carboni C, Lerone M, Valente M, Sidorini B, Ricotti G, Bianco P: Tecniche e strategie di screenings di massa delle microcitemie. Atti VI Congr Intern su "La Prevenzione delle Malattie Microcitemiche." Minerva Med, 1981.
5. Silvestroni E, Bianco I: Il metodo di Simmel per lo studio delle resistenze globulari. Il Policlinico Sez Prat 51:153, 1945.
6. Silvestroni E, Bianco I: Sull'esistenza nella popolazione italiana di soggetti non microcitemici portatori di un'elevata quota di emoglobina adulta lenta (Hb A_2) e sui loro rapporti con i malati di anemia microcitica. Il Policlinico Sez Prat 64:1869, 1957.
7. Silvestroni E, Bianco I: Screening for microcythemia in Italy: Analysis of data collected in the past 30 years. Am J Hum Genet 27:198, 1975.
8. Bianco I, Graziani B, Carboni C: Genetic patterns in thalassemia intermedia (constitutional microcytic anemia) - Familial, hematologic and biosynthetic studies. Hum Hered 27:257, 1977.

Thalassemia Types in Calabria (Southern Italy)

Carlo Brancati, MD, and Antonio Tagarelli

It is interesting to remember that the general epidemiology of thalassemia in Calabria (the investigation has concerned 250,000 subjects [1]) has shown marked correspondence between the areas which, in the 8th-6th centuries BC, were Greek colonies, and the areas where the percentage of people subject to thalassemia is the highest, as can be seen in Figure 1.

A more recent study which has tried to identify the various thalassemia genotypes in Calabria has allowed us to determine frequency. Of 3,252 carriers of the thalassemia trait, the various heterozygote genotypes are reported in Table 1.

The data in Table 1 show that the β-genotypes with increased level of A_2 prevail over others, but some other genotypes, such as the $\delta\beta$-genotypes and the genotype which conditions the variant with "increased levels of A_2 and F," are to some extent also present. The δ, α, and Lepore (Boston) types are also present.

The fact that Calabrian people are carriers of several thalassemic genes has made possible several forms of homozygosity and for several different types of thalassemia genes to be present in the same subject simultaneously. The above has been confirmed by a genetic study of "severe types of thalassemia" which has covered all members of the families investigated. We think that the expression "severe types of thalassemia" is the most appropriate one to identify these hemopathies, but it is also necessary to identify the specific genotypes. The hemopathies which we have investigated can be classified as shown in Table 2.

The presence or complete absence of Hb A in our patients has allowed us to infer the presence of β^+- and β°-genes. The number of patients with β° has turned out to be more or less equal to the number of patients with β^+.

The presence of Hb A in relatively high quantities in some of the most severe types of thalassemia has not changed the course of the illness very much. Some other considerations regarding the patients who are described in Table 2 can be synthesized as follows:

Birth Defects: Original Article Series, Volume 18, Number 7, pages 147–155
© 1982 March of Dimes Birth Defects Foundation

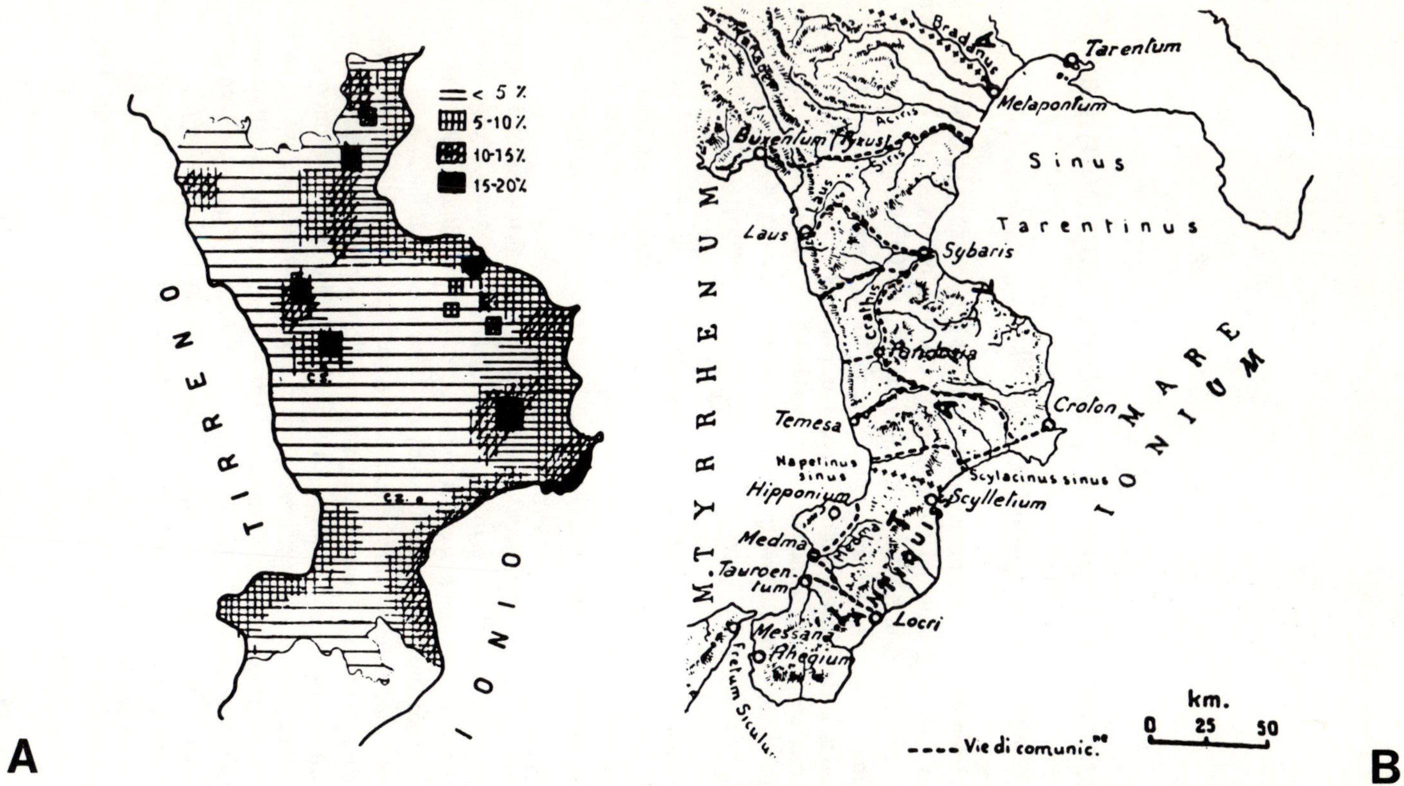

Fig. 1. Comparison of the 2 figures shows the correspondence between distribution of thalassemia and old Greek colonies (8th-6th centuries BC). A) The distribution of thalassemia in Northern Calabria. B) Communication network in Magna Graecia (from E. Pais "Storia dell'Italia antica").

TABLE 1. Frequencies of the Different Varieties of Thalassemic Heterozygotes

Genotypes	No.	%
β-thalassemia with increased level of A_2	2,905	89.33
$\delta\beta$-thalassemia	160	4.92
β-thalassemia with increased levels of A_2 and F	127	3.91
β-thalassemia with increased level of A_2 only	5	0.15
Hb Lepore (Boston)	2	—
δ-thalassemia	6	0.18
α-thalassemia	47	1.45
Total	3,252	

TABLE 2. Frequencies of "Severe Types of Thalassemia" (ie Cooley Anemia Transfusion-Dependent)

Genetic Constitution	No.	%
β-thalassemia with increased level of A_2 homozygosity	86	74.1
β-thalassemia with increased level of A_2 + thalassemia with increased levels of A_2 and F	13	11.2
β-thalassemia with increased level of A_2 + $\delta\beta$-thalassemia	11	9.5
β-thalassemia with increased level of A_2 and F homozygosity	5	4.3
$\delta\beta$-thalassemia homozygosity	1	—
Total	116	

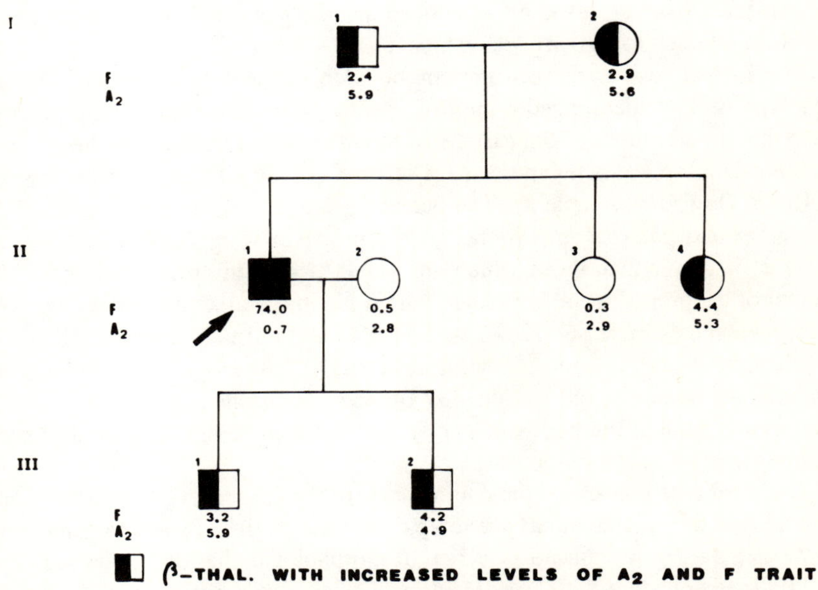

Fig. 2. Family pedigree showing homozygous state β-thalassemia with increased levels of A_2 and F.

1) Out of 13 patients affected by β-thalassemia + thalassemia with increased levels of A_2 and F, 3 who are now between 11 and 16 years of age, have shown a less severe syndrome and have rarely had blood transfusions.
2) Of the 5 patients affected by "β-thalassemia homozygosity with increased levels of A_2 and F" one is particularly interesting. This patient, aged 24, married a woman who is not affected, and who has given birth to 2 children. Both children are carriers of the same type of thalassemia (Fig. 2).

This latter case recalls a similar case investigated by Schokker et al [2], and gives us the opportunity to make some brief remarks. The percentage of Hb F in the thalassemic heterozygotes of the above-described type have turned out to have lower percentages than those noticed by other authors. As a matter of fact, in 127 carriers of this genotype, the values of Hb F vary between 2.20–7.20%, the average being 4.12%. We may hypothesize that this special trait among Calabrian people depends on the presence of a particular gene.

As for the distribution of the various genotypes in the areas under investigation, we should like to point out that some genotypes, eg the δβ-genotypes, are relatively more frequent in some areas along the Tyrrhenian Sea (the Savuto Valley) and along the Ionian Sea (the Sybaris Plain).

In the course of our investigation we have identified subjects who have shown unusual combinations of genes that have not been the cause of any illness.

The first case concerned the combination of the β-genotype and the δ-genotype, which, as we had expected, did not modify the hematologic picture of the subject. However, it should be noticed that the percentage of A_2 in the carriers of double heterozygosity was rather low.

The second case concerned the combination of the δ-genotype and the δβ-genotype in 2 brothers, aged 8 and 6 respectively, whose hematologic pictures were the same as those of the carriers of the thalassemia trait, while their hemoglobinic data showed a high percentage of Hb F (12–13%) and complete absence of Hb A_2 (Fig. 3 and Table 3). The percentages of Hb A_2 which were found in the father and paternal grandfather of the propositi were 1.6% and 1.7%, ie about 50% lower than those which are usually found in normal subjects. The mother of the propositi and her father, who were δβ-thalassemia carriers, showed high percentages of Hb F (12.0% and 11.3%) and normal values of Hb A_2. In conclusion, in the 2 propositi the absence of A_2 (phenotypically similar to δ-thalassemia homozygosity) depended on the coexistence of the δ- and δβ-thalassemic genes. The high values of F and the hematologic picture depended on the presence of the δβ-gene.

The third case concerned the combination of the δβ-genotype and a very rare genetic type of β-thalassemia, phenotypically characterized by a high percentage of "isolated" A_2, ie with no evidence of morphologic changes in the red cells [3, 4]. It is held that the above-mentioned type in association with typical β-thalassemia may cause a severe syndrome similar to Cooley anemia [5]. This

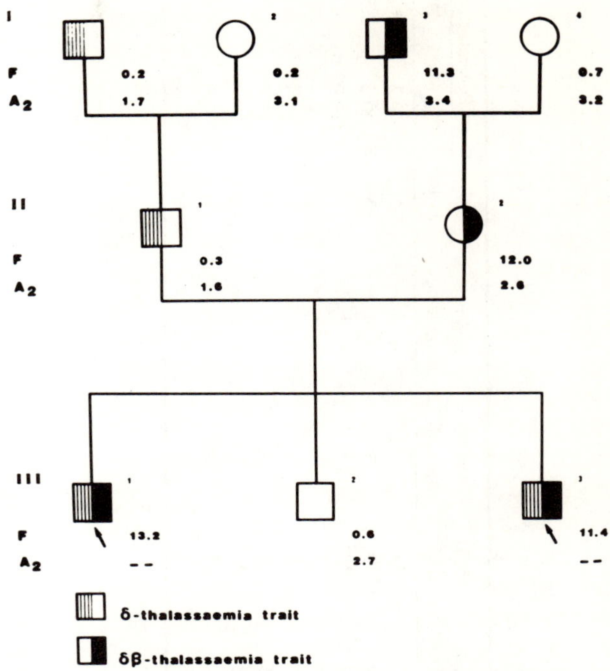

Fig. 3. Family pedigree showing interaction of δ-thalassemia and δβ-thalassemia.

unusual combination (Fig. 4 and Table 4) was observed in a 4-year-old girl (the proposita) who was growing normally, enjoyed good health, and whose clinical findings and hematologic picture were not different from those of the carriers of the thalassemia trait. The hemoglobin pattern was characterized by the presence of Hb F (60.1%) and A_2 (2.8%) while the non-α/α globin synthesis ratio was 0.41. The father and a brother of the proposita turned out to be carriers of the δβ-genotype, while 2 maternal uncles, 1 maternal aunt, and 1 maternal cousin showed increased levels of "isolated" A_2, normal values of F, and a normal hematologic picture, except for a slight decrease of MCH in some of them.

It is important to note that the values of A_2 were rather high. There is no doubt that this type should be further investigated from the genetic and biochemical points of view, so that it would be possible to give it its proper place among β-thalassemias.

The following are some of the epidemiologic findings we should like to point out, namely, the complete absence of Hb Barts hydrops and the extreme infrequency of Hb H disease among Calabrian people, even though forms of the α-thalassemia carrier state may be found. However, these latter forms are not infre-

TABLE 3. Findings Concerning Family Shown in Figure 3

Subject	Age (yr)	Hb (gm/dl)	RBC (10^{12}/1)	PCV (%)	MCV (fl)	MCH (pg)	MCHC (gm/dl)	Red cell morphology	OF*	Percentage of Hb F	Percentage of Hb A_2
I.1	70	17.1	5.25	49	93	33	35	− − −	N	0.2	1.7
I.2	72	17.2	5.69	49	86	30	35	− − −	N	0.2	3.1
I.3	55	15.8	6.97	50	72	23	32	+ + +	D	11.3	3.4
I.4	59	16.2	5.68	50	88	29	32	− − −	N	0.7	3.2
II.1	39	17.9	6.03	53	88	30	34	− − −	N	0.3	1.6
II.2	32	13.6	5.74	38	66	24	36	+ + +	D	12.0	2.6
III.1	8	13.1	6.07	37	61	22	35	+ + +	D	13.2	—
III.2	6	13.6	4.99	38	76	27	36	− − −	N	0.6	2.7
III.3	5	13.0	5.60	35	63	23	37	+ + +	D	11.4	—

*Osmotic fragility: N = normal; D = decreased

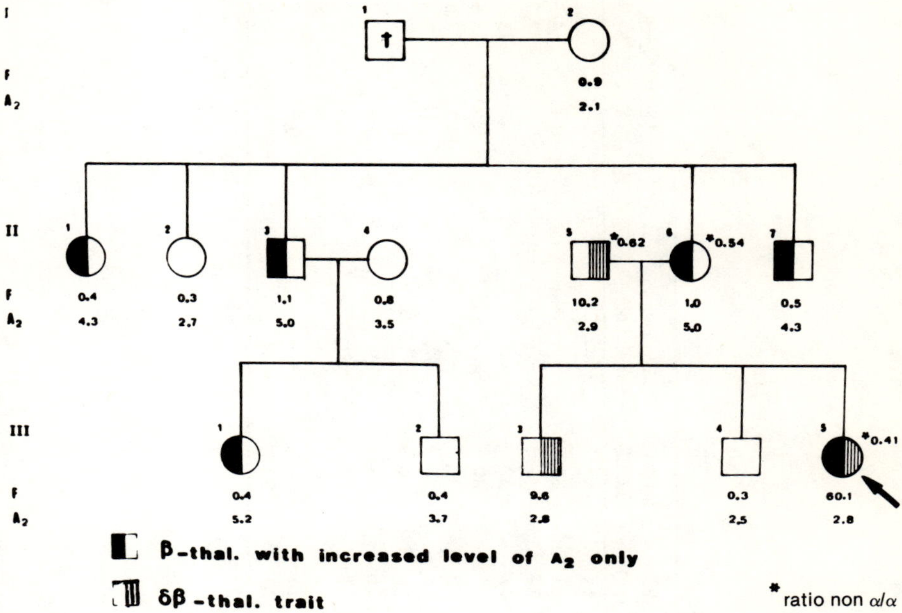

Fig. 4. Family pedigree showing interaction of $\delta\beta$-thalassemia and β-thalassemia with "increased levels of A_2 only."

quent. This has been confirmed by an ongoing study of the presence of Hb Barts at birth, which has shown that 1.2% of newborn babies have this type of hemoglobin, in agreement with the percentage of α-heterozygosity found in adult people. The percentages of Hb Barts show a bimodal distribution (one group with 1.3–2.2%, and another group 2.5–8.0%).

The epidemiologic aspect of what has been described may be explained (in agreement with the results of research recently carried out with the restriction endonuclease mapping of DNA) [6], if we hypothesize that the genotypes present among our population, as well as among the black population, belong to the types $-\alpha/\alpha\alpha$ (heterozygosity) and $-\alpha/-\alpha$ (homozygosity for the $-\alpha/$ haplotype), while the genotypes $--/\alpha\alpha$ are extremely rare.

It is interesting to note the presence among the Calabrian population of abnormal hemoglobins (S, J Oxford, J Norfolk, G San José, J Calabria, B_2) and their not infrequent association with several types of thalassemia. It is useful to remember that the allelism between the thalassemia gene and the gene responsible for abnormal hemoglobins is not always the cause of illnesses (for example, in the case of β-thalassemia + G San José) [7]. Rather, illnesses may depend on the

TABLE 4. Findings Concerning Family Shown in Figure 4

Subject	Age (yr)	Hb (gm/dl)	RBC (10^{12}/1)	PCV (%)	MCV (fl)	MCH (pg)	MCHC (gm/dl)	Red cell morphology	OF*	Percentage of Hb F	Percentage of Hb A_2
I.2	77	13.5	5.42	42	77	25	32	− − −	N	0.9	2.1
II.1	48	14.6	5.47	43	79	27	34	− − −	N	0.4	4.3
II.2	45	14.7	5.22	43	82	28	34	− − −	N	0.3	2.7
II.3	43	14.2	6.88	47	68	21	30	− − −	N	1.1	5.0
II.4	40	10.8	4.03	36	89	27	30	− − −	N	0.8	3.5
II.5	40	13.9	6.19	44	71	22	32	+ + −	D	10.2	2.9
II.6	37	11.5	4.77	38	80	24	30	− − −	N	1.0	5.0
II.7	36	13.8	6.48	48	74	21	29	− − −	N	0.5	4.3
III.1	7	11.1	5.21	33	63	21	33	+ − −	N	0.4	5.2
III.2	5	13.4	4.96	38	77	27	35	− − −	N	0.4	3.7
III.3	14	12.8	6.10	42	69	21	30	+ + −	D	9.6	2.8
III.4	10	12.8	5.04	43	85	25	30	− − −	N	0.3	2.5
III.5	4	10.8	5.27	34	65	20	32	+ + −	D	60.1	2.8

*Osmotic fragility: N = normal; D = decreased

physicochemical and functional characteristics of abnormal hemoglobins in genetic compounds.

Finally, we should like to underline the percentages (varying between 26% and 40%) of α-abnormal hemoglobins not associated with α-thalassemia (J Oxford, J Norfolk) which were clearly shown, in the cases investigated, and which may suggest the existence of a quantitative polymorphism of the α-haplotypes [8].

REFERENCES

1. Brancati C, Tagarelli A: Genotipi microcitemici (o thalassemici) in Calabria. Atti VI Congr. Intern. Ass. Naz. lotta contro le microcitemie in Italia, Ed Minerva Medica, Roma, 1980, p 101.
2. Schokker RC, Went LN, Bok J: A new genetic variant of β-thalassemia. Nature 209:44, 1966.
3. Silvestroni E, Bianco I: Sull'esistenza nella popolazione italiana di soggetti non microcitemici portatori di una elevata quota di emoglobina adulta lenta (HbA2) e sui loro rapporti con i malati di anemia microcitica. Policlinico-Sez Prat 64:1868, 1957.
4. Ceppellini R: Atti VII Congr. Intern. Ematologia, Symposium Genet Haemat Roma. Acta Genet Med Gemellol (Roma) (Suppl II):47, 1959.
5. Lucci R, Soffritti R, Borgatti L, Cabassa N: Malattia da Hb A2 elevata-microcitemia. Acta Genet Med Gemellol (Roma) 11, 71, 1962.
6. Higgs DR, Old JM, Clegg JB, Pressley L, Hunt DM, Weatherall DJ: Negro α-thalassemia is caused by deletion of a single α-globin gene. Lancet 2:272, 1979.
7. Brancati C, Marinucci M, Borghesi V, Tentori L: Doppia eterozigosi tra HbG San José (β7 Glu $\rightarrow$Gly) e β°-microcitemia in una famiglia Calabrese. Atti del XXVI Congr. Naz. della S.I.E. Torino, 10–11 giugno 77.
8. Modiano G, Brancati C, Marinucci M, Massa A, Mavilio F, Tentori L: Genetic polymorphism of the α-globin haplotypes in a population from Calabria (Southern Italy). Studies with variants of the α-globin chain. Hum Hered 29:337, 1979.

Thalassemia Types in Southern Sardinia

Antonio Cao, MD, Renzo Galanello, MD, and Mario Furbetta, MD

In the last few years, several studies have been carried out either in the Kan laboratory or in ours on the frequency, distribution, heterogeneity, and molecular pathology of thalassemias in southern Sardinia [1–12].

This report reviews these studies in order to give a comprehensive picture of the different types of thalassemias so far observed and characterized on this island.

β-THALASSEMIAS

Incidence

A mass screening directed at the adult population, using the diagnostic scheme reported in Figure 1, showed the frequencies summarized in Table 1.

The β-thalassemia carrier frequency of 12.9% gives a gene frequency of 0.0645, which is one of the highest so far observed in white populations [1]. With this frequency, the couples at risk are 1:60, and the expected incidence at birth of homozygous β-thalassemia is 1:240. This value is very close to the figure of 1:213 observed in a survey of all inpatient and outpatient admissions in the different hospitals on the island in 1976 before antenatal testing was being done.

The $\delta\beta^0$-thalassemia carrier rate was found to be 0.00164, which gives a gene frequency of 0.00088 [9]. Considering that the gene frequency of β-thalassemia in southern Sardinia is 0.0645, the expected number of double heterozygous individuals is 1.1/10,000. The ratio of $\delta\beta$-thal/β-thal to β-thal/β-thal patients should therefore be 1:38.

Carriers of β-thalassemia with normal levels of Hb A_2 and F ($\gamma\delta\beta$-thalassemia or associated δ- and β-thalassemias) should be very rare, since among 638 obligate carriers (parents of children with β-thal major or intermedia) only one was identified [1, 4].

Birth Defects: Original Article Series, Volume 18, Number 7, pages 157–164
© 1982 March of Dimes Birth Defects Foundation

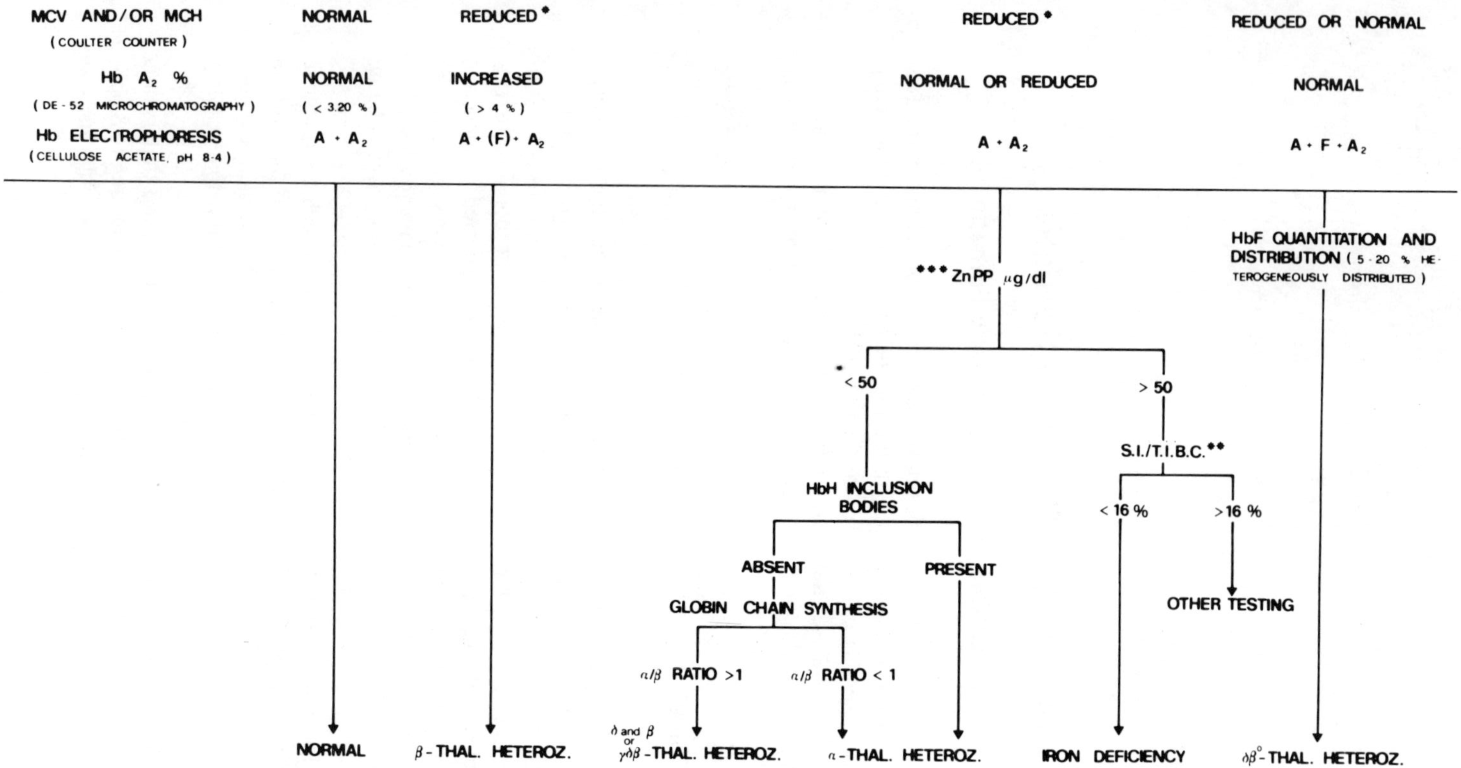

* VALUES LESS THAN NORMAL MEAN VALUES MINUS 2 STANDARD DEVIATIONS

** S.I. = SERUM IRON; T.I.B.C. = TOTAL IRON BINDING CAPACITY

*** ZnPP = ZINC PROTOPORPHYRIN

Fig. 1. Scheme for mass screening for thalassemia syndromes.

TABLE 1. Incidence of Thalassemia Syndromes and Hereditary Hemoglobinopathies in Southern Sardinia

	No.	%
Normal Subjects	1,918	
β-Thalassemia Heterozygotes	310	12.9
α-Thalassemia Heterozygotes	160	6.7
$\delta\beta^0$-Thalassemia Heterozygotes	3	0.12
HPFH Heterocellular Heterozygotes	6	0.25
Hb J Sardinia Carriers	2	0.08
Sickle Cell Trait	1	0.04

HPFH - Hereditary persistence of fetal hemoglobin

Hematologic Aspects

In the southern part of the island (Cagliari and Oristano provinces), where our studies were carried out, apart from 6 subjects with $\delta\beta^0/\beta^0$-thal genotype and 8 with β^0/β^+- or, less likely, β^+/β^+-thal, all patients (900) presenting with thal major or intermedia at our hematology service turned out to be β^0-thal homozygotes [5].

The α/γ-globin chain synthesis ratios found in these patients are reported in Table 2. It can be seen that the α/γ-ratio is highly variable with no statistically significant difference in the mean values between transfusion-dependent (thalassemia major) and nontransfusion-dependent patients (thalassemia intermedia). From these data it seems that in this population the degree of α/γ-globin chain synthesis imbalance in β^0-thal homozygotes cannot predict the severity of the clinical course.

The β-thalassemia carriers have the commonly recognized characteristics of thalassemia-like red cell indices and increased Hb A_2 levels (4.9±0.5%) [4]. Hemoglobin F was found to be elevated in the range of 0.1–3.4% in only one-third of the carriers. The α/β-globin chain synthesis ratio showed a mean of 1.51±0.26 with a range from 0.62 to 3.24 (Fig. 2) ([4] and unpublished results). A prospective study of β-thalassemia carriers from birth to one year demonstrated that carrier screening with MCV or MCH determination is feasible from 3 months on with few false negatives (2.7%), while with Hb A_2 quantitation, this identification seems to be possible at 3 months with slight overlap and is clear-cut from 4 months [12].

The $\delta\beta^0$-thalassemia carriers, although in many respects showing the usual picture of $\delta\beta^0$-thalassemia as abnormal red cell indices, normal Hb A_2, Hb F heterogeneously distributed in the erythrocytes, and slightly unbalanced $\alpha/\beta+\gamma$ synthesis ratios (1.46±0.37), have unusually high levels of Hb F (range 10–20%), and particularly low glycine content (range 0.02–0.14) in the isolated γ-CB3 peptide [9].

TABLE 2. α/γ-Globin Chain Synthesis Ratio in Patients With Homozygous β^0-Thalassemia

	No.	Mean ± SD
Transfusion-dependent	102	2.39 ± 1.08
Nontransfusion-dependent	15	2.09 ± 0.47

Clinical Aspects

Most of the patients (870 of 900) with homozygous β^0-thalassemia have the clinical features of transfusion-dependent thalassemia major with presentation usually at 3–24 months. The others (30 of 900) have the phenotypic aspects of nontransfusion-dependent thalassemia intermedia, with clinical presentation slightly delayed in comparison with thalassemia major subjects, minor facial modifications, normal or subnormal growth, normal or slightly retarded puberty, and mean annual Hb levels varying from 8.0 to 10.0 gm/dl (unpublished observations). On the whole, it seems that in a patient with homozygous β^0-thalassemia presentation over 2 years with a hemoglobin level of about 9 gm/dl, may predict a milder course of the disease with no transfusion dependence [12].

As far as β^0/β^+-genetic compound or β^+/β^+-thalassemia homozygotes are concerned, the clinical picture was variable, being mild in 5 cases (thalassemia intermedia) and severe in 3 (thalassemia major).

Molecular Pathology

The molecular pathology mechanism has been studied in a few patients by cloning and sequence analysis of a β-globin cDNA [10]. At the position corresponding to amino acid number 39, a single nucleotide mutation converted a glutamine codon (CAG) to an amber termination codon (UAG). Thus, β^0-thalassemia in Sardinia represents the second example of a nonsense mutation [10], the first being a Chinese patient with an amber nonsense mutation at amino acid 17 [13].

In this and other Sardinian patients with β^0-thalassemia, there is a uniform decrease (β/α-mRNA ratio of ≤ 0.05) of β-globin mRNA in the reticulocytes (Kan and Cao, unpublished results). This may be due to nuclease degradation of the large section of the mRNA lacking ribosomal binding. Recently, a polymorphism of DNA sequences in the β-globin gene region in linkage disequilibrium with the β^0-mutation was found in the southern Sardinian population. Briefly, when the human DNA is digested with the restriction enzyme Bam HI, the β-globin gene is cleaved into 2 portions: the 5′ portion is contained in a fragment of DNA 1.8 kilobase (kb) in length, while the 3′ portion is in a fragment of 9.3 kb. A variation in the nucleotide sequence affecting the site recognized by this en-

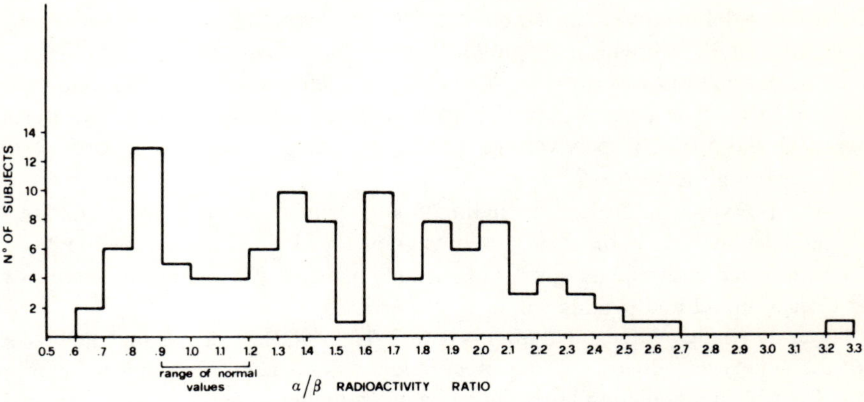

Fig. 2. α/β Globin synthetic ratio in β-thalassemia heterozygotes.

zyme on the 3′ side of the β-globin gene results in a longer fragment, 22 kb in length. In Sardinian subjects without β-thalassemia, the frequency of the 9.3 kb fragment was found to be 0.67, while that of the 22 kb fragment was 0.33. In contrast, all the β^0-thalassemia genes in Sardinia were exclusively associated with the 9.3 kb fragment [7].

The most probable explanation for this finding is that the mutational event which gave rise to the β^0-thalassemia lesion in the Sardinian population occurred in a chromosome containing the normal 9.3 kb Bam site.

This conclusion supports the hypothesis, based on historical and biochemical evidence, that β^0-thalassemia in Sardinia most likely arose as a single mutational event.

DNA analysis, by restriction endonuclease mapping of several patients with thalassemia intermedia due to homozygous β^0-thalassemia, suggests that the mild course of this disease may be caused by the coexistence of heterozygous ($-\alpha/\alpha\alpha$) or homozygous α-thalassemia ($-\alpha/-\alpha$) (Weatherall and Cao, unpublished results).

Finally, in $\delta\beta^0$-thalassemia no abnormal restriction pattern has been found using several enzymes (Kpn I, Bam HI, Hind III, Eco RI, Bgl II, Pst I, Hpa I, Xba I) [8].

These results are compatible with the absence of any gross rearrangement in the G_γ - A_γ -δ-β-cluster, although small deletions cannot be ruled out.

α-THALASSEMIAS

Incidence

A hemoglobin survey carried out in 2,291 newborn infants showed an overall incidence of 12.9% with hemoglobin Barts of more than 1% [3] (Table 3).

The distribution was trimodal: low (1–2%), intermediate (2–10%), and high (about 25%). The percentage of subjects with low and intermediate Hb Barts was 7% and 5.6%, respectively; 5 infants, including a couple of monozygotic twins had high levels (~25%).

At follow-up examination, including globin chain synthesis analysis and family studies, subjects in the 25% group had developed Hb H disease, while those in the low and intermediate groups manifested hematologic findings indicative of α-thalassemia-2 and α-thalassemia-1, respectively.

Family studies suggest that infants with 2–10% Hb Barts levels may have one of the genotypes: -α/-α or --/αα. Restriction endonuclease mapping, as seen in the USA black population [14], showed a much higher frequency (Kan, personal communication), ie -α 33.3%, -α/-α 1.5%, while among 69 subjects analyzed, the genotype --/αα was not detected.

In our population, Hb H disease is rather frequent with a prevalence of 1:1,250 in adults attending voluntary screening sessions, while hydrops fetalis has never been found.

Clinical and Hematologic Aspects

Hemoglobin H disease in the Sardinian population was found to have a high degree of variability in clinical severity, usually being intermediate between that found in Oriental and black populations [2, 14].

The α/β-globin chain synthesis ratio was 0.40±0.12, indicating a globin chain imbalance in the same range as that described in Orientals (Fig. 3).

Two genetic transmission patterns were found: 1) the more prevalent, with one parent showing α-thal-1 trait and the other α-thal-2, and 2) much rarer, with both parents with hematologic and biosynthetic measurements compatible with α-thal-1 [2].

TABLE 3. Incidence of Hb H Barts at Birth

	No.	%
Newborns without Hb Barts	1,998	
Newborns with low Hb Barts (1–2%)	160	7.0
Newborns with intermediate Hb Barts (2–10%)	128	5.6
Newborns with high Hb Barts (~25%)	5	0.2

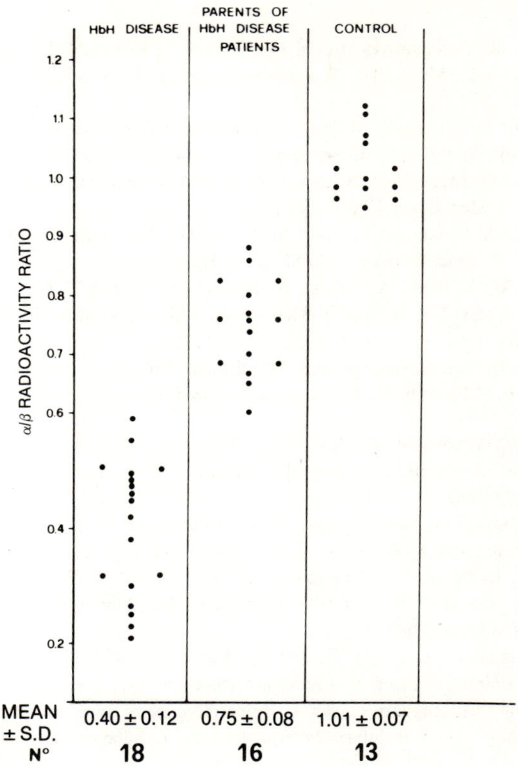

Fig. 3. α/β-Radioactivity ratios in Hb H disease patients and their parents.

Molecular Pathology

So far, the molecular basis of Hb H disease has been investigated by hybridization and restriction endonuclease mapping of the DNA in 8 patients [6].

The genotypes seen in these patients were as follows: a combination of a deletion and nondeletion defect (--/$\alpha\alpha^{th}$) in 2 patients, a deletion defect involving 3 of the 4 α-globin structural genes (-α/--) in 6. Thus, the deletion genotype predominates.

From the results reported in this review it seems that fetal hydrops, although never identified, must occur albeit with a very low frequency.

This depends on the very low incidence of α-thalassemia carriers with the two α-structural genes deleted in cis (--/$\alpha\alpha$), which makes the occurrence of the genotype --/-- with all four α-globin structural genes deleted very rare.

REFERENCES

1. Cao A, Galanello R, Furbetta M, Muroni PP, Garbato L, Rosatelli C, Scalas MT, Addis M, Ruggeri R, Maccioni L, Melis MA: Thalassemia types and their incidence in Sardinia. J Med Genet 6:443–445, 1978.
2. Galanello R, Melis MA, Furbetta M, Angius A, Rosatelli C, Cao A: Hemoglobin H disease in Sardinia: Phenotypic and genetic observations. Hemoglobin 2(4):333–349, 1978.
3. Galanello R, Diana G, Furbetta M, Angius A, Melis MA, Rosatelli C, Cao A: α-Thalassemia in Sardinian infants. J Med Genet 17:357–362, 1980.
4. Galanello R, Melis MA, Ruggeri R, Addis M, Scalas MT, Maccioni L, Furbetta M, Angius A, Tuveri T, Cao A: β^0-Thalassemia trait in Sardinia. Hemoglobin 3(1):33–46, 1979.
5. Cao A, Furbetta M, Ximenes A, Angius A, Rosatelli C, Tuveri T, Scalas MT, Falchi AM, Maccioni L, Melis MA, Galanello R: β-Thalassemia types in Southern Sardinia. J Med Genet 18:196–199, 1981.
6. Kan YW, Dozy AM, Stamatoyannopolos G, Hadjiminas MG, Zachariades R, Furbetta M, Cao A: Molecular basis of hemoglobin H disease in the Mediterranean population. Blood 54:1423, 1979.
7. Kan YW, Lee KW, Furbetta M, Angius A, Cao A: Polymorphism of DNA sequence in the β-globin gene region: Application to prenatal diagnosis of β^0-thalassemia in Sardinia. N Engl J Med 302:185–188, 1980.
8. Ottolenghi S, Giglioni B, Taramelli R, Comi P, Mazza U, Saglio G, Camaschella C, Izzo R, Cao A, Galanello R, Gimferrer E, Baiget M, Gianni AM: Molecular comparison of $\delta\beta$-thalassemic and HPFH DNA: Evidence for a regulatory area? Proc Natl Acad Sci (In press)
9. Cao A, Melis MA, Galanello R, Angius A, Furbetta M, Giordano P, Bernini LF: $\delta\beta$(F) Thalassemia in Sardinia. J Med Genet (In press)
10. Trecartin RF, Liebhaber SA, Chang JC, Lee KY, Kan YW, Angius A, Furbetta M, Cao A: β^0-Thalassemia in Sardinia is caused by a nonsense mutation. J Clin Invest 68:1012–1017, 1981.
11. Galanello R, Melis MA, Ruggeri R, Cao A: Prospective study of red blood cell indices, hemoglobin A_2 and hemoglobin F in infants heterozygous for β-thalassemia. J Pediatr 99:105–107, 1981.
12. Galanello R, Cossu P, Pirastu M, Cao A: Clinical presentation of thalassemia major due to homozygous β^0-thalassemia. Nouv Rev Fr Hematol 23:101–106, 1981.
13. Chang JC, Kan YW: β^0-Thalassemia: A nonsense mutation in man. Proc Natl Acad Sci USA 76:2886–2889, 1979.
14. Dozy AM, Kan YW, Embury SH, Mentzer WC, Wang WC, Lubin B, Davis JR Jr, Konig HM: Alpha globin gene organization in Blacks precludes the severe form of α-thalassemia. Nature 280:605–607, 1979.

Thalassemia Phenotypes in Sardinia*

Ugo Carcassi, MD, Enrico Cacace, MD, Quirico Mela, MD, Guiseppe Passiu, MD, Guiseppe Perpignano, MD, and Aldo Pintus, MD

In the last few years many screening programs have been carried out to determine the distribution of glucose-6-phosphate dehydrogenase (G6PD) deficiency and the incidence and severity of the thalassemias in Southern Sardinia [1-3].

The incidence of the β-thalassemia trait is highly variable, from 11.9% on the east coast of the Cagliari province to 19.4% in the coastal areas of the Oristano province. A high incidence (34.3%) of G6PD deficiency, especially in some villages of the Oristano province, has been found; therefore, the incidence of β-thalassemia associated with G6PD deficiency proves to be 5.4%.

The diagnosis of β-thalassemia trait was based on the presence of abnormal red cell morphology, MCV < 79 fl, MCH < 27 pg/cell, hemoglobin electrophoretic pattern, and Hb A_2 levels above 4% (determined by DE52 microchromatography according to Huisman and co-workers).

The last 298 β-thalassemia carriers examined (163 females and 135 males aged 15–72 years) showed mean red cell counts of 5.78±0.4 and 5.25±0.7, mean hemoglobin levels of 12.57±1.5 and 11.59±1.5, mean corpuscular volumes (MCV) of 66.28±8.3 and 68.02±10 fl with mean corpuscular hemoglobins (MCH) of 22.14±3.3, and 22.10±3.1 pg/cell, respectively. The mean Hb A_2 levels were 5.25±0.7% and 5.12±0.8% and Hb F 1.15±0.5% and 1.29±1%, respectively.

A very high incidence of anemia (Hb < 14 gm/dl in the males and Hb < 12 gm/dl in the females, as defined by the Committee on Iron Deficiency) was found: 79.4% in the males and 57% in the females. 6.48% of the anemic males showed normochromic-normocytic red cells, 6.48% hypochromic-normocytic red cells, and 87% hypochromic-microcytic red blood cells. Iron deficiency was

*This work was partially supported by funds of Istituto di Ricerche sulle Talassemie ed Anemie Mediterranee-CNR, by Assessorato Regionale Igiene e Sanità della Sardegna, and by Ministero della Pubblica Istruzione.

Birth Defects: Original Article Series, Volume 18, Number 7, pages 165–168
© 1982 March of Dimes Birth Defects Foundation

present in 8.33% of anemic males. No iron deficiency was found in any of the nonanemic males; 3.2% of anemic females showed normochromic-normocytic anemia, 5.3% hypochromic-normocytic anemia, and 91.4% hypochromic microcytic anemia. Iron deficiency (serum ferritin < 10 ng/ml - transferrin saturation $< 15\%$) was present in 16.12% of these anemic females. Iron deficiency was also found in 7.14% of the nonanemic females.

Our β-thalassemia carriers are very likely to be heterozygous for $\beta°$-thalassemia, since, to date no Hb A_1 or β-globin chains have been seen in our β-thalassemia intermedia patients.

Many β-thalassemia carriers with G6PD deficiency living on the east coast of Cagliari province showed RBC indices within the normal range which were significantly higher than those of β-thalassemia carriers without G6PD deficiency (MCV = $p < 0.01$; MCH = $p < 0.05$). Anemia was present in 44% of carriers of both genes (β-thalassemia/G6PD deficiency).

The interaction between α- and β-thalassemia genes, especially between α-thalassemia$_1$ and β-thalassemia, may cause an increase in red cell indices [4-6]: at least one of the parents of many $\beta°$-thalassemia intermedia patients has a β-thalassemia gene in association with RBC indices within the normal range (MCV in particular) and the same hematologic findings are often found in a first-degree relative.

Heart involvement was studied by noninvasive methods: ECG, dynamic ECG (continuous magnetic tape recording of ECG for 24 hours, by Holter), echocardiographic evaluation (M-mode), polycardiography (simultaneous registration of: ECG, phonocardiogram, carotid and jugular pulse, apexcardiogram), watt test, myocardial scintigraphy with thallium 201, vectorcardiography and chest roentgenogram in 10 β-thalassemia carriers ranging in age from 20-40 years. No patient showed clinical evidence of cardiac disease. The incidence of angina pectoris and myocardial infarction in β-thalassemia carriers hospitalized in the 1st Institute of Clinical Medicine (1975-1980) was 2.77% (2/72); this incidence is not significantly different from that of the hospitalized controls, 2.8% (292/10,279). None of the subjects examined showed endocrine disorders, evaluated by assessment of GH, FSH, LH, LH after GN-RH, TSH, TSH after TRH, T_3, T_4, prolactin, PTH, ACTH (17 hydroxysteroid and 17 ketosteroid excretion), insulin and testosterone in serum or plasma.

The incidence of diabetes mellitus in the hospitalized β-thalassemia carriers was 5.55% (4/72), not significantly different from that of the control subjects, 6.76% (695/10,279). The incidence of the impaired glucose tolerance test in β-thalassemia carriers was 4.16% (3/72), higher, but not significantly, than that of the control subjects, 1.55% (160/10,279). The incidence of rheumatoid arthritis in β-thalassemia carriers was 6.72% (8/119), significantly higher ($p < 0.001$) than in noncarrier patients: 1.9% (198/10,279) [7].

The incidence of α-thalassemia carriers was 10% in some villages of the Cagliari province, and slightly higher, 13.2%, in the coastal areas of Oristano; and the association of α-thalassemia/G6PD deficiency was 2.7%. Alpha thalassemia trait was established as follows: parents of subjects with Hb H disease, and/or subjects with MCV < 79 fl, MCH < 27 pg/cell, normal or reduced Hb A_2 levels with normal Hb F, normal serum iron, and Hb H inclusion bodies in erythrocytes. Using these criteria only 27.2% of undefined thalassemia carriers (with hypochromic microcytic red blood cells, normal Hb A_2 and F and normal iron stores) required globin-chain synthesis for diagnosis. The Hb H inclusion bodies' study represents a test of diagnostic value in the Sardinian population [8]. Approximately 1 of 100,000 red blood cells shows Hb H inclusion bodies in α-thalassemia$_1$ trait, while they are rarely found in α-thalassemia$_2$ carriers.

Hematologic data on α-thalassemia$_1$ carriers (including obligate α-thalassemia carriers) indicate a slight anemia: mean hemoglobin levels of 13.4± 0.7 and 12.5±0.6 gm/dl in males and females, respectively, with significantly reduced MCV (70.2±5.8 and 63.5±6.4 fl) and MCH (24.1±1.8 and 22.8±1.9 pg/cell).

In Southern Sardinia iron stores, using serum ferritin determination, were evaluated in 40 α-thalassemia$_1$ carriers (21 males and 19 females) aged 10–50 years. No subject with liver disease and/or infection was included in this study. Serum ferritin levels were not significantly different from those of controls; 5 female α-thalassemia$_1$ carriers showed serum ferritin levels < 10 ng/ml [9].

Our patients with Hb H disease show the mild clinical picture of thalassemia intermedia with mean hemoglobin levels of 11.6±1 gm/dl. Repeated infections (particularly respiratory tract) may cause an exacerbation of anemia but we have not observed mean hemoglobin < 9 gm/dl. Mean red cell counts were 5.52±0.5 with mean RBC indices of 66±11 (for MCV) and 23.2±6.2 (for MCH).

The amount of Hb H is highly variable, 2.4–36% of total hemoglobin, with Hb A_2 levels significantly decreased.

Iron stores, evaluated by serum ferritin measurement, showed a high variability in Hb H patients: the mean serum ferritin levels were 301±243 ng/ml and 35.16±31.67 in males and females, respectively. Thus, in Hb H disease, iron overload and iron deficiency *may* be found, whereas in β-thalassemia intermedia iron overload is *always* present.

In many of our Southern Sardinian patients the picture of β-thalassemia intermedia is the result of the interaction of different genes such as homozygous β°-thalassemia (Hb A_1, or β-chains have never been shown by electrophoresis and chromatography) with α-thalassemia genes or β°-thalassemia heterozygosity with a β-chain mutant gene (eg β°-thal/β-Leslie) [4-6,10]. These patients show mean hemoglobin levels ranging from 8.5 to 11 gm/dl, and often require no regular transfusion therapy.

REFERENCES

1. Cao A, Galanello R, Furbetta M, Muroni PP, Garbato L, Rosatelli C, Scalas MT, Ruggeri RR, Laccione L, Melis MA: Thalassemia types and their incidence in Sardinia. J Med Genet 15:443, 1978.
2. Carcassi U: The interaction between beta-thalassemia, G-6-PD deficiency and favism. Ann NY Acad Sci 232:297, 1974.
3. Silvestroni E, Bianco I: Screening for microcytemia in Italy: Analysis of data collected in the past 30 years. Am J Hum Genet 27:198, 1975.
4. Furbetta M, Galanello R, Ximenes A, Angius A, Melis MA, Serra P, Cao A: Interaction of alpha and beta thalassemia genes in two Sardinian families. Br J Haematol 41:203, 1979.
5. Kan YW, Nathan DG: Mild thalassemia: The result of interactions of alpha and beta thalassemia genes. J Clin Invest 49:635, 1970.
6. Weatherall DJ, Clegg JB, Wood WG, Old JM, Higgs DR, Pressley BL, Darbre PD: The clinical and molecular heterogeneity of the thalassemia syndromes. Ann NY Acad Sci 344:83, 1980.
7. Carcassi U: Aspetti internistici della talassemia minor. Aspetti cardiologici, endocrinologici e clinici generali. Atti 81° Congr. Naz. Soc. It. Medicina Interna, Roma, 27-30 Ottobre 1980.
8. Melis MA, Rosatelli C, Falchi AM, Angius A, Furbetta M, Galanello R, Cao A: Haematological characteristics of Sardinian alpha-thalassemia carriers detected in a population study. Acta Haematol 63:32, 1980.
9. Mela Q, Pintus A, Cacace E, La Nasa G, Cirillo R, Montaldo P, Perpignano G, Carcassi U: Serum ferritin in alpha-thalassemia. The 6th Meet. Internat. Soc. Haematol. Europ. Afr. Div. Athens, Greece, August 30 - September 4, 1981.
10. Carcassi U, Pintus A, Gravely ME, Huisman THJ: β°-thalassemia in association with Hb Leslie ($\alpha_2\beta_2$ 131 gln → 0) in a Sardinian family. Hemoglobin 4(2):195, 1980.

A Tentative Systematization of β-Thalassemia Syndromes Present in Northern Sardinia*

Maurizio Longinotti and Bruno Masala

Beta and alpha thalassemia are characterized by a variable degree of β- and α-globin chain suppression, respectively, and the resulting total globin chain imbalance can be accurately measured by in vitro hemoglobin synthesis.

Without doubt, Sardinia is the Italian region with the highest incidence of thalassemia. Recent studies [1] have fixed the frequency of β-thalassemia in the entire Sardinian population at about 13%. However, the effective incidence of α-thalassemia is less clear-cut. Depending on the screening method it may range from 4% [2] to 14% [3], at least in northern Sardinia.

Phenotypically, homozygous β-thalassemia is rather heterogeneous, and it has been proposed that the severity of the disease in homozygotes can be predicted by studying the globin chain ratio in parents [4].

In northern Sardinia, the presence of different β-thalassemia genes and their eventual association with α-thalassemia may contribute, more than anywhere else, to the heterogeneity of thalassemia syndromes. Hence, it seemed useful to summarize the biosynthetic and hematologic data collected from a great number of α-thalassemic patients and their parents from this area.

SUBJECTS AND METHODS

Patients

This study involved 57 Sardinian patients with homozygous β-thalassemia; 36 of them (6 months–12 years of age) were randomly selected from 195 children with classic transfusion-dependent Cooley anemia attending therapy in the city of Sassari; 21 patients (5-62 years of age), who were never, or were irregularly

*Supported in part by CNR, Program of Preventive Medicine (M.E.E. project) grant no. 80.2268.83.

Birth Defects: Original Article Series, Volume 18, Number 7, pages 169–176
© 1982 March of Dimes Birth Defects Foundation

transfused, and presenting a clinical picture of thalassemia intermedia (Table 1) were also studied. Six subjects with thalassemia intermedia were discovered by chance during routine laboratory investigation, and 4 by postproband family examination. In addition, 25 parents of patients with Cooley anemia and 18 of intermediate subjects were also examined.

Methods

Red cell indices were measured by a Coulter counter Model S. Hemoglobin electrophoresis was carried out on Titan III (Helena, Beaumont, Texas) in Tris-EDTA-borate buffer, pH 8.6. Hemoglobin A_2 was quantified by DE-52 microchromatography [5] and the Hb F level was determined by an alkali denaturation method [6]. Red cell Hb H inclusion body test was performed by the brilliant cresyl blue standard method.

In vitro hemoglobin synthesis was performed on samples of peripheral blood obtained at least 2 weeks after the last transfusion in the polytransfused patients. In 6 cases with Cooley anemia this study was done prior to any transfusion. The method was essentially that of Weatherall et al [7] and, briefly, was as follows: samples of peripheral blood (enriched for reticulocytes by centrifugation at 20,000 g for 30 minutes in the case of heterozygous thalassemic subjects) were incubated with 100 μC of ^{3}H-leucine for 2 hours at 37° C in the incubation mixture of Lingrel and Borsook [8]. The washed cells were lysed and globin precipitated with the acid-acetone method. The constituent chains were separated on a CM-cellulose column (32 × 1.5 cm) in 8 M urea 2 mercaptoethanol using a linear gradient of Na phosphate, pH 6.7, generated by an Ultrograd (LKB, Bromma, Sweden). The α/β, α/γ and $\alpha/\beta + \gamma$ ratios were expressed as ratios of total counts taken up by each chain.

RESULTS

The biosynthetic analysis of 57 homozygous β-thalassemic patients showed that β^0- and β^+-genotypes coexist in the northern Sardinian population (Fig. 1),

TABLE 1. Main Clinical Findings in 21 β-Thalassemic Homozygous Patients With Thalassemia Intermedia

	Age (yrs) $\bar{x}$	Hb (gm/dl) $\bar{x}$	Never Transfused	Irregularly Transfused	Transfusion-Dependent Until Splenectomy
β^0-Homozygotes (7)	26 (5-35)	8.9	1	5	1 (5 splenectomized)
β^+-Homozygotes (14)	36 (5-62)	10.2	9	3	2 (4 splenectomized)

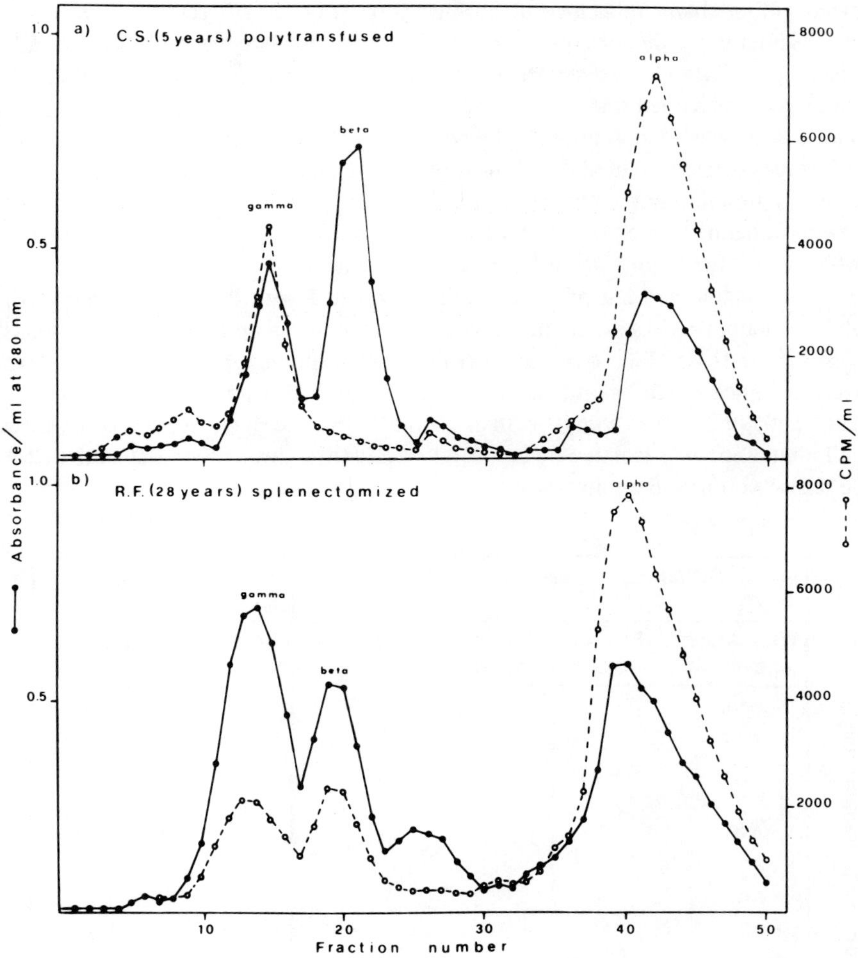

Fig. 1. Typical CM-cellulose chromatograms of globin (100 mg) from a) β^0- and b) β^+-homozygous thalassemic patients. The small peaks eluting after the β-chains are δ-chains.

even though the relative gene frequency in this ethnic group cannot be definitely established from the present data owing to the small sample of homozygotes examined. Further biosynthetic studies of all the 350 β-thalassemic homozygotes at present undergoing clinical treatment in the whole district of Sassari will help to elucidate this point.

The β^0-genotype is certainly more frequent as it is present in 75.4% of the examined homozygotes and, when it occurs with classic Cooley anemia, shows a mean globin chain imbalance of 3.01 ± 0.63 (Fig. 2, left section). Thus, β^0-thalassemia is the most frequent cause of the severest form of the illness. In this case, the obligatory heterozygotes have a mean α/β ratio of 1.97 ± 0.25. It should be underlined that the α/β ratio in these β^0-heterozygotes may be lower than 1.5, as was seen in only 3 subjects of the present series. Seven of 43 (16%) β^0-homozygotes presented the clinical picture of thalassemia intermedia (Fig. 2, central part). These patients showed a lower mean globin chain imbalance, the α/γ ratio being 1.58 ± 0.51, while in their parents the α/β ratio had a markedly wide range, the values being less than 1 in 2 cases.

A reasonable amount of radioactivity associated with the elution peak of β-globin chain was found in the CM-cellulose chromatographies of peripheral blood (Fig. 1b) of 14 out of the 57 β-thalassemic homozygotes. Similar results were obtained when "nonthalassemic" cold Hb A was added to their hemolysates and, in 2 cases, when "β-thalassemic" Hb A derived from bone marrow cell incubation was isolated by gel filtration and then chromatographed on a CM-cellulose column (data not shown).

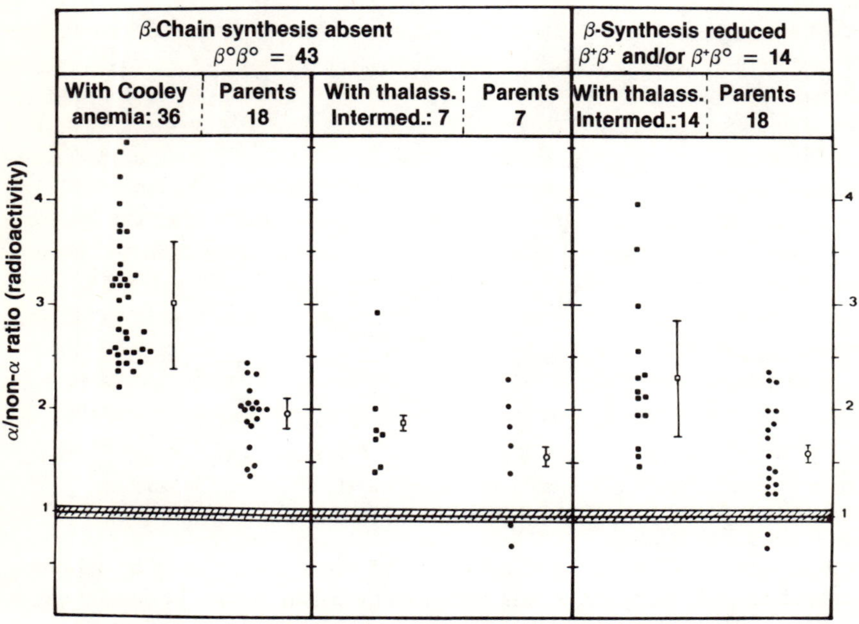

Fig. 2. Behavior of α/non-α-globin chain ratios in 57 β-thalassemic homozygotes and in 43 of their parents of northern Sardinian origin. According to their biosynthetic findings, 75.4% of homozygotes had the β^0 form of thalassemia while 25.5% displayed the β^+ type. This series represents a limited sample of the 350 β-thalassemic homozygotes at present undergoing clinical treatment in the district of Sassari.

Thus, these findings demonstrate that at least 24.5% of the northern Sardinian β-thalassemic homozygotes, the subjects of the present study, are affected by the β^+ form of thalassemia. It should be underlined that all β^+ homozygotes, except 2 cousins tentatively classified as having a thalassemia intermedia owing to their transfusion dependency (necessary until splenectomy in the oldest), presented a clinical picture compatible with the diagnosis of thalassemia intermedia.

On the whole, β^+ homozygotes displayed an Hb A production ranging from 10–36%, the Hb F value varying from 55–89% ($\bar{x}$ = 60%), while the Hb A_2 level was rather elevated ($\bar{x}$ = 5.13 ± 1.83). The total globin chain imbalance expressed by the $\alpha/\beta + \gamma$ ratio (Fig. 2, right section) is 2.29 ± 0.73, the individual values ranging from 1.47 to 3.99 without any correlation to the severity of the illness.

Moreover, neither the Hb A or Hb F amounts, nor the chain-ratio distribution allowed us to distinguish the β^+/β^+ from the β^+/β^0 form of thalassemia, the latter certainly present in Sardinia and probably also in the present series.

Eighteen parents of β^+ homozygotes, all being carriers of the typical high Hb A_2 β-thalassemia traits, showed a mean α/β ratio notably lower than that found in parents of β^0 patients with Cooley anemia (1.59 ± 0.47 vs 1.99 ± 0.25), but very similar to the value observed in parents of intermediate β^0 homozygotes (Fig. 2), the individual figure being below 1.5 or actually lower than 1 in as many as 9 cases.

From a practical point of view, β^+ homozygotes have a clinical course very similar to that occurring in β^0 patients with thalassemia intermedia; their mean hemoglobin level remaining between 9 and 10 gm/dl (Table 1).

On the whole, even if some of the oldest β^+ patients may have iron overload as assessed by the serum ferritin test (probably owing to an increased iron absorption), β^+ homozygotes do not manifest overt gonadal, thyroid, and hypothalamic dysfunction (unpublished results). Therefore, they have normal physical growth and several of them are able to procreate.

The hematologic data of the 45 parents, divided into 3 groups according to the clinical and biosynthetic findings in homozygotes, are compared in Figure 3.

Although the individual identification of β^0 and β^+ genotype in a heterozygous state might be considered useful in order to offer more accurate genetic counseling, the comparison of several hematologic indices did not permit such a distinction. However, the mean MCV value tends to increase steadily in the 3 groups of β-thalassemic heterozygotes together with the decreasing α/β ratio, suggesting an association with α-thalassemia probably more frequent in the series of parents of intermedia thalassemia affected patients, whether of β^0 or β^+ type.

The double heterozygosity for α- and β-thalassemia seems characterized by a mean cellular volume higher than that displayed by the β-thalassemia trait alone in Sardinia [9]. It has been well known for some time that the α/β-ratio in this association is more balanced or even lower than one [10].

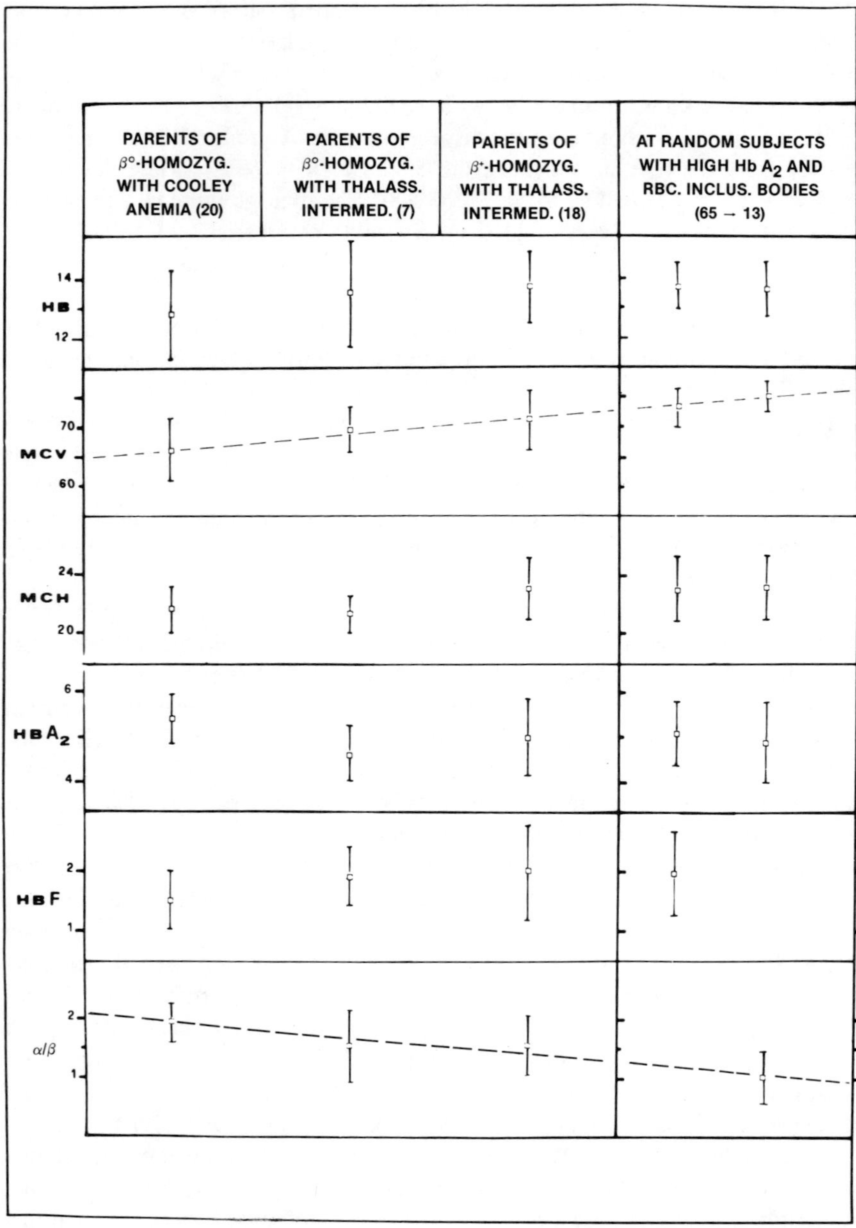
PARENTS OF
β°-HOMOZYG.
WITH COOLEY
ANEMIA (20)
PARENTS OF
β°-HOMOZYG.
WITH THALASS.
INTERMED. (7)
PARENTS OF
β⁺-HOMOZYG.
WITH THALASS.
INTERMED. (18)
AT RANDOM SUBJECTS
WITH HIGH Hb A2 AND
RBC. INCLUS. BODIES
(65 → 13)
HB
14
12
MCV
70
60
MCH
24
20
HB A2
6
4
HB F
2
1
α/β
2
1

This suggested that we test 450 high Hb A_2 individuals attending voluntary screening for erythrocyte Hb H inclusion bodies: the hematologic data found in the 65 positive cases (14.4%) (Fig. 3, right section) not only demonstrated a further increase of the MCV value ($\bar{x} = 73.4 \pm 7.9$ fl) but 13 of them, chosen at random, also showed a balanced α/β ratio ($\bar{x} = 1.06 \pm 0.44$), or even a manifest α-chain deficiency with MCV values ranging from 61 to 89 fl. Therefore, they could be considered carriers of α/β-thalassemia even if such an association, while suspected on finding higher red cell volume during mass screening, still needs traditional family study and biosynthetic investigation.

CONCLUSIONS

In this study, 57 of the 350 β-thalassemic homozygotes undergoing treatment in the district of Sassari in northern Sardinia were examined by means of in vitro hemoglobin synthesis and classified according to their clinical aspects. Forty-three of them (75.4%) had the β^0 form of thalassemia, and 14 (24.5%) had the β^+ type. From a clinical point of view, 36 β^0 homozygotes presented the classic transfusion-dependent Cooley anemia, while 7 β^0 homozygotes showed the clinical picture of thalassemia intermedia. However, all β^+ homozygotes had a milder form of the disease, so that the majority of them did not need transfusion therapy. Northern Sardinian parents of β^0 and β^+ homozygotes with thalassemia intermedia often showed an α/β-chain ratio typical of α/β-thalassemia and, given the high frequency of α-thalassemia here, this observation is not rare even in β-thalassemic heterozygotes attending voluntary mass screening. Mapping of α-globin genes in intermediate β-thalassemic homozygotes would be helpful to prove — or disprove — if the α-thalassemia gene segregation in homozygous β-thalassemia, particularly of β^+ type, is really the main molecular cause of a much milder disease. If this is the case, the probability that offspring homozygotes conceived by α/β-thalassemia at-risk couples will manifest a very mild form of the disease should be kept in mind during genetic counseling and antenatal diagnosis.

Fig. 3. Hematologic and biosynthetic data in 45 obligatory β-thalassemic heterozygote parents of β^0 and β^+ patients with different severities of disease. The data were compared with that found in 65 subjects with high Hb A_2 and presence of Hb H inclusion bodies in their erythrocytes. These latter subjects, in 13 of whom the α/β ratio was also calculated, were selected by testing 450 β-thalassemic heterozygotes found during voluntary screening for Hb H inclusion bodies.

ACKNOWLEDGMENTS

The authors thank F. Dore, M. Tidore, S. Pardini, L. Oggiano, P. Demuro, and P.P. Falchi-Delitala, all co-workers in this investigation.

REFERENCES

1. Cao A, Galanello R, Furbetta M et al: Thalassemia types and their incidence in Sardinia. J Med Genet 15:443, 1978.
2. Bianco I, Graziani B, Salvini P et al: Fréquence e caractères de l'alpha-microcytémie dans les populations de la Sardaigne septentrionale. Nouv Rev Fr Hematol 12:191, 1972.
3. Demuro P, Masala B, Longinotti M et al: Il fenotipo ematologico dei neonati portatori di Hb Bart's Abstracts XIII^{0} Riun. Gruppo Studio Eritrocita, pp 42–45, Roma, 1980.
4. Nathan DG, Oski FA: "Hematology in Infancy and Childhood." Philadelphia: WB Saunders, 1974, p 475.
5. Huisman TH, Schroeder WA, Brodie AN et al: Microchromatography of hemoglobins. III. A simplified procedure for the determination of hemoglobin A_2. J Lab Clin Med 86:700, 1975.
6. Pembrey ME, McWade P, Weatherall DJ: Reliable routine estimation of small amounts of foetal haemoglobin by alkali denaturation. J Clin Pathol 25:738, 1972.
7. Weatherall DJ, Clegg JB, Na-Nakorn S et al: The pattern of disordered haemoglobin synthesis in homozygous and heterozygous beta-thalassaemia. Br J Haematol 16:251, 1969.
8. Lingrel HE, Borsook GJ: A comparison of amino-acid incorporation into hemoglobin and ribosomes of marrow erythroid cells and circulating reticulocytes of severely anemic rabbits. Biochemistry 2:309, 1963.
9. Longinotti M, Masala B, Tidore M et al: Hematological and biosynthetic features of beta^{0}-thalassemia with an associated alpha-thalassemia heterozygosity in Sardinia. Hemoglobin 5(6):619, 1981.
10. Kan YW, Nathan DG: Mild thalassemia: The result of interaction of alpha and beta-thalassemia genes. J Clin Invest 49:635, 1970.

The Pattern of Thalassemia in Naples

Guglielmina Pepe, MD, Leo Lupi, MD, Antonella Mastrobuono, MD, Concetta Carestia, MD, Arturo Lania, and Lucio Luzzatto, MD

The genetic heterogeneity of thalassemia syndromes has been widely investigated in many parts of the world [1].

Analysis of the mutant genes underlying various clinical phenotypes is of interest on the one hand because each one of them may offer a new clue to the pathogenesis of reduced globin-chain synthesis. On the other hand, such studies in a particular locale are a requirement for appropriate public health measures, including screening, genetic counseling, and prenatal diagnosis.

In Naples (Campania), southern Italy, at least three conditions have polymorphic frequencies: $\beta°$-thalassemia, β^{+}-thalassemia [2], and α-thalassemia (personal communication: L. Luzzatto, L. Lania). In addition Hb Lepore is common [3].

In this paper we report studies on three clinically important conditions arising from various interactions among these genes: Cooley anemia, thalassemia intermedia, and homozygous Hb Lepore.

THE INCIDENCE OF THALASSEMIA IN A RANDOM SAMPLE OF THE POPULATION OF THE CITY OF NAPLES

From 2,068 cord blood samples, representing a random sample of the newborn population of Naples, Hb Barts (detected by gel electrophoresis) had been found in trace amounts in 34 cases and between 1% and 16% in 5 more cases. These data give a minimum estimate for heterozygote frequency of the α-thalassemia gene of 0.25%. On 535 random blood samples from primary school children, 13 had elevated Hb A_2 (3.7–6.7%; normal range is 2.2–3.4%), and abnormal red blood cell indices, which gave an estimate of the β-thalassemia heterozygote frequency of 2.4%. We have studied 32 children from Naples, Italy with Cooley anemia. These patients presented typical clinical and hematologic findings. They had an absolute requirement for transfusions and all of the parents

Birth Defects: Original Article Series, Volume 18, Number 7, pages 177–184
© 1982 March of Dimes Birth Defects Foundation

had elevated Hb A_2. Globin biosynthesis studies on peripheral blood samples showed that 5 children (2 sets of sibs) were $\beta°$. The others had β^+-thalassemia (Fig. 1a). Thus, the frequency of the β^+-thalassemic globin gene among unrelated patients was about 90% and the β/α ratio showed a wide range between 0.01 and 0.016, which is the same as that found in the literature [2].

We have investigated 45 heterozygous β-thalassemics, most of whom were parents of the patients (obligate heterozygotes) (Fig. 1b). The β/α ratio showed a wide range of values between 0.24–0.75. The lowest values, as seen in Figure 1b, have never been reported in the literature [2].

In collaboration with Dr. N. Quattrin, we have studied 9 patients homozygous for Hb Lepore, belonging to 5 unrelated families from the Campania region. Globin chain biosynthesis studies have been carried out in peripheral blood reticulocytes in 4 of these cases [3]. The Hb Lepore percentage ranged between 8 and 15%. The β/α biosynthetic ratio was between 0.03 and 0.12. In 2 cases, the Hb Lepore studied was identified as Lepore Boston by fingerprint analysis.

We have studied some intermedia thalassemic patients. Two of these families have been further studied. The first family showed an interaction between a milder β^+-thalassemic gene and probably a Swiss type of HPFH gene, perhaps with an α-thalassemia [4].

METHODS

Hematologic values and indices, Hb A_2 and Hb F determinations, globin chain synthesis studies in peripheral blood cells have been carried out as previously described elsewhere [2].

RESULTS AND DISCUSSION

Cooley Anemia and β-Thalassemia Heterozygotes

Figure 1a shows the plurimodal distribution of the β/α globin chain biosynthetic ratios in patients with Cooley anemia. Since by our techniques we can detect as little as 1% β-chain synthesis, our operational definition of $\beta°$-thalassemia is a patient who synthesizes less than that amount. About 90% of our patients are β^+-thalassemic. Forty obligate heterozygotes plus 5 diagnosed heterozygotes are represented in Figure 1b. The distribution of the β/α ratio appears to be plurimodal here too, and the range of β/α ratios is quite wide. The sample at the extreme right is from a family that will be discussed below. The samples on the extreme left (β/α=0.23–0.30) have a very low ratio, but clinically and hematologically they do not show any difference when compared to other heterozygotes (data not shown).

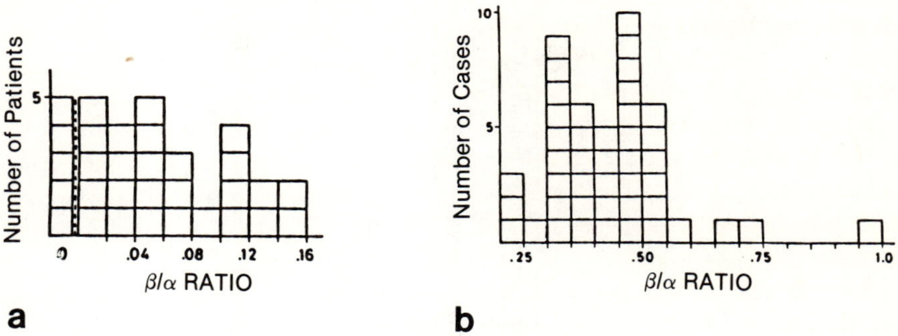

Fig. 1. Distribution of globin chain biosynthetic β/α ratios in a) 32 patients with Cooley anemia, and b) 45 subjects heterozygous for β-thalassemia.

Hemoglobin Lepore

Two brothers with homozygous Lepore have been studied [5]. Fingerprint analysis characterized this hemoglobin as Lepore Boston, the most common form [1,3,6].

Although these 2 brothers must have inherited the same Lepore genes, they appear clinically different (Table 1). The younger has a Cooley phenotype which has improved significantly after splenectomy. The older has an intermedia thalassemic phenotype. For ethical reasons, we cannot study the bone marrow which might explain the differences between these 2 patients.

Biosynthetic ratios in the peripheral blood, obtained in 1975 by B. Luppis and V. Ventruto [7], were found to be highly reproducible on repeat runs carried out in 1977. Whereas it has often been stated in the literature that δ- or $\delta\beta$-chain synthesis is not detectable in peripheral blood reticulocytes [1], we found, in fact, that it could be measured in these patients at a time when there were no circulating normoblasts. The $\delta\beta/\alpha$ and γ/α globin chain ratios in the peripheral blood reticulocytes reflect the amount of individual mRNA as measured by translation in a wheat germ cell-free system [5,8].

Thalassemia Intermedia

In Figure 2 and Table 2, respectively, are represented the pedigree and the hematologic data of a family which show an interaction between α- and β-thalassemia. The proposita (*III-3*) is homozygous for β-thalassemia and potentially could be a carrier for α-thalassemia. The reason for this hypothesis is that in this family, which is included in the study described in Figure 1, the proposita

TABLE 1. Two Brothers Homozygous for Hb Lepore

			Hematologic Data						Globin Chain Synthesis and mRNA Ratios					
		Hb	RBC	MCV	Rts	Serum			$\delta\beta/\alpha$		$\delta\beta/\alpha$	γ/α		γ/α
	Age	gm/dl	$\times 10^6/\mu l$	fl	%	iron	Bilirubin		1975	1977*	mRNA	1975	1977	mRNA
Patient 1	5	13	4.2	72	3.8	135	6	Patient 1	0.10	0.12	0.10	0.46	0.42	0.70-1.0
Patient 2	13	8	2.4	70	4.5	145	2.7	Patient 2	0.06	0.06	0.025	0.32	0.38	0.25

*Patient 2 after splenectomy.

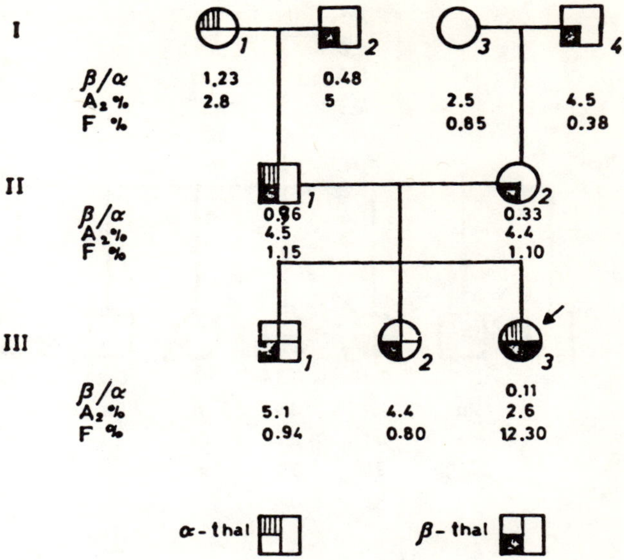

Fig. 2. Pedigree of *Family R.*

TABLE 2. ***Family R:*** **Hematologic and Biochemical Data.**

Subjects	Hb G/dl	RBC $\times 10^6/\mu l$	Hct %	MCV fl	MCH pg	MCHC %	A_2 %	F %	β/α Ratio	Rt. %
I-1.	15.0	5.60	36.0	64.2	26.7	41.6	2.8		1.23	0.6
I-2.	15.0	5.80	43.0	74.1	25.8	34.8	5.0		0.48	0.3
I-3.	13.1	5.90	43.9	74.0	22.2	29.7	2.5	0.85		0.2
I-4.	14.8	6.20	53.7	87.0	23.8	27.4	4.5	0.98		0.6
II-1.	14.1	7.10			19.8		4.5	1.15	0.96	1.0
II-2.	11.2	5.00			22.4		4.4	1.10	0.33	1.6
III-1.	12.5	6.70	45.0	67.0	18.6	27.7	5.1	0.94		0.8
III-2.	11.5	7.50	43.5	58.0	15.3	26.7	4.4	0.80		3.5
III-3.	8.32	3.50			23.7		2.6	12.30	0.11	

has one of the highest β/α ratios in our Cooley population. In the second generation, *II-2* has β-thalassemia trait and a β/α ratio in the low range of our histogram (Fig. 1b). The patient's father (*II-1*), with elevated Hb A_2 and a β/α ratio almost equal to one, carries both genes for α- and β-thalassemia. The paternal grandmother shows a probable α-thalassemia 1 trait [1].

Figure 3 shows a case in which an anemic pregnant woman and all of her family were found to carry β-thalassemic genes. Clinically (see Table 3) the 3

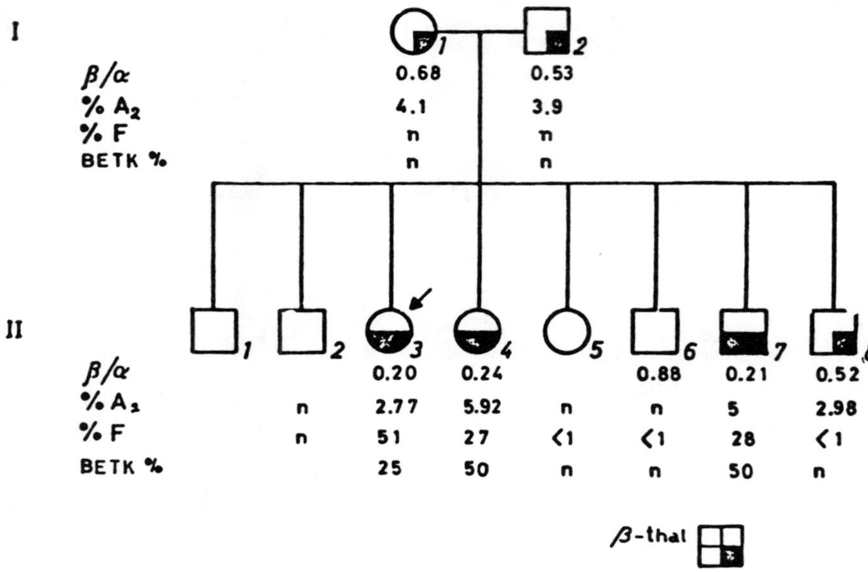

Fig. 3. Pedigree of *Family B.*

sibs (*II-3,II-4,II-7*) have a thalassemia intermedia. They were never transfused, except once when the proposita (*II-3*) was pregnant. The proposita and her 2 sibs (*II-4* and *II-7*) have a β/α ratio between 0.20 and 0.24. The proposita and her brother (*II-7*) have 50% Hb F and normal Hb A_2, while the sister shows 25% Hb F and elevated Hb A_2. Another brother (*II-8*) has a β/α ratio of 0.52 but normal Hb A_2 (in this last case iron deficiency was strictly ruled out). The parents' F cells have been studied with the immunofluorescent antibodies technique. The father (*I-2*) has 11% F cells, a value higher than our normal range, and the mother (*I-1*) has 8% F cells, the highest value in the normal range (data not shown). The mother shows an elevated β/α ratio which is in the range of those carrying an α-thalassemic gene(s). The father is a carrier for the β-thalassemic gene and probably for a heterocellular Swiss-type HPFH. The brother (*II-7*) and the sister (*II-4*) of the proposita present high Hb F percentages (27% and 28%) but lower than that of *II-3,* and high β/α ratio because they have inherited the β-thalassemic gene from the father and both α- and β-thalassemic genes from the mother. This is in agreement with the fact that patients, homozygous for β-thalassemia gene and carrying an α-thalassemic gene, often show an elevated Hb A_2 [1]. The proposita has received the β-thalassemic gene from both parents and

TABLE 3. ***Family B:*** **Hematologic and Biochemical Data.**

Subjects	Hb G/dl	RBC $\times 10^6/\mu l$	Hct %	MCV fl	MCH pg	MCHC %	A_2 %	F %	Betke %	β/α	γ/α Ratio	non-α/α
I-1.	10.5	4.70	31.7	66	22.3	33.1	4.1	1	n	0.68		0.79
I-2.	14.8	6.00	41.7	70	24.6	35.4	3.9	1	n	0.53		0.75
II-3.	9.4	4.10	26.4	64	22.9	35.6	2.8	51	85	0.20	0.24	0.45
II-4.	9.9	4.80	31.6	66	20.6	31.3	4.3	27	50	0.24	0.13	0.38
II-6.							n	1	n	0.88		1.39
II-7.	10.5	5.20	31.2	60	20.1	33.6	5.2	28	50	0.21	0.12	0.33
II-8.	14.7	6.70	45.7	68	21.9	32.1	3.0	1	n	0.52		0.58

the HPFH gene from the father. This could explain why she does not have elevated Hb A_2 and has a higher percentage of Hb F.

SUMMARY

1. The expected number of patients with Cooley anemia in Naples, as predicted from heterozygote frequencies, is about 300 which is more than that found from hospital statistics.

2. Considering the presence of at least two β-thalassemic alleles and the coexistence of a significant incidence of the Lepore gene in the population of the area surrounding Naples (the maximum incidence is thought to be in the neighboring province of Caserta), there are at least 6 different genotypes (3 true homozygotes and 3 genetic compounds) that can give rise to clinically important thalassemia syndromes, ranging from thalassemia intermedia to classic Cooley anemia.

3. Since an α-thalassemic gene is also present at polymorphic frequency in this population, this gene may coexist by random assortment in subjects who also have a β-thalassemia syndrome, thus accounting for part of the variability of globin gene expression.

4. It is remarkable that 2 brothers homozygous for Hb Lepore present differences in the non-α/α ratio. The clinical differences could be explained by the γ/α mRNA ratio close to 1 in one of them.

REFERENCES

1. Weatherall DJ, Clegg JB: "The Thalassemia Syndromes." London: Blackwell Scientific Publications, 1981.
2. Pepe G, Lupi L, Luzzatto L: Genetic and biochemical heterogeneity of β-thalassemia in Naples. Br J Haematol 45:417, 1980.

3. Quattrin N, Camardella L, Cimino R, D'Avino R, diPrisco G, Luzzatto L, Mastrobuono A, Pepe G: Homozygous hemoglobin Lepore condition, clinical and biochemical studies in nine patients. France-Italy Meeting of Erythrocyte Study Group. Paris, July 1978.
4. Pepe G: Studio genetico e biochimico della β-talassemia in Campania. Doctoral Thesis in Medicine, II University of Naples, Italy, October 1978.
5. Ramirez F, Mears JG, Nudel U, Bank A, Luzzatto L, diPrisco G, D'Avino R, Pepe G, Camardella L, Gambino R, Cimino R, Quattrin N: Defects in DNA and globin mRNA in homozygotes for hemoglobin Lepore. J Clin Invest 63:736, 1979.
6. Efremov GD: Hemoglobins Lepore and anti-Lepore. Hemoglobin 2(3):197, 1978.
7. Luppis B, Ventruto V: The synthesis of α, $\delta\beta$ and γ-chains by reticulocytes from two brothers homozygous for hemoglobin Lepore. Acta Haematol 61:216, 1979.
8. Forget BG, Cavallesco C, Benz EJ Jr, McClure PD, Hillman DG, Krieger H, Clarke B, Housman D: Studies of globin chain synthesis and globin mRNA content in a patient homozygous for hemoglobin Lepore. Hemoglobin 2(2):117, 1978.

Types of Thalassemia in Sicily

Guiseppe Russo, MD

Thalassemias are by far the most common disorders of hemoglobin synthesis in Sicily [1].

Both α- and β-thalassemias are present. Epidemiologic studies by many researchers and by ourselves have demonstrated that β-thalassemia in Sicily has a mean prevalence in the general population of about 7-8% in heterozygous carriers. This figure is higher (12%) in the southeastern province of Ragusa and lower (4%) in the interior province of Caltanissetta. The prevalence of α-thalassemia is not known.

In the last 7 years (1974-1980), we have studied 210 consecutive subjects, and their relatives, with various forms of thalassemia. There is a wide variety of clinical expression, from the severe transfusion-dependent thalassemia major to various forms of thalassemia intermedia (Table 1). We have calculated the relative gene frequency of various thalassemia genes (Table 2) from the above families.

Although this gives an idea of the relative frequency of various types of thalassemia, the figures do not exactly represent their real incidence, because the milder forms of the disease certainly escape pediatric observation and are recognized only in adolescence and in adulthood.

The diagnosis of $\beta°$-thalassemia has been carried out by means of CMC chromatographic separation of the various chains. This does not allow one to distinguish between $\beta°/\beta^+$ and β^+/β^+. Although it would seem plausible to distinguish between the above two conditions on the basis of the amount of β-chains present, we did not find the expected bimodal distribution. Probably this is due to a wide range of the amounts of β-chains, so that a heterozygous condition with high β-chain synthesis could give the same results as the homozygous condition with low β-chain synthesis.

In vitro hemoglobin synthesis has shown the following values of the ratio $(\gamma + \beta)/\alpha$: "silent" type 0.77 ± 0.10, β-trait 0.56 ± 0.11, β-intermedia 0.46 ± 0.14, thalassemia major 0.23 ± 0.10. The differences between these groups have been statistically significant, with the exception of that between $\beta°$- and β^+-thal major.

Birth Defects: Original Article Series, Volume 18, Number 7, pages 185–188
© 1982 March of Dimes Birth Defects Foundation

TABLE 1.

Thalassemia Major	
$\beta^{\circ}/\beta^{\circ}$	60
β°/β^{+} β^{+}/β^{+}	124
β°/Lepore	4
β^{+}/Lepore	2
	190

Thalassemia Intermedia	
β^{+}/β^{+}	5
$\beta^{\circ +}/(\delta\beta)^{\circ}$	3
$(\delta\beta)^{\circ}/(\delta\beta)^{\circ}$	1
$\alpha+\beta^{\circ +}/\beta^{\circ +}$	1
$\beta^{sil}/\beta^{\circ +}$	10
	20

β^{sil} - presumably silent.

TABLE 2. Relative Gene Frequency as Calculated From the Analysis of 210 Consecutive Patients With β-Thalassemia Major and Intermedia and Their Parents

Type	%
β°	53.2
β^{+}	39.2
β^{++}	2.4
$\delta\beta$	1.2
β^{sil}	2.4
Lepore	1.4

It is interesting to point out that, in 3 out of 10 subjects considered carriers of silent β-thalassemia on genetic grounds, even the β/α ratio fell within the normal limits.

After transfusion, the $(\gamma + \beta)/\alpha$ ratio in β-thalassemia major has shown an increase toward normal values, but no new β-chains were noted in β°-thalassemia cases [2].

Owing to a relatively high (1.8%) prevalence of β-hemoglobin variants, the most common being Hb S, a number of double heterozygous genotypes (β-thal/β-variant) have been observed (Table 3) [3].

In a unique case of β-thalassemia major + Hb J Oxford ($\alpha_2^{15\ gly\rightarrow asp}\ \beta_2$) a new alkali-resistant hemoglobin ($\alpha_2^{J\ Oxford}\ \gamma_2^{F}$) has been observed [4].

As for molecular defects, δβ-thalassemia has been shown to be due to a gene deletion [5,6].

TABLE 3. Double Heterozygosities for β-Thalassemia and β-Variant

β°thal/Hb S	30
β^{+}thal/Hb S	55
β°thal/Hb C	2
β^{+}thal/Hb C	1
β°thal/Hb Lepore Boston	4
β^{+}thal/Hb Lepore Boston	2
β^{+}thal/Hb G-San José	1
β°thal/Hb G-San José	1
β^{+}thal/Hb J. Baltimore	1

TABLE 4. Parents of Subjects With Hb H

Red cell morphology	N	A	N	A
α/β	N	N	↓	↓
Number	2	5	2	5

In a few cases of homozygous β°-thalassemia it was shown that both β-DNA and β-mRNA were present, so the molecular defect lies probably either in the fine structure of DNA or in the processing of mRNA.

In agreement with other observations in the literature, a reduced amount of β-mRNA has been found in β^{+}-thalassemia.

α-Thalassemia is also present in Sicily, but thus far no case of hydrops fetalis has been observed.

To date, we have seen 7 families in which the propositus presented as thalassemia intermedia with Hb H.

We have carefully studied the parents of these subjects. By comparing the two most sensitive parameters, ie red cell morphology and α/β ratio, we found (Table 4) that only 2 parents were completely normal; the other 12 were identified as carriers by either abnormal red cell morphology or reduced α/β ratio, or by both of these parameters. But we were unable to distinguish between α_1-thal and α_2-thal, either by routine hematologic parameters or by α/β ratios [7].

REFERENCES

1. Schilirò G, Musumeci S, Pizzarelli G, Di Gregorio L, Fischer A, Russo G: β-Thalassemia in Sicily. Acta Haematol 60:193, 1978.
2. Russo G, Musumeci S, Schilirò G, Pizzarelli G, Fischer A, Romeo MA: In vitro globin chain synthesis after blood transfusion in Sicilian homozygous β-thalassemia. Ann NY Acad Sci 344:305, 1980.

3. Schilirò G: Sicily: The world reservoir for thalassemias and haemoglobinopathies. Nature 276:761, 1978.
4. Schilirò G, Musumeci S, Pizzarelli G, Russo A, Marinucci M, Bruni E, Russo G: A new alkali-resistant hemoglobin $\alpha_2^{J\ Oxford}\ \gamma_2^{F}$ in a Sicilian baby girl with homozygous $\beta°$-thalassemia. Blood 48(5):639–651, 1976.
5. Ramirez F, O'Donnell JV, Marks PA, Bank A, Musumeci S, Schilirò G, Pizzarelli G, Russo G, Luppis B, Gambino R: Abnormal or absent β mRNA in $\beta°$-Ferrara and gene deletion in $\delta\beta$-thalassemia. Nature 263:471, 1976.
6. Ottolenghi S, Comi P, Giglioni B, Tolstoshev P, Lanyon WG, Mitchell GJ, Williamson R, Russo G, Musumeci S, Schilirò G, Tsistrakis GA, Charache S, Wood WG, Clegg JB, Weatherall DJ: $\delta\beta$-Thalassemia is due to a gene deletion. Cell 9:71, 1980.
7. Musumeci S, Schilirò G, Pizzarelli G, D'Agata A, Fischer A, Russo G: α-Thalassemia in Sicily: Haematological and biosynthetic studies. Br J Haematol 43:413, 1979.

Geographic Distribution and Heterogeneity of Thalassemias in the Italian Population*

Gennaro Sansone, MD, Guiseppina Villy Sciarratta, Sarah Agosti-Vallerino, Giovanni Ivaldi, Maria Isola Parodi, and Daniela Leone-Da Passano

In the last 10 years the industrial areas of northern Italy have been the convergent point of a remarkable internal migration of ethnic groups with a high incidence of thalassemia trait (Fig. 1). Consequently thalassemia has emerged in Genoa as an important medico-social problem in which we have become more interested, both for research and service.

We present here a brief analysis of the clinical and genetic heterogeneity of the thalassemia syndromes and an epidemiologic study of the ethnic origin of our cases.

α-THALASSEMIA

In the last few years an extensive screening program has been carried out in 4 Genoa hospitals. From a total of 9,205 cord blood samples 542 Hb Barts were detected (5.88%). It is worth noting that in one of the hospitals in which the number of migrant patients was larger, the percentage reached 11%. However, it has been very difficult to extrapolate the absolute incidence of the defect in relation to the areas of origin.

Screening for Hb Barts has also been carried out in other Italian regions (Table 1). As far as Pordenone is concerned, we should like to explain that this is a town in northeastern Italy with an insignificant migration.

In the course of screening for β-thalassemia trait, we identified 300 adults with α-thalassemia. In this group there was a predominance of Sardinian subjects (28.8%).

*Supported in part by the Consiglio Nazionale delle Ricerche No. 7903279.04.

Birth Defects: Original Article Series, Volume 18, Number 7, pages 189–193
© 1982 March of Dimes Birth Defects Foundation

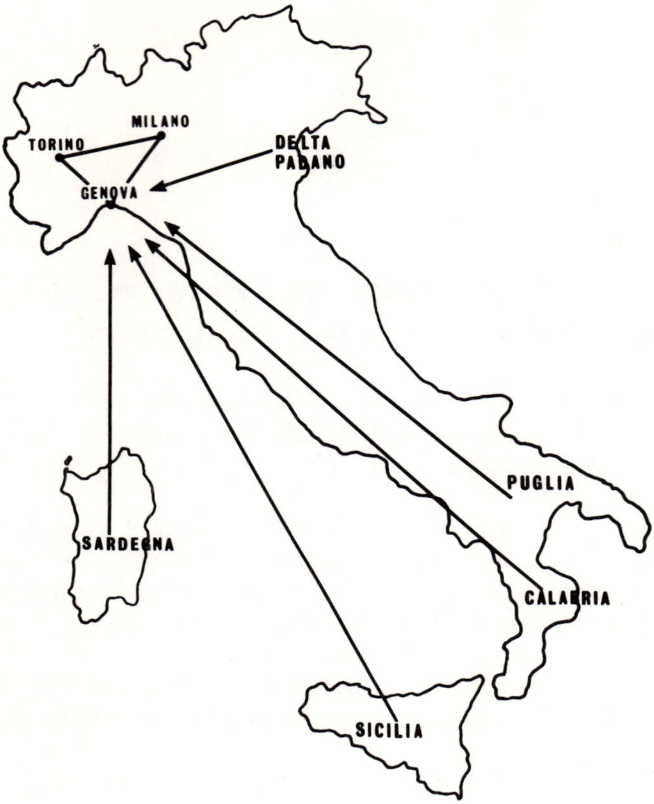

Fig. 1. Migratory flux toward the industrial areas of northern Italy (so-called "industrial triangle").

Furthermore, we studied 16 families with 26 patients affected by Hb H disease. Half of the families were of Sardinian origin.

In one case, α-thalassemia was associated with Hb Hasharon, an α-chain variant frequently occurring in the Po River Delta population.

β-THALASSEMIA

In the last 15 years, we have had the opportunity of studying 193 cases of classic thalassemia major. During this time, 50 cases were classified as thalassemia intermedia.

TABLE 1. Screening for Hb Barts in the Italian Population.

Area	Samples (No.)	Hb Barts %	References
Northern Sardinia	465	4.30	Bianco I et al [1]
Northern Sardinia	5054	4.27	Longinotti M et al [2]
Southern Sardinia	2291	12.9	Galanello R et al [3]
Naples	319	2.7	Pinto L et al [4]
Bari	550	1.6	Izzo P (personal communication)
Bari	900	2.3	Putignano A et al [5]
Milan	2000	3.1	Sciariada L (personal communication)
Turin (Torino)	3200	1.9	Mazza U (personal communication)
Pordenone	4467	0.38	Molaro GL (personal communication)
Genoa	9205	5.88	Sansone G et al [6]

Biosynthetic investigations were performed on 20 patients with thalassemia major. All 8 Sardinian subjects examined were of $\beta°$ type. Of the 12 subjects originating from other Italian regions, half were $\beta°$ and half β^+.

Almost all cases of thalassemia intermedia were investigated by biosynthesis. They showed a remarkable clinical and genetic heterogeneity. In 12 patients, the homozygous β-thalassemia was associated with an α-thalassemia gene, which resulted in a less severe course.

This additional defect may be demonstrated by careful family investigations.

In addition, 5 patients apparently homozygous for β-thalassemia were studied. In all instances, one of the parents appeared completely normal by standard laboratory examinations. The biosynthesis of the globin chains in vitro showed an imbalance of the α/non-α-ratio. Therefore, the presence of a silent gene for the β-thalassemia was postulated [7].

In the majority of cases of β-thalassemia carriers all classic parameters are clearly abnormal. However, in some subjects hematologic alterations are minimal, and one or more laboratory findings may result in the normal range. In a small not well-defined percentage all examinations are normal, except the biosynthesis. This is the phenotype of the silent gene.

In recent years we have observed 39 cases of sickle cell/thalassemia in 33 families. Biosynthetic studies were performed in only 10 of them: 5 resulted in β^+-th/Hb S and 5 $\beta°$-th/Hb S. In one case, sickle cell/thalassemia was associated with the hereditary persistence of Hb F.

TABLE 2. Geographic Origin of Hb Lepore Families

Area	Families	Subjects
Sicily	5	6
Calabria	10	15
Campania	10	15
Puglia	1	5
Marche	1	1
Abruzzo	1	1
Total	28	43

It is interesting to mention that Hb S, frequently occurring in Sicily and southern Italy, is almost unknown in Sardinia (we observed only one case of sickle cell/thalassemia in a young woman of Sardinian ancestry), and it has never been described in the Po River Delta population.

OTHER THALASSEMIAS

We detected only a few cases of delta-beta thalassemia: 6 heterozygous subjects and 4 cases of delta-beta/beta thalassemia. In 2 cases, delta-beta, beta, and alpha-thalassemia were combined [6].

In 7 patients belonging to 3 families the β-thalassemia was associated with hereditary elliptocytosis. It is difficult to explain why this association causes a chronic hemolytic anemia.

In addition to the previously mentioned case in which heterozygous β-thalassemia and sickle cell trait were associated with hereditary persistence of Hb F, we have also detected 2 familial cases of β-thalassemia trait/hereditary persistence of Hb F, and 10 subjects in 5 families with only hereditary persistence of Hb F.

Finally, we have investigated 28 families with Hb Lepore with 43 heterozygous subjects, and 3 unrelated cases of Hb Lepore/β-thalassemia. In Table 2 the geographic origin is reported. Hb Lepore has never been described in subjects originating from Sardinia or from the Po River Delta.

CONCLUSION

We have briefly called attention to the wide spectrum of genetic and clinical variability of the thalassemia syndromes. We have also shown that the different defects are not homogeneously distributed in the Italian population. The industrial areas of northern Italy, owing to internal migrations, present a unique place for these studies.

To further complicate the study of our patients we have to mention some other possible combinations, such as enzymatic defects of red cell, especially G6PD, with structural anomalies of Hb, other than Hb S, with genetic nonhemoglobinopathic erythropathies, deficiencies of various exogenous factors (iron, folate, etc).

In conclusion, only a very careful analysis of the propositi and of a large number of their relatives allows a better insight into the nature of the defects responsible for so many different phenotypes. In this regard biosynthesis of globin chains in vitro, in addition to the battery of all pertinent laboratory examinations, appears to be a very useful technique. However, the recent and more sophisticated methodologies will make possible the discovery of new genetic polymorphisms in this field in the future.

REFERENCES

1. Bianco I, Graziani P, Salvini P, Mastromonaco I, Silvestroni E: Fréquence et caractères de l'alpha-microcytémie dans les populations de la Sardaigne septentrionale. Nouv Rev Fr Hematol 12:191–200, 1972.
2. Longinotti M, Masala B, Meloni T, Dore F, Pranzetti P, Campus S: Hb Bart's, sintesi globinica e alfa-talassemia in neonati del nord-Sardegna. Proc Natl Congress of the Italian Society of Hematology, Torino, 1977.
3. Galanello R, Diana G, Furbetta M, Angius A, Melis MA, Rosatelli G, Cao A: Alpha-thalassaemia in Sardinian infants. J Med Genet 17:357–362, 1980.
4. Pinto L, Vitale R, Scarano G, Esposito L, Cicale F, Nobili B: L'alfa talassemia in Campania: Risultati di una indagine condotta su 319 neonati. Pediatria (Napoli) 86:637–645, 1978.
5. Putignano A, Colasuonno G, Pietrapertosa A, Tannoia N: L'alfa talassemia: Studio ematologico e biochimico di 14 nuclei familiari. Lab J Res Lab Med 7:609–613, 1980.
6. Sansone G, Sciarratta GV, Agosti-Vallerino SF: A thalassaemia syndrome resulting from the interaction of delta-beta and alpha-beta thalassaemia genes. A case report. Pathologica 72:715–721, 1980.
7. Aicardi G, Naselli A, Sciarratta GV, Sansone G: The silent carrier of beta thalassemia: Interaction with the typical beta thalassemic trait. Blood 38:473–478, 1979.

Thalassemia Types in Puglia

Nunzia Tannoia, MD, Michele Monaco, MD, Filippo Muratore, MD, Francesco Battista, MD, Anna Pietrapertosa, MD, Guiseppe Malcangi, MD, and Angelo Putignano, MD

Puglia (Apulia) is in the southeastern region of Italy which is divided into 5 provinces: Bari (BA), Lecce (LE), Foggia (FG), Taranto (TA), and Brindisi (BR).

The incidence and distribution of thalassemia syndromes in Puglia have been previously investigated. Screening indicated that from 5% (FG) to 8% (LE) of the population are carriers of β-thalassemia [1–3], while the frequency of α-thalassemia is about 2% [4]. However, our systematic screening for α-thalassemia and β-thalassemia syndromes has not been completed.

In 1978, an epidemiologic study showed that there were 553 cases of Cooley anemia in Puglia: 149 of these were in the area of Bari, 113 in the province of Taranto, 133 in the province of Lecce, 57 in the province of Foggia, and 101 in the province of Brindisi. However, if we relate these figures of Cooley anemia to the actual population figure, we can see that the highest incidences of Cooley anemia are in fact in the provinces of, first, Brindisi, then Taranto, then Lecce, followed by Bari and Foggia with a much lower incidence figure [5].

Although we do not know the frequency of β^+-thalassemia or β^0-thalassemia among these patients, isolated data show a predominance of β^0-thalassemia forms. A systematic study is being carried out to establish these frequencies.

From 1962 to 1981 in the Department of Clinical Medicine at the University of Bari and in the Centers for Thalassemia Research at Foggia, Taranto, and Lecce, 49,258 subjects were examined.

For the diagnosis of thalassemia syndromes all of the following parameters were used: red cell counts, Hb determination, PCV, MCH, MCV. MCV values were obtained by Microcell Counter model 1800 Toa. Morphologic red blood cell modifications, including inclusion bodies, were estimated by observation of blood film. The hematologic techniques employed for the diagnosis of thalassemia syndromes were described in our previous study [4].

The distribution of Hb F in red cells was evaluated by the acid elution technique. Red cell osmotic fragility was determined by the method of Simmel.

Birth Defects: Original Article Series, Volume 18, Number 7, pages 195–198
© 1982 March of Dimes Birth Defects Foundation

TABLE 1. Frequency of Thalassemia Variants and Hemoglobinopathies in Puglia

	Provinces				
	Bari	Foggia	Taranto	Lecce	Total
Normals	11,991	11,671	5,311	10,744	39,717
β-Thal Heterozygotes	2,339	3,109	1,945	1,645	9,038
β-Thal Heterozygotes with High Hb F	72	110	4		186
δβ-Thal Heterozygotes	36		5		41
α-Thal Heterozygotes	105	35	10	15	165
HPFH Heterozygotes	4	4	3		11
Double Heterozygotes for HPFH and Thal	3				3
Hb Lepore Heterozygotes	10	14			24
Hb S Trait	7	31	5	3	46
Double Heterozygotes for Hb S and β-Thal	5				5
Hb D Punjab Heterozygotes	3				3
Double Heterozygotes for Hb D and β-Thal	1				1
Hb C Trait	2		1		3
Variants Unclassified		15			15
Total	14,578	14,989	7,284	12,407	49,258

Hb A_2 was quantitated by cellulose acetate electrophoresis with elution, and in the last few years by microchromatography. Hb F was estimated by the method of Betke and the pattern of hemoglobinopathies in collaboration with Istituto Superiore di Sanità, Rome. Serum iron was determined with a Boehringer Mannheim kit.

The results from the Centers for Thalassemia Research are shown in Table 1. In the Department of Clinical Medicine at the University of Bari, 14,578 subjects were examined; 2,587 of these were carriers of thalassemia syndromes or other hemoglobin disorders; 2,339 had β-thalassemia, and 72 had β-thalassemia with high Hb F levels. These β-thalassemia heterozygotes with high levels of Hb F had values ranging from 5–19% with heterogeneous distribution of this hemoglobin in the peripheral blood; 36 had $\delta\beta^0$-thalassemia; Hb H disease was found in 19 cases; and 105 were by definition α-thalassemia (biosynthetic studies are underway for most of these subjects). The thalassemia heterozygotes with normal Hb A_2 and Hb F values were not included in this study, because measurement of hemoglobin synthesis, and parents were not available. Furthermore, in 4 subjects there was HPFH, and in 3 HPFH was associated with β-thalassemia.

Of 28 cases of hemoglobinopathies 10 had Hb Lepore Boston, 3 Hb D Punjab, 7 Hb S, 5 sickle cell thalassemia, 1 Hb D with β-thalassemia, and 2 Hb C.

Dr. Monaco studied the thalassemia syndromes in the province of Foggia (Table 1) from 1967 to 1981. He examined 14,989 subjects, 3,109 of whom had

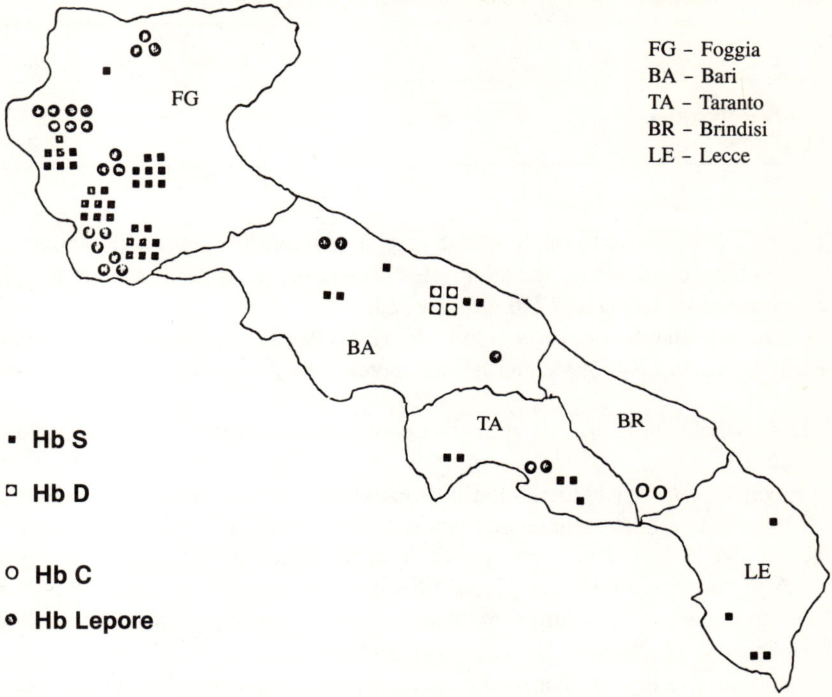

Fig. 1. Distribution of some hemoglobinopathies in Puglia (Apulia).

β-thalassemia, 110 β-thalassemia with elevated Hb F, 35 were obligate α-thalassemia carriers, 4 with HPFH, 14 with Hb Lepore, and 31 with Hb S.

No classification was made in the 15 cases of slow β-variant hemoglobin.

Dr. Battista has studied the thalassemia syndromes in the province of Taranto: 7,284 subjects were examined: of these 1,945 were β-thalassemia, 4 β-thalassemia with elevated Hb F, 5 $\delta\beta^0$-thalassemia, 10 with α-thalassemia, 3 HPFH, 5 Hb S, 1 Hb C.

We have no data for the province of Brindisi.

In the province of Lecce, Professor Muratore studied 12,407 subjects of whom 1,645 had β-thalassemia, 15 α-thalassemia, and 3 Hb S.

In our study, there were 9,038 β-thalassemia heterozygotes, 186 β-thalassemia with high Hb F, 41 $\delta\beta^0$-thalassemia, 165 by definition α-thalassemia, 11 HPFH, 3 HPFH and β-thalassemia, and 24 Hb Lepore (Table 1).

It is noteworthy that Hb Lepore was found almost exclusively in the province of Foggia, especially in the northwestern area, bordering Campania which is the Italian area with the largest incidence of Hb Lepore. α-Thalassemia, however, is

TABLE 2. β-Thalassemia Homozygotes and Hb H Disease in Puglia

	Bari	Foggia	Taranto	Lecce	Brindisi	Total
β-Thal Homozygotes	149	57	113	133	101	553
Hb H Disease	19	1	1			21

uniformly distributed throughout the region. Among the hemoglobinopathies, the most frequent is Hb S, and again, this is more frequent in the area of Foggia. The presence of Hb D and Hb C is sporadic (Fig. 1).

β-Thalassemia homozygotes and Hb H in Puglia are reported in Table 2 which shows 553 β-thalassemia homozygotes, and 21 subjects with HB H disease.

The birthplace of subjects with Hb Lepore and hemoglobinopathies is shown in Figure 1.

In conclusion, our epidemiologic investigation shows: 1) a higher incidence of β-thalassemia homozygous and heterozygous forms were found in the provinces of Brindisi, Taranto, and Lecce, namely in the area that roughly corresponds to the area known as "Magna Grecia," one of the major areas of ancient Greek colonization; 2) a larger incidence of Hb Lepore in the province of Foggia; and 3) some cases of Hb H disease and Hb S.

The objective of our investigation, carried out in collaboration with the Centers for Thalassemia Research at Bari, Lecce, Foggia, and Taranto, was to obtain epidemiologic data. Our purpose has been to draw up a map of Puglia showing the probable variants of thalassemia and hemoglobinopathies, as we had already done for Cooley anemia [5].

This study represents the starting point for further studies both of Hb and thalassemia variants. It is our plan to present a map indicating biochemical, biosynthetic, and genetic variants to be found in Puglia.

REFERENCES

1. Bini L, Tannoia N, Pesce M, Fatone A: Frequency and meaning of some red blood cells and haemoglobin abnormalities in a sample of the population from Apulia. Blut 13:305, 1966.
2. Borgia T: Contributo allo studio della frequenza delle microcitemie in provincia di Lecce. Atti Giornate sulla Microcitemia, Cagliari 1968, pp 519–521.
3. Lucentini L, Monaco M, Placentino M, Faleo D: Incidenze del trait talassemico nella popolazione di Puglia. Arch Casa Soll Soff II:138–144, 1967.
4. Putignano A, Colasuonno G, Pietrapertosa A, Tannoia N: L'alfa-talassemia: Studio ematologico e biochimico di 14 nuclei familiari. L.A.B.I., Res Lab Med (7) 6:609–613, 1980.
5. Tannoia N, Bonomo L: L'epidemiologia del morbo di Cooley in Puglia. Atti VI Congresso Internazionale, "La Prevenzione delle Malattie Microcitemiche," Roma, Ed. Minerva Medica, 81, 1980.

Thalassemia in Ferrara

Calogero Vullo, MD

Thalassemias are fairly uncommon in northern Italy, but are frequently found in the area of the Po River Delta, where Silvestroni and Bianco found that mean values of carriers were 7% with peaks around 20% [1]. The data refer to the results of the Simmel test, which is positive when osmotic resistance is increased, so cumulative data for β- and α-carriers are obtained.

Causes of the high frequency of thalassemia in the Delta area are unknown, however 2 points deserve attention, namely: 1) the area was endemic for malaria for many centuries before World War II; 2) a distortion of segregation or a high mutation rate are not the causes of the high gene frequency of β-thalassemia, since neither of them has been found by Papi et al [2].

The molecular defect of Ferrara β-thalassemia has been studied by Conconi and his co-workers since 1968. These authors have demonstrated that Ferrara β-thalassemia is a β°-thalassemia and has particular characteristics which are indicated in Table 1.

The defect causes a very severe syndrome. Symptoms appear usually within the first 6 months of life, and death within the first year was very common in untreated children.

Recently, Conconi and co-workers have found that β^+ rather than β° is the more common form of β-thalassemia in the northern area of the Po River Delta [8] (Table 2).

The β^+- defect found in the Po River Delta also results in a severe syndrome in the homozygote. A comparison between the syndromes due to the β°- and β^+-defects is not yet available.

Since β-thalassemia is so common in the Po Delta area, a program of genetic counseling was started by Silvestroni and Bianco in 1955, and is still in progress. The efficacy of the program, which has not been good in the past [9,10], has improved dramatically in the last few years, both as a consequence of the availability of prenatal diagnosis, and of a change in the reproductive behavior of the population [11].

Birth Defects: Original Article Series, Volume 18, Number 7, pages 199–202
© 1982 March of Dimes Birth Defects Foundation

TABLE 1. Characteristics of Ferrara $\beta°$- Thalassemia

1) Absence of β-globin synthesis [3]
2) Presence of β-globin mRNA as indicated by:
   a) hybridization studies [4]
   b) in vitro translation of β-globin mRNA (homologous and heterologous systems) [5]
   c) in vivo translation of β-globin mRNA (presence of β-globin synthesis after blood transfusion) [6]
3) Normal arrangement of δ- and β-globin genes [7]

TABLE 2. Characteristics of β^+-Thalassemia in the Po River Delta

1) Normal arrangement of δ- and β-globin genes
2) β-globin synthesis varies between 5—30% (with a mean value of 14.9 ± 6.5 and unimodal distribution)
3) β-globin mRNA is stable, so that a defect of β-globin mRNA transcription or processing may be postulated
4) β^+- heterozygotes have higher MCV values than $\beta°$- heterozygotes

In the Po River Delta area, hydrops fetalis due to α-thalassemia and Hb H disease have never been observed. As a consequence, little attention was given to α-thalassemia in the past. At the Centro della Microcitemia of Ferrara during the 1970-1974 period hematologic studies were carried out in about 12,000 subjects for the detection of thalassemia trait. About 4% of these subjects showed alterations of red cell morphology and increased red cell osmotic resistance but normal Hb A2 levels. Studies performed in 63 of these subjects showed decreased MCV and MCH values (mean values 68 ± 3.73 fl and 21.69 ± 1.82 pg, respectively) and a mean α/β ratio of 0.77 ± 0.05. Subsequent studies done by Del Senno and co-workers confirmed the reduced α/β ratios, and by means of restriction enzyme analysis, showed a restriction pattern identical to that of normal subjects, suggesting a nondeletion type of α-thalassemia. Since the amount of α-globin synthesis and of mRNA are equally reduced and since α-globin is stable, a molecular defect at mRNA transcription or processing level has been postulated by these authors [12].

Several abnormal hemoglobins, both α- and β-variants, have been found in the Po River Delta population. Among those observed, Hb Hasharon deserves special mention because of its high incidence and genetic peculiarities [13]. This hemoglobin, identified as hemoglobin L Ferrara in 1963 [14], was recognized as Hb Hasharon in 1970 by Tentori et al [15]. The amount of Hb Hasharon found in Italian heterozygotes is 30-40% of the total Hb [15]. This is higher than the amount found in Ashkenazi heterozygotes which is between 14-22% [16,17]. These data suggest that gene arrangement is different in Italian and Ashkenazi

Hb Hasharon subjects. Restriction enzyme analysis of DNA demonstrated that, in Italians, Hb Hasharon is associated with an α-globin gene deletion [18,19].

Double heterozygosity for Hb Hasharon and β-thalassemia is characterized by amounts of Hb Hasharon lower than those found in Hb Hasharon carriers. This is due to the fact that abnormal α-chains in excess are removed at a faster rate than normal α-chains in excess [20].

CONCLUSION

In the Po River Delta: both β- and α-thalassemia are present; β-thalassemia is heterogeneous; α-thalassemia does not cause Hb H disease or hydrops fetalis and is due to a nondeletion type defect; and finally, subjects carrying Hb Hasharon have a peculiar gene arrangement.

REFERENCES

1. Silvestroni E, Bianco I: Screening for microcytemia in Italy: Analysis of data collected in the past 30 years. Am J Hum Genet 27:198, 1975.
2. Papi C, Prampolini B, Vullo C, Barrai I: Segregation analysis of thalassemia in Ferrara. Am J Hum Genet 29:627, 1977.
3. Conconi F, Bargellesi A, Pontremoli S, Vigi V, Volpato S, Gaburro D: Absence of β-globin synthesis and excess of α-globin synthesis in homozygous β-thalassaemic subjects from the Ferrara region. Nature 217:259, 1968.
4. Ottolenghi S, Comi P, Giglioni B, Williamson R, Vullo C, Del Senno L, Conconi F: Direct demonstration of β-globin mRNA in homozygous Ferrara $\beta°$-thalassaemia patients. Nature 266:232,1977.
5. Conconi F, Rowley PT, Del Senno L, Pontremoli S, Volpato S: Induction of β-globin synthesis in the β-thalassaemia of Ferrara. Nature (New Biol) 238:83, 1972.
6. Conconi F, Del Senno L, Ferrarese P, Menini C, Borgatti L, Vullo C, Labie D: Appearance of β-globin synthesis in erythroid cells of Ferrara $\beta°$ thalassaemic patients following blood transfusion. Nature 254:256, 1975.
7. Del Senno L, Conconi F, Little PFR, Williamson R: Restriction enzyme analysis of the β-globin gene in DNA from $\beta°$-thalassaemie subjects from Ferrara. Biochem Biophys Res Commun 91(2):548–553, 1979.
8. Del Senno L, Bernardi F, Busin M, Marchetti G, Perrotta C, Conconi F, Capellozza G, Vullo C: Genotipi α e β-talassemici nel delta del Po. Minerva Med 72(11):684–689, 1981.
9. Aguzzi S, Vullo C, Barrai I: Reproductive compensation in families segregating for Cooley's anaemia in Ferrara. Am J Hum Genet 42:150, 1978.
10. Barrai I, Vullo C: Assessment of prospective genetic counseling in the Ferrara area. Am J Med Genet 6:195, 1980.
11. Barrai I, Vullo C: Screening for beta-thalassaemia heterozygotes. Lancet 2:1256, 1980.
12. Del Senno L, Bernardi F, Buzzoni D, Marchetti G, Perrotta C, Conconi F: Molecular characteristics of a non deletion α-thalassaemia of the Po River Delta. Eur J Biochem 116:127, 1981.
13. Alberti R, Mariuzzi GM, Marinucci M, Bruni E, Tentori L: Haemoglobin Hasharon in a north Italian community. J Med Genet 12:294, 1975.

14. Bianco I, Modiano G, Bottini E, Lucci R: Alteration in the α-chain of haemoglobin L Ferrara. Nature 198:395, 1963.
15. Tentori L, Bruni E, Marinucci M, Vullo C, Cristofori G, Salsini G: The relationship between hemoglobin L Ferrara and haemoglobin Hasharon: Is haemoglobin L Ferrara really 47 Asp → Gly? Haematologica 59:250, 1974.
16. Lemmann H, Vella F: Haemoglobin Hasharon. Humangenetik 25:237, 1974.
17. Mavilio F, Marinucci M, Massa A, Fontanarosa PP, Tentori L, Cappellozza G: Haemoglobin Hasharon E [α 47 (CD5) Asp → His B_2] linked to α thalassaemia in northern Italian carriers. Hematological and biosynthetic studies. Acta Haematol 63:305, 1980.
18. Giglioni B, Comi P, Taramelli R, Ottolenghi S, Ciocca-Vasino MA, Ane' C, Cappellini MD, Gianni AM: Organization of α-globin genes in Hb Hasharon (α 47 asp → His) carriers. Blood 56:1145, 1980.
19. Del Senno L, Bernardi F, Marchetti G, Perrotta C, Conconi F, Vullo C, Salsini G, Cristofori G, Cappellozza G, Bellinello F, Bedendo B, Mercuriali M: Organization of α-globin genes and mRNA translation in subjects carrying haemoglobin Hasharon (47 Asp → His) from the Ferrara region (Northern Italia). Eur J Biochem 111:129, 1980.
20. Conconi F, Alberti R, Mariuzzi GM, Guglielmini C, Vullo C, Del Senno L: Decrease of α-Hasharon globin in β-thalassemia. Br J Haematol 39:529, 1978.

β-Thalassemia in Southern Italy: A Preliminary Approach*

Leonardo Tentori, MD, Marino Marinucci, PhD, Adriana Massa, PhD, Fulvio Mavilio, PhD, Raffaella Guerriero, PhD, Marco Gabbianelli, PhD, Adele Giampaolo, PhD, Paolo Cianciulli, MD, Nadia M. Sposi, PhD, M. Masi, MD, M. Cecconi, MD, M. Antimi, MD, and G. Pratesi, MD

In the last few years, increasing evidence has been provided for marked heterogeneity of the molecular defects underlying the various forms of both β^0- and β^+-thalassemia. These defects may involve virtually every step in the biosynthesis of the β-globin chain, that is, DNA transcription, nuclear RNA processing, and mRNA translation.

In Italy, 2 forms of β-thalassemia at present have been characterized in detail, including their geographic distribution. They are the Sardinian β^0-thalassemia and the Ferrara β^0-thalassemia, the latter being due to a defect in a soluble factor required for β-mRNA translation [1]. On the contrary, little is known at the molecular level of β-thalassemias in other Italian areas, particularly southern Italy, where β-thalassemia is very prevalent.

We have under examination now a number of southern Italian patients affected by Cooley anemia, who have been admitted to the Hematological Division of Sant'Eugenio Hospital in Rome. They originate from 6 Italian regions, namely, Latium, Campania, Basilicata, Puglia, Calabria, and Sicily.

The aim of our research is to provide more information about the molecular heterogeneity of β-thalassemia in Italy, permitting future studies to ascertain the existence of linkage disequilibrium between the non-α-globin genes and polymorphic restriction sites in β-thalassemia subjects, in view of applications to antenatal diagnosis of β-thalassemia on fibroblast DNA obtained by amniocentesis.

*This work supported in part by a CNR grant Progetto Finalizzato Medicina Preventiva (contr. no. 81.00332.83).

Birth Defects: Original Article Series, Volume 18, Number 7, pages 203–210
© 1982 March of Dimes Birth Defects Foundation

This communication is concerned with the results of a preliminary approach consisting of biosynthetic studies on peripheral blood reticulocytes from 47 patients.

The relative proportion among these different geographic groups reflects only the peculiar composition of the sample which is currently under treatment in the Sant'Eugenio Hospital in Rome, and whose geographic origin is as follows: Latium (8.5%), Campania (8.5%), Basilicata (8.5%), Puglia (19.2%), Calabria (19.1%), Sicily (23.4%), mixed southern Italian origin: (12.8%). The age of the patients ranges from 5 to 23 years.

Reticulocytes were obtained immediately before blood transfusion and enriched by centrifugation on Percoll density gradients [2], in order to minimize WBC contamination. Biosynthesis was carried out according to Alter et al [3]. All of the patients were affected with a severe clinical picture, and all but 5 were splenectomized.

The overall non-α/α chain synthesis ratio is shown in Figure 1. The distribution is roughly normal around a mean of 0.37.

Figure 2 shows the distribution of β/α chain synthesis ratios, which range from 0.002 to 0.34, around a mean of 0.097. This is surely not due to a technical bias, since no traces of radioactivity were found under the β-chain chromatographic peak in an adequate sample of both Sardinian and Ferrara β^0-thalassemia homozygotes.

The spectrum of variability in the β/non-α ratios observed in these patients, which ranges from 0.006 to 0.73 with an abnormal distribution and a mean of 0.27, is shown in Figure 3.

The distribution of the β/γ synthetic ratios is roughly exponential (Fig. 4), indicating a considerable prevalence of subjects having low amounts of β-chain synthesis with respect to the γ-chain synthesis. On the other hand, the distribution of the γ/α ratios (Fig. 5) is roughly normal, ranging from 0.05 to 0.75, around a mean of 0.27. The distributions shown in Figures 3-5 are the graphic expression of well-known phenomena, namely the complete independence of the β from the γ-chain synthesis in peripheral blood, the latter depending only on the proportion of red cells surviving ineffective bone marrow erythropoiesis, as well as on its extent. That is better represented in Figure 6 which indicates no correlation between β-chain synthesis, expressed as the β/α ratio, and the overall chain imbalance, expressed as non-α/α ratio. Consequently, the correlation between the amount of β-chain synthesis, expressed as β/α ratio, and that expressed as β/non-α ratio, is significant (Fig. 7).

Some preliminary conclusions may be drawn from these data. The first is that the distribution of values indicating the relative amount of β-chain synthesis is neither unimodal nor clearly plurimodal. This type of distribution in our sample of southern Italian subjects indicates the presence of much phenotypic heterogeneity in β-thalassemia, which does not allow an unambiguous identification of

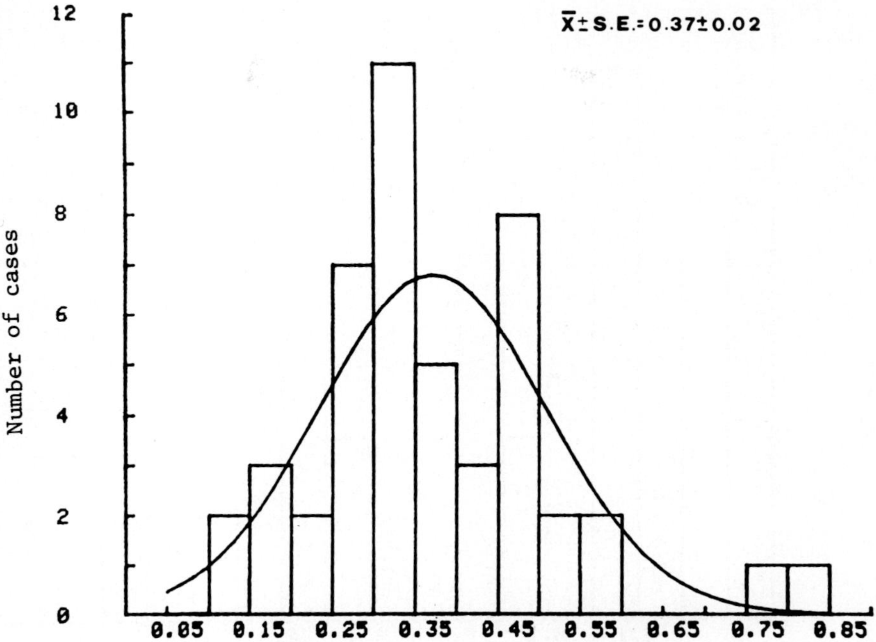

Fig. 1. Distribution of the non-α/α chain synthetic ratios.

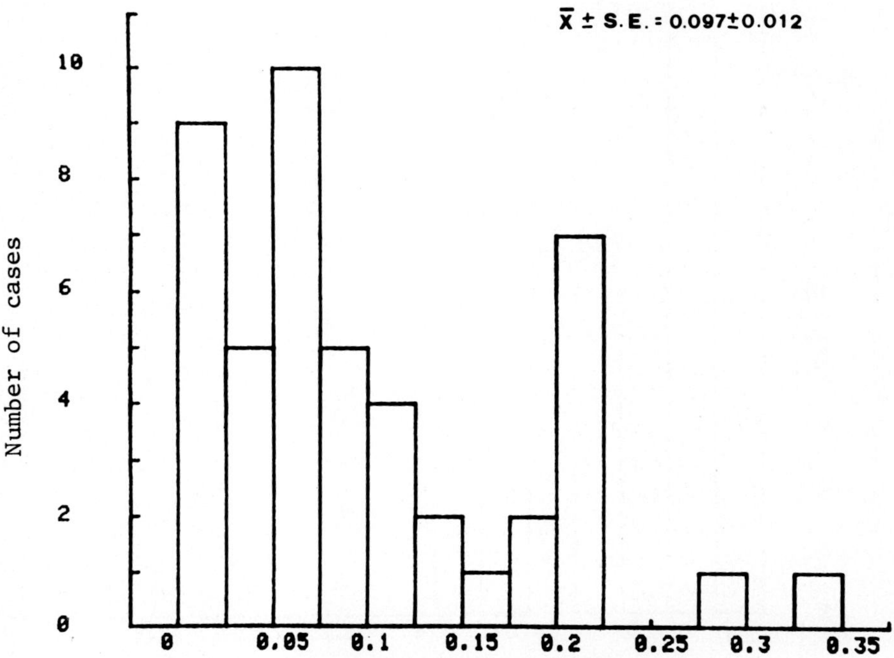

Fig. 2. Distribution of the β/α chain synthetic ratios.

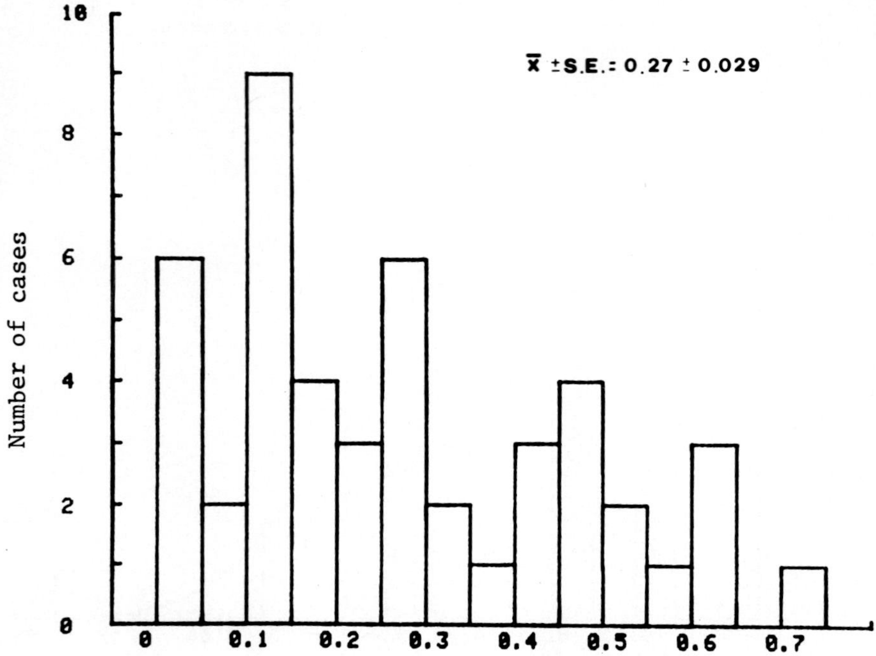

Fig. 3. Distribution of the β/non-α chain synthetic ratios.

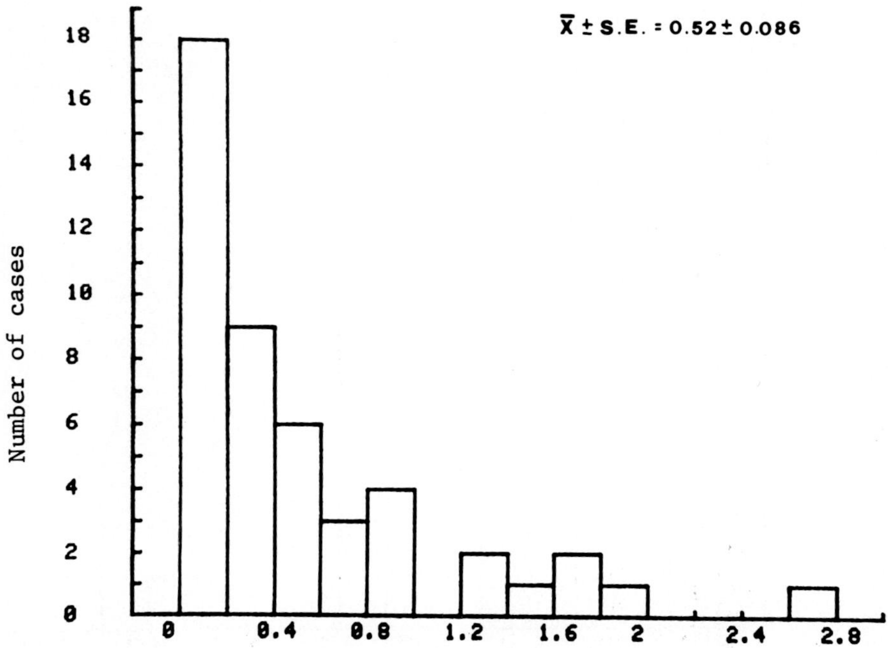

Fig. 4. Distribution of the β/γ chain synthetic ratios.

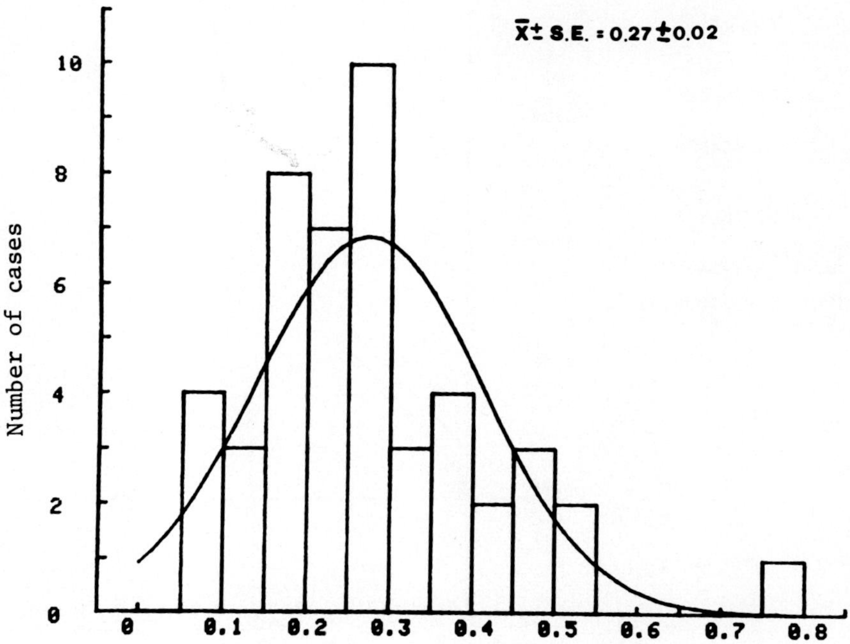

Fig. 5. Distribution of the γ/α chain synthetic ratios.

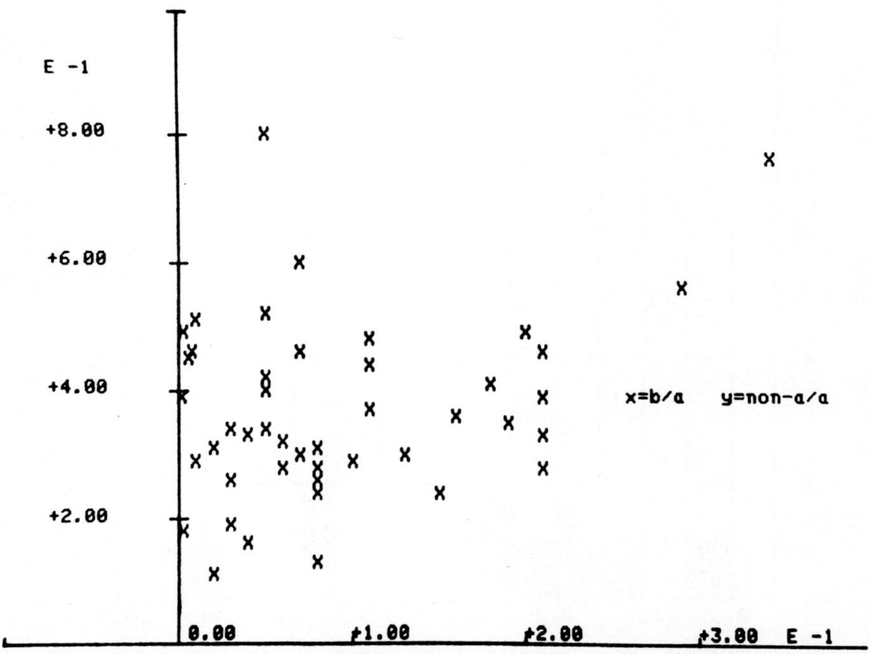

Fig. 6. Correlation between β/α ratio (in abscissa) and non-α/α ratio (simple linear regression).

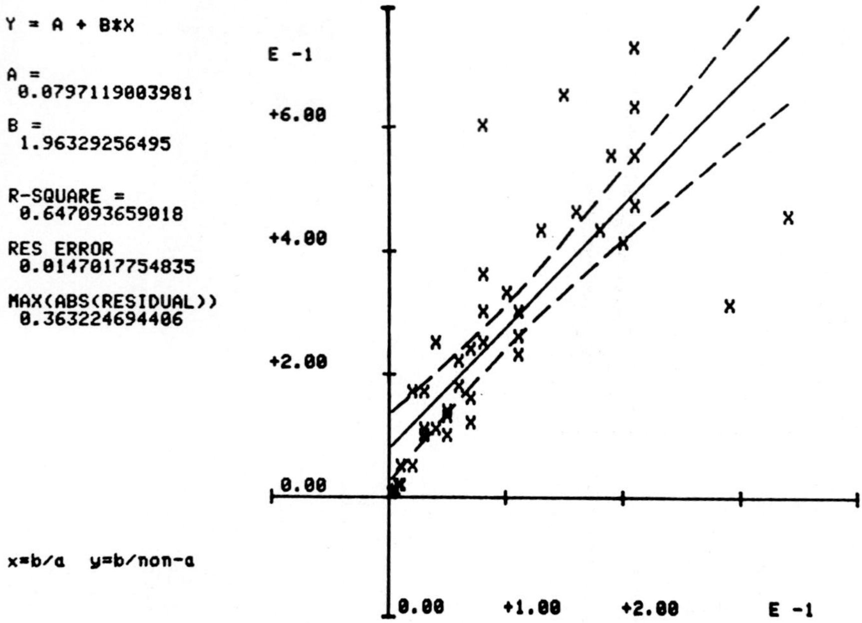

Fig. 7. Correlation between β/α ratio (in abscissa) and β/non-α ratio (simple linear regression).

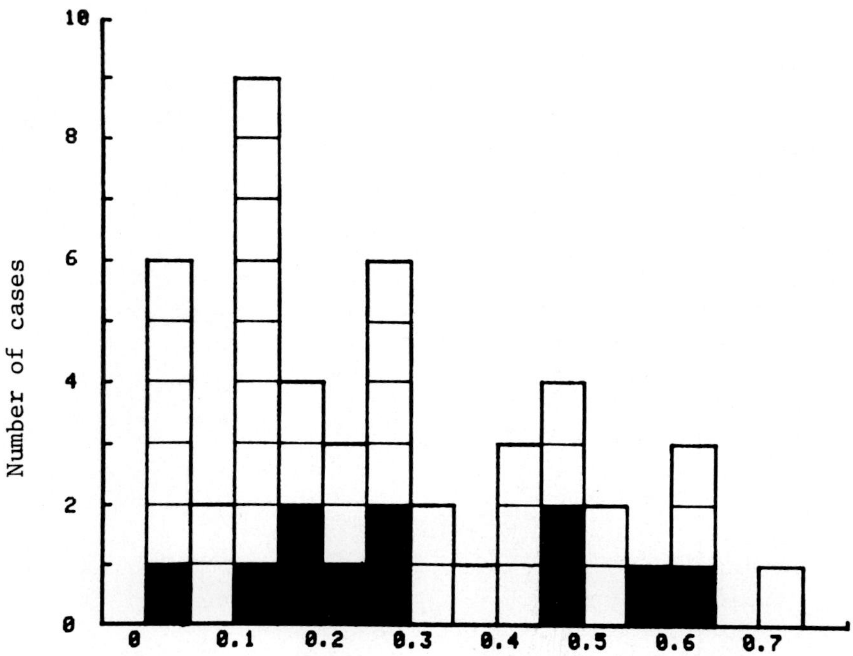

Fig. 8. Distribution of the α/non-α chain synthetic ratios. The dark squares indicate the β-thalassemia patients from Sicily.

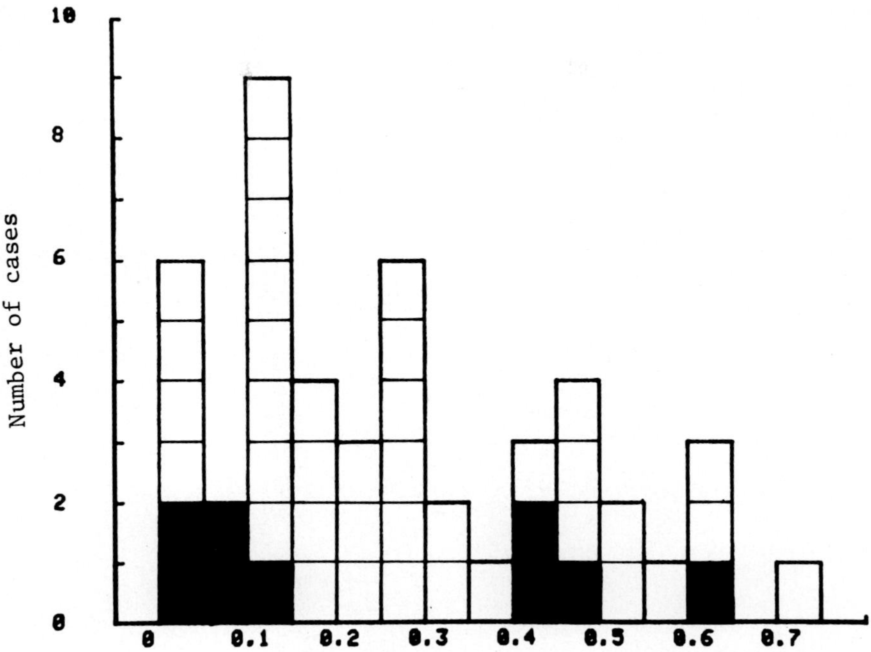

Fig. 9. Distribution of the β/non-α chain synthetic ratios. The dark squares indicate the β-thalassemia patients from Calabria.

genotypes. Indeed, if we consider some better delimited populations with a significant number of subjects (and precisely Sicilians and Calabrians, as shown in Figures 8 and 9, respectively), some suggestion of clustering in at least 2 classes arises, which might roughly indicate the presence of β^0/β^+- and of β^+/β^+-genotypes. Another point of interest is that in the present sample, subjects with β/α ratios lower than 0.002 have not been found.

If we define β^0-thalassemia as complete absence of β-chain synthesis, this type of β-thalassemia appears to be lacking in the homozygous state in our sample, but the relatively small number of subjects examined to date does not allow us to rule out its existence in southern Italy. However, it can be statistically calculated that our findings are not compatible with a frequency of β^0-thalassemia traits higher than approximately 25%, with a confidence of 95%.

On the other hand, if one takes as the cut-off point a value of β/α ratio different from zero, for instance the 0.01 value proposed by Pepe and co-workers [4], the incidence of β^0-thalassemia trait in our sample approaches 36%, which is in good agreement with the data of these authors for the Campanian population.

An immediate consequence of such a high prevalence of β^+-thalassemia trait in southern Italy is that great care must be taken in the evaluation of the chain synthesis ratios in the prenatal diagnosis of homozygous β-thalassemia.

REFERENCES

1. Conconi F, Rowley PT, Del Senno L, Pontremoli S, Volpato S: Induction of β-globin synthesis in β-thalassemia of Ferrara. Nature (New Biol) 238:83, 1972.
2. Vettore L, De Matteis MC, Zampini P: A new density gradient system for the separation of human red blood cells. Am J Hematol 8:291, 1980.
3. Alter BP, Model CB, Fairweather D, Hobbins JC, Mahoney MJ, Frigoletto FD, Sherman AS, Nathan DJ: Prenatal diagnosis of hemoglobinopathies. A review of 15 cases. N Engl J Med 295:1437, 1976.
4. Pepe G, Lupi L, Luzzatto L: Genetical and biochemical heterogeneity of β-thalassemia in Naples. Br J Haematol 45:417, 1980.

PATHOPHYSIOLOGY AND CLINICAL ASPECTS OF THALASSEMIA SYNDROMES

Hypoxemia in Thalassemia*

Prawase Wasi, MD, PhD, Suthat Fucharoen, MD, Praparn Youngchaiyud, MD, and Dhira Sonakul, MD, ChB, DTM

Hypoxemia is a newly discovered and important feature in thalassemia. In 1977, a 16-year-old patient with β-thalassemia/Hb E disease was noted to be cyanotic without apparent causes. Her partial arterial oxygen saturation (PaO_2) was 62.5 mmHg and had been persistently low over the years. Examination of a large number of thalassemic patients revealed that most splenectomized cases had low PaO_2 with normal $PaCO_2$ [1]. Figures 1 and 2 illustrate PaO_2 values in 65 patients with β-thalassemia/Hb E disease. Thirty-five patients had had splenectomy 1 to 26 years previously (average 14.3). These patients received no or few blood transfusions. The splenectomized and nonsplenectomized patients had comparable ages and severity (Table 1). While PaO_2 was low in 31 out of 35 splenectomized patients (89%), it was reduced in 6 out of the 30 nonsplenectomized cases (20%).

Independently, Keens et al [3] and Cooper et al [4], respectively, found low PaO_2 in 10 out of 12, and 15 out of 17 cases of thalassemia, presumably homozygous β-thalassemia. Extensive lung function studies were performed by these two groups of workers; their findings and interpretation differed. Keens et al [3] found normal total lung capacity (TLC), increased residual volume, and abnormal expiratory flow rates at lower percentages of TLC. They interpreted these and other findings as showing small airway obstruction, probably due to iron deposition in the lungs or other factors. Cooper et al [4], on the contrary, found reduced TLC; this, with normal expiratory flow rates, indicated a restrictive type of defect and they believed that it was due to defective growth of alveolar airspaces.

Why differing lung functions were obtained by the two United States groups is not clear. Lung function study in our patients reveals restrictive defect in most cases (to be reported in detail by Youngchaiyud et al). To compare salient fea-

*This study was supported by a USPH research grant AM 09801 from the National Institute of Arthritis, Metabolism and Digestive Diseases.

Birth Defects: Original Article Series, Volume 18, Number 7, pages 213–217
© 1982 March of Dimes Birth Defects Foundation

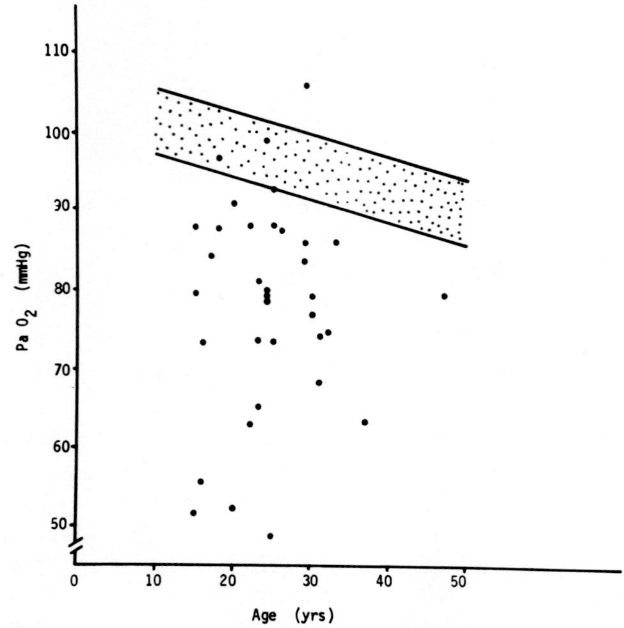

Fig. 1. Partial arterial oxygen pressure in 35 splenectomized thalassemic patients. The expected normal values were calculated according to Melemgaard [2].

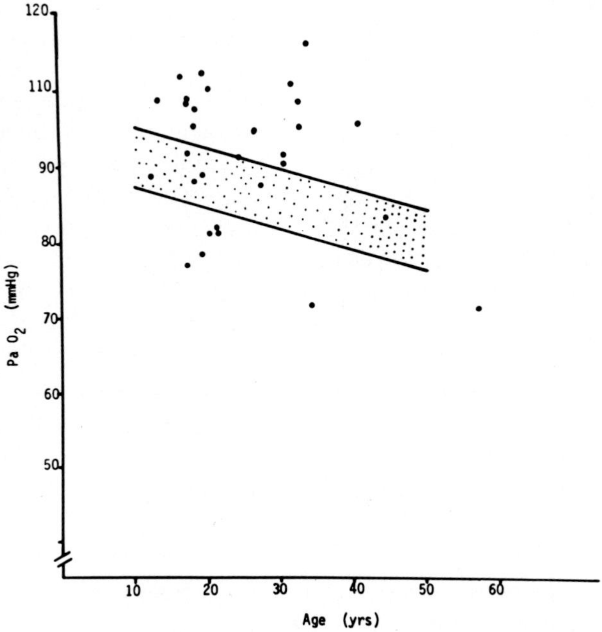

Fig. 2. Partial arterial oxygen pressure in 30 nonsplenectomized thalassemic patients.

TABLE 1. Comparison of Mean Ages, Hemoglobin Concentrations and PaO_2 in the Splenectomized and Nonsplenectomized Patients

Groups	No.	Age yr	Hb gm/dl	PaO_2 mmHg
Splenectomized	35	24.8	6.57	77.9
Nonsplenectomized	30	24.7	6.48	100.8

TABLE 2. Summary of Salient Features Concerning Hypoxemia in the Thalassemic Patients

	UCLA Keens et al [3]	New York Cooper et al [4]	Bangkok This study
Disease	Homoz. β-thal	Homoz. β-thal	β-thal/Hb E
No. of patients	12	17	35
Mean age (yr.)	18.2	11.7	24.8
Splenectomy	not known	not known	yes
Blood transfusions	Hyper	Hyper	No, minimal
Iron chelation	—	3 yrs	—
Mean Hb (gm/dl)	11.9	11.5	6.6
Hypoxemia (cases)	10	15	31
Lung function	Small airway obstruction	Restrictive	Restrictive

tures, findings in the three series are summarized in Table 2. Hypoxemia is a common feature, regardless of differences in ages, hemoglobin levels, amounts of blood transfusion, and whether or not the patients had been chelated. Iron deposition in the lungs in our patients is minimal. It is thus unlikely that iron deposition in the lungs causes small airway obstruction as suggested by Keens et al [3]. The restrictive defect could be contributed by various factors, ie abnormal thoracic cages, hepatomegaly, cardiomegaly, intrathoracic extramedullary hematopoietic masses, or defective development of airspaces as suggested by Cooper et al [4]. Pulmonary fibrosis which can cause restrictive defect is not a general feature of thalassemia.

While causes for restrictive defect remain to be delineated, other findings, however, suggest that hypoxemia in thalassemia may be multifactorial. Recently, Sonakul et al [5] found that of the 43 patients with β-thalassemia/Hb E disease autopsied in our hospital, 19 (44%) showed obstructive lesions in the pulmonary arteries (Fig. 3). These consisted of organized, recanalized thromboemboli completely occluding the lumens of muscular arteries of 100-800 μ in size. The obstructive lesions varied in number from 1-2/cm^2 to 14/cm^2 averaging 6/cm^2. Right ventricular hypertrophy was evident in the majority of the patients with these pulmonary artery obstructive lesions. No doubt this newly observed phenomenon is an additional factor contributing to common cardiac failure in

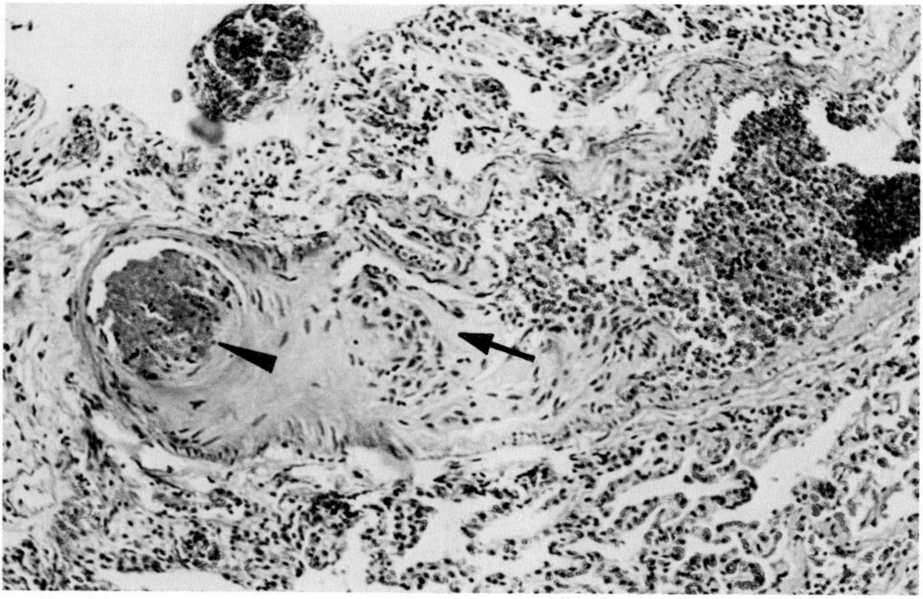

Fig. 3. Lung section obtained at autopsy from a patient with β-thalassemia/Hb E disease showing recanalized thrombosis in a large pulmonary artery with recent thrombosis in a newly formed channel (thick arrow), and polyploid structure (thin arrow) (H & E × 100).

thalassemia. When extensive, it can contribute to hypoxemia in thalassemia through defective perfusion.

Of the 19 patients found to have pulmonary artery occlusion, 17 were splenectomized cases, while there were 28 splenectomized and 15 nonsplenectomized patients in the series. Thus, it appears that splenectomy is commonly related to both pulmonary artery occlusion and hypoxemia in thalassemia. Thrombocytosis is found in splenectomized cases. We found a mean platelet count of 571 × 10^9/liter in splenectomized thalassemic patients against 189 × 10^9/liter in the nonsplenectomized ones [6]. Circulating platelet aggregates also were demonstrated in the splenectomized thalassemic patients. These suggest that after splenectomy the resulting thrombocytosis and increased platelet aggregation may contribute to pulmonary artery thromboembolism and hypoxemia.

We treated 12 thalassemic patients with low PaO_2 (average 67.1 mmHg) with aspirin and/or Persantin and 10 showed a significant rise of PaO_2 (average 85.04 mmHg) [1]. This suggests that hypoxemia in splenectomized thalassemic patients is attributable to reversible platelet aggregation in a majority of cases. It should be pointed out that the platelets are particularly abundant in the lung and the pulmonary circulation [7].

It appears that there are many ramifications of hypoxemia in thalassemia. While detailed studies concerning its pathogenesis and various related features are in progress, the findings on the platelets and results of treatment with aspirin and/or Persantin warrant institution of antiplatelet aggregation therapy in thalassemic patients after splenectomy.

REFERENCES

1. Fucharoen S, Youngchaiyud P, Wasi P: Hypoxaemia and the effect of aspirin in thalassaemia. Southeast Asian J Trop Med Public Health 12:90, 1981.
2. Mellemgaard K: The alveolar arterial oxygen difference; its size and components in normal man. Acta Physiol Scand 67:10, 1966.
3. Keens TG, O'Neal MH, Ortega JA, Hyman CB, Platzker CG: Pulmonary function abnormalities in thalassemia patients on a hypertransfusion program. Pediatrics 65:1013, 1980.
4. Cooper DM, Mansell AL, Weiner MA, Berdon WE, Chetty-Baktaviziam A, Reid L, Mellins RB: Low lung capacity and hypoxemia in children with thalassemia major. Am Rev Respir Dis 121:639, 1980.
5. Sonakul D, Pacharee P, Laohapand T, Fucharoen S, Wasi P: Pulmonary artery obstruction in thalassaemia. Southeast Asian J Trop Med Public Health 11:516, 1980.
6. Winichagoon P, Fucharoen S, Wasi P: Increased circulating platelet aggregates in thalassaemia. Southeast Asian J Trop Med Public Health 12:556, 1981.
7. Tavassoli M: Megakaryocyte-platelet axis and the process of platelet formation and release. Blood 55:537, 1980.

Pathologic Changes of Red Blood Cell Membranes in Thalassemia

Eliezer A. Rachmilewitz, MD

MORPHOLOGIC, METABOLIC, AND BIOCHEMICAL CHANGES IN THALASSEMIC RBC MEMBRANES

One of the most impressive observations shared by everyone dealing with thalassemia is the severe morphologic change in the shape and appearance of the red blood cells (RBC), particularly in homozygotes. The poor hemoglobinization of the cells due to the basic genetic defect could not account for the morphologic changes, since the RBC in severe hypochromic anemia due to iron deficiency do not appear so markedly distorted. Ultrastructural studies have provided additional observations on the characterization and magnitude of the pathologic changes in the RBC [1]. The ultimate conclusion from all these studies is that the membrane of thalassemic RBC is severely damaged. The damaged membrane could explain metabolic changes, particularly K^+ efflux, which is the main defect that has been found in cation permeability. These metabolic changes can contribute to additional alterations in RBC shape, such as reduction in size, increased rigidity, and increased resistance to osmotic lysis [2, 3].

What could be the mechanism for the severe membrane changes of the thalassemic RBC? Thus far, there are no available data to suggest a basic abnormality in membrane components in addition to the primary genetic defect in the synthesis of one of the major globin chains. Therefore, one must assume that all membrane changes are secondary to the major hemoglobin abnormality, and they may be common to other congenital hemolytic anemias resulting from a primary hemoglobin defect, such as sickle cell disease.

Several changes in the intracellular environment of the thalassemic RBC may account for some of the membrane defects that have been observed and characterized. One possible factor could be excess production of free-oxygen radicals, which are highly deleterious to all cellular and membrane components. Autoxidation of the unstable hemoglobin subunits to precipitated hemichromes can gen-

Birth Defects: Original Article Series, Volume 18, Number 7, pages 219–222
© 1982 March of Dimes Birth Defects Foundation

erate excess free-oxygen radicals, of which the hydroxyl radical seems to be the most active and potent [4]. Moreover, the large intracellular excess of iron which has been found within thalassemic RBC [5], probably resulting from the denaturation of the unstable hemoglobin chains, can serve as a potent catalyst of lipid membrane peroxidation by reacting with unsaturated fatty acids to form peroxide and ferric iron. The lack of normal quantities of hemoglobin concentration (MCHC), which can serve as a substrate for the potent oxygen radicals, could result in an easier excess of the free radicals to oxidize several membrane components.

While the exact deleterious role of free radicals has yet to be verified, evidence for peroxidative damage to the lipid component of the thalassemic RBC membrane has been documented by the following observations: 1) increased levels of malonyldialdehyde (MDA), a secondary breakdown product of lipid peroxidation, following exogenous oxidant stress [6], 2) lower percentage of phosphatidylethanolamine, and 3) a considerable decrease in the level of the unsaturated arachidonic acid while the level of the saturated palmitic acid was slightly higher than the controls [7].

Following the same oxidant stress used to generate MDA, cross-linking of several membrane proteins was more prominent in the sodium dodecyl sulfate gel of thalassemic RBC [8]. In addition, the number of titratable sulfhydryl groups was significantly decreased to 50% in thalassemic RBC membranes [9]. These data indicate that membrane proteins were also peroxidized, although the evidence is less convincing when compared to the lipids.

Further support for the idea of peroxidative damage to the thalassemic RBC membrane emerged from the finding of markedly decreased serum vitamin E levels, which protects a nonenzymatic attack of molecular oxygen on polyunsaturated fatty acids, mainly in untransfused patients with β-thalassemia intermedia [10]. In view of negative evidence for dietary insufficiency or malabsorption of the vitamin, it is conceivable that the low serum levels could result from increased consumption, which is required for neutralization of free-oxygen radicals, and their deleterious effects on the RBC membrane. Daily administration of large doses of vitamin E for several months failed to change significantly the pretransfusion hemoglobin levels and transfusion requirements, although MDA levels decreased and some inconsistent prolongation of RBC survival has been observed in the treated patients [10]. It seems, therefore, that vitamin E by itself is insufficient to correct the variable changes in the thalassemic RBC membrane. Nevertheless, vitamin E administration is recommended to replenish the empty reservoirs and to prevent additional changes that might be attributed to the deficiency by itself.

ALTERATIONS IN THALASSEMIC RBC MEMBRANE AS A MODEL FOR AGING NORMAL RBC

The process of aging of normal RBC is associated with a loss of 10–20% of membrane sialic acids (SA). Whether the removal of SA and exposure of new antigenic sites on the surface of the RBC is a major factor, resulting in their eventual phagocytosis, has still to be determined [11]. Thalassemic RBC, as well as other congenital hemolytic anemias with a higher percentage of young RBC in the peripheral circulation, were found to have a 25% decrease in their membrane SA content [12]. Moreover, the SA residues are distributed in an uneven manner along the membrane and are less abundant when compared to normal RBC [13]. The loss of SA was located on the receptor domain of glycophorin(s) on the outer surface of the membrane and occurred after the younger RBC emerged from the bone marrow into the peripheral blood [12]. The mechanism of the SA changes is presently still unknown. A possible indirect etiologic relationship may be connected to the excess of intracellular free-oxygen radicals. On the other hand, extracellular factors in the serum or in macrophages and endothelial cells may be responsible for these changes. However, regardless of the cause of the decrease and uneven distribution of the SA along the RBC membrane, the average phagocytosis of thalassemic RBC from splenectomized patients by mouse macrophages was 22-fold higher than that of normal RBC [14]. Human macrophages also showed a tendency to phagocytize thalassemic RBC more readily [15]. In a recent study, it was shown that thalassemic RBC bear autologous IgG antibodies, with antigalactosyl specificity on their surface. These antibodies were also found to be present in normal as well as in thalassemic serum. When SA residues are decreased, the new exposed antigenic site is galactose, which is recognized by the natural antigalactosyl antibody in the serum (U. Galili et al, unpublished observations). This RBC antibody complex then becomes bound to human macrophages via an Fc receptor [16]. This mechanism could also apply to the physiologic process of aging of normal RBC. Ways and means to correct the SA defect in young pathologic RBC have yet to be explored.

In summary, the RBC membrane in thalassemia and in other congenital hemolytic anemias is severely damaged. The damage affects all membrane components. While excess formation of intracellular free-oxygen radicals can account for alterations in membrane lipids and proteins, and for the low serum vitamin E levels, it does not explain the decreased levels of SA that have been found. The latter changes could be the underlying mechanism by which macrophages recognize and phagocytize the damaged cells, and result in the shortened survival of the RBC in the peripheral circulation.

REFERENCES

1. Polliack A, Rachmilewitz EA: Ultrastructural studies in β thalassaemia major. Br J Haematol 24:319, 1973.
2. Vettore L, Falezza GC, Cetto GL, De Mateis ML: Cation content and membrane deformability of heterozygous β thalassemic red blood cells. Br J Haematol 27:429, 1974.
3. Gunn RB, Silvers DN, Rosse WF: Potassium permeability in β thalassemia minor red blood cells. J Clin Invest 51:1044, 1972.
4. Brunori M, Falcioni G, Fiorreti E, Giardina B, Rotilio J: Formation of superoxide in the autoxidation of the isolated α and β chains of human hemoglobin and its involvement in hemichrome precipitation. Eur J Biochem 54:99, 1975.
5. Bauminger ER, Cohen SG, Ofer S, Rachmilewitz EA: Quantitative studies of ferritin-like iron in red blood cells of thalassemia, sickle cell anemia and hemoglobin Hammersmith, using Mossbauer spectroscopy. Proc Natl Acad Sci USA 76:939, 1979.
6. Stocks J, Offerman EL, Modell CB, Dormandy TL: The susceptibility to autoxidation of human red cell lipids in health and disease. Br J Haematol 23:713, 1972.
7. Rachmilewitz EA, Lubin BM, Shohet SB: Lipid membrane peroxidation in β thalassemia major. Blood 47:495, 1976.
8. Kahane I, Shifter A, Rachmilewitz EA: Cross-linking of red blood cell membrane proteins induced by oxidative stress in β thalassemia. FEBS Lett 85:267, 1978b.
9. Kahane I, Rachmilewitz EA: Alterations in red blood cell membrane and the effect of vitamin E on osmotic fragility in β thalassemia major. Isr J Med Sci 12:11, 1976.
10. Rachmilewitz EA, Shifter A, Kahane I: Vitamin E deficiency in β thalassemia major. Blood 47:495, 1976.
11. Durocher JR, Payne RC, Conrad ME: Role of sialic acids in erythrocyte survival. Blood 45:11, 1975.
12. Kahane I, Ben-Chetrit E, Shifter A, Rachmilewitz EA: The erythrocyte membranes in β thalassemia: Lower sialic acid levels in glycophorin. Biochem Biophys Acta 596:10, 1980.
13. Kahane I, Polliack A, Rachmilewitz EA, Bayer EA, Skutelsky E: Distribution of sialic acids on the red blood cell membrane in β thalassaemia. Nature 271:674, 1978.
14. Knyszynski A, Dannon D, Kahane I, Rachmilewitz EA: Phagocytosis of nucleated and mature β thalassaemic red blood cells by mouse macrophages in vitro. Br J Haematol 43:251, 1979.
15. Rachmilewitz EA, Treves A, Treves AJ: Susceptibility of thalassemic red blood cells to phagocytosis by human macrophages in vitro. Ann NY Acad Sci 344:314, 1980.
16. Kay MMB: Role of physiologic autoantibody in the removal of senescent human red cells. J Supramol Struct 9:555, 1978.

Comparison of Sickle Cell $\beta°$-Thalassemia and Sickle Cell β^+-Thalassemia in Black Populations

Graham R. Serjeant, MD, FRCP, **and Beryl E. Serjeant,** FIMLS

Two forms of β-thalassemia genes are commonly recognized in black populations, the β^+-thalassemia gene resulting in a decreased synthesis of β-chains and the $\beta°$-thalassemia gene associated with absence of β-chain synthesis. Inheritance of these genes along with that for sickle hemoglobin results in the formation of sickle cell β^+-thalassemia (Sβ^+-thalassemia), and sickle cell $\beta°$-thalassemia (S$\beta°$-thalassemia), respectively. Sβ^+-thalassemia in black populations is generally associated with 18–30% Hb A, resulting in a mild condition, whereas the absence of normal β-chains and hence of Hb A in S$\beta°$-thalassemia results in a condition which is electrophoretically, hematologically, and clinically similar to homozygous sickle cell (SS) disease. The extent of clinical and hematologic differences in the two conditions does not appear to be widely recognized and the experience in Jamaican black patients with Sβ^+-thalassemia and S$\beta°$-thalassemia is therefore reviewed.

PATIENTS AND METHODS

The patients attended the sickle cell clinic at the University Hospital of the West Indies and a group of peripheral sickle cell clinics operated by the staff of the MRC Laboratories. There were 59 patients (30 male, 29 female) with S$\beta°$-thalassemia with ages ranging from 5–62 years (median age 14 years), and 76 patients (34 male, 42 female) with Sβ^+-thalassemia with ages ranging from 5–70 years (median age 22 years). Patients below 5 years were excluded in order to avoid the rapid age-related changes in Hb F levels and red cell indices which may occur in this age group.

The diagnosis of S$\beta°$-thalassemia was based on the presence of only Hbs S, F, and A_2 on hemoglobin electrophoresis, on cellulose acetate, and agar gel, and the demonstration of the β-thalassemia trait in a parent or offspring in 48 of the 59 patients. In the 11 patients without confirmation by family study the diagnosis was based on Hb A_2 levels over 5.0% in 8 patients, and α/β-globin chain ratios of 1.15 or greater in the remaining 3 patients with Hb A_2 levels below 5.0%. The

Birth Defects: Original Article Series, Volume 18, Number 7, pages 223–229
© 1982 March of Dimes Birth Defects Foundation

diagnosis of Sβ^+-thalassemia was based on the characteristic electrophoretic pattern with hemoglobin bands in the position of Hbs A, F, S, and A_2, with Hb A representing between 18–30% of the total hemoglobin on elution or column chromatography. A subgroup of patients with Hb A levels between 5–15% had all inherited the β-thalassemia gene from Indian ancestors; these were excluded as being unrepresentative of Sβ^+ in black populations. Of the 76 patients with Sβ^+-thalassemia, the diagnosis was supported by the finding of the β-thalassemia trait in a parent or offspring in 46 patients.

Hemoglobin (Hb), red cell count (RBC), and mean cell volume (MCV) were measured in an electronic cell counter (Coulter ZBI6, Coulter Electronics, Hialeah, Florida) regularly calibrated with a commercial standard (Coulter 4C, Coulter Electronics). Packed cell volume (PCV) was measured by the microhematocrit after 5 minutes centrifugation at 12,000 g. Mean cell hemoglobin concentration (MCHC) was calculated from the Hb and PCV, and mean cell hemoglobin (MCH) from the Hb and RBC. Reticulocytes were counted as a proportion of 500 red cells after 30 minutes incubation with brilliant cresyl blue and irreversibly sickled cells (ISCs) counted as described by Serjeant et al [1]. Hb A_2 was measured by elution after electrophoresis on cellulose acetate, as described by Millard et al [2] and Hb F by the alkali denaturation method of Betke et al [3]. Hematologic analyses were based on mean steady-state values and their distributions in the two genotypes were compared by Student's *t* test. This statistical procedure assumes indices to be normally distributed and, as the frequency distributions of Hb F, and reticulocytes, were positively skewed, the transformed values $\log_e$ (%Hb F + 4), and $\log_e$ (%retics + 1), were used to give approximately normal distributions. The constants 4, and 1 added before taking logarithms, were chosen to improve the approximation.

Clinical data were obtained by retrospective review of the patients' dockets and the frequency of clinical features in the two genotypes was compared using the χ^2 test or the difference between normal distributions assessed by the Student's *t* test.

RESULTS

Modes of presentation of the two genotypes (Table 1) indicated the most common presenting manifestation to be episodes of bone pain, the mean age of presentation with this complication being 8.2 years in Sβ°-thalassemia and 13.2 years in Sβ^+-thalassemia. In the 76 patients with Sβ^+-thalassemia not diagnosed by neonatal screening, the diagnosis was made by family study, or incidental to other conditions in 17 (26%).

The clinical features in 59 patients with Sβ°-thalassemia and in 71 patients with Sβ^+-thalassemia, in whom adequate documentation was available, are compared in Table 2. Leg ulceration, hepatomegaly, and splenectomy were all more common in Sβ°-thalassemia. Puberty was more delayed and pregnancies were less common in this sample of patients with $S\beta°$-thalassemia. Painful crisis appeared to affect equal proportions of patients in the two genotypes, but more patients were admitted to hospital for painful crises and the number of admissions per patient admitted appeared greater in $S\beta°$-thalassemia. The extent of these differences was likely to have been reduced by the greater mean age of patients with $S\beta^+$-thalassemia and the prevalence of severe painful crisis has

TABLE 1. Modes of Presentation of $S\beta^+$-Thalassemia and of $S\beta°$-Thalassemia

Mode of Presentation	$S\beta°$-Thalassemia	$S\beta^+$-Thalassemia
Painful crisis	36 (61%)	37 (52%)
Family study	3 (5%)	13 (18%)
Incidental	2 (3%)	4 (6%)
Pneumonia	3 (5%)	4 (6%)
Pallor	6 (10%)	0
Diagnosed at birth	6 (10%)	5 (7%)
Other	3 (5%)	8 (11%)
Total	59 (99%)	71 (100%)

Figures in parentheses refer to percentages within genotypes.

TABLE 2. Comparison of Some Clinical Features in $S\beta°$-Thalassemia and in $S\beta^+$-Thalassemia

	$S\beta°$-Thalassemia (59)	$S\beta^+$-Thalassemia (71)	Significance
Painful crisis			
Patients affected	47 (80%)	54 (75%)	NS
Patients admitted	24 (44%)	14 (19%)	$p < 0.01$
Adm/pt admitted	77/24 (3.0)	16/14 (1.3)	—
Leg ulcers (pts > 10 yrs)	9/40 (23%)	5/59 (8%)	NS
Acute pulmonary episode	14 (24%)	10 (14%)	NS
Priapism	4/28	0/27	NS
Aplastic crisis	2	0	NS
Proliferative retinopathy	2/21 (10%)	8/44 (18%)	NS
Age at menarche	15.35 ± 1.39	14.18 ± 1.33	$p < 0.05$
No. of pregnancies	18/14 (1.3)	75/31 (2.4)	—
Fetal loss	1/18 (6%)	10/75 (13%)	—
Hepatomegaly 3 cm	6	1	$p < 0.05$
Splenomegaly	17/51 (33%)	22/70 (31%)	NS
Splenectomy	8 (14%)	1 (1%)	$p < 0.05$
Media age	14 years	22 years	—

Number in parentheses at head of column = n except where denominator appears in Table. Denominators for priapism represent total males; for proliferative retinopathy represent all patients with detailed peripheral retinal examination; for pregnancy represent total postpubertal females; and for splenomegaly represent total patients not subjected to splenectomy.

TABLE 3. Comparison of Rates for Hospital Admissions for Painful Crisis in the 2 Genotypes, Expressed as Admissions/100 Observation Years

	Sickle Cell $\beta°$-Thalassemia			Sickle Cell β^+-Thalassemia		
Age Group (years)	Total Admissions	Observation Years	Admissions/100 Observation Years	Total Admissions	Observation Years	Admissions/100 Observation Years
0–9	26	495	5.25	6	635	0.94
10–19	18	293	6.14	3	459	0.65
20–29	25	145	17.24	6	259	2.32
30–39	8	66	12.12	1	134	0.75
40+	0	40	—	0	89	—
Total	77	1039	7.41	16	1576	1.02

been more readily compared by expressing hospital admissions in relationship to the number of observation years (Table 3). From this it may be seen that severe painful crises are most common in the 3rd decade and are consistently and significantly more common in S$\beta°$-thalassemia.

The prevalence of splenomegaly was difficult to compare in the two genotypes because of the higher frequency of splenectomy in S$\beta°$-thalassemia. Of the 8 splenectomies performed in S$\beta°$-thalassemia, 7 were for hypersplenism and 1 for recurrent splenic infarction. The one splenectomy in Sβ^+-thalassemia was for hypersplenism. In those patients not having had splenectomy, splenomegaly tended to be of greater size in S$\beta°$-thalassemia (mean size 3.3 cm below costal margin in S$\beta°$-thalassemia, 2.0 cm in Sβ^+-thalassemia), and a spleen $\geq$ 4 cm occurred in 7/17 patients with S$\beta°$-thalassemia compared with 2/22 patients with Sβ^+-thalassemia ($\chi^2 = 5.56$, $p < 0.05$). However, the age patterns of splenomegaly also differed in the 2 groups, those in S$\beta°$-thalassemia resembling that seen in SS disease with a high prevalence (61%) in the 1st decade, and falling in subsequent decades. In Sβ^+-thalassemia, on the other hand, splenomegaly was not observed in children under 10 years in this cross-sectional study except for one child requiring splenectomy at 9. It reached a high prevalence (39%) in the 2nd decade, and remained at 27% in subsequent decades.

Growth in height and weight during childhood and adolescence did not show any significant difference between the genotypes although only small numbers of observations were available. Patients aged 17 years and over showed no difference in height, although male patients with S$\beta°$-thalassemia were of generally lower weight (Fig. 1).

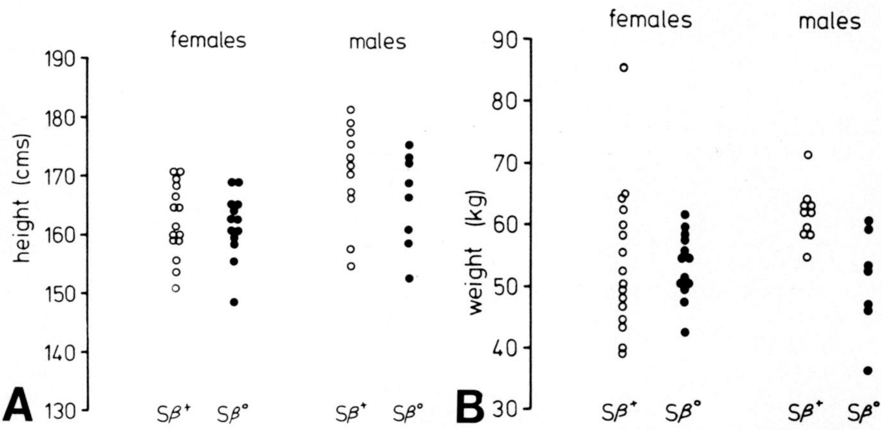

Fig. 1. A) Height in adult patients with Sβ^+-thalassemia and S$\beta°$-thalassemia. B) Weight in adult patients with S$\beta°$-thalassemia and Sβ^+-thalassemia.

Hematologic indices in the 2 genotypes are compared in Table 4. Preliminary analysis indicated that significant sex-related differences within genotypes did not occur except in Hb A_2 levels in Sβ^+-thalassemia (males 4.83 ± 0.56, females 4.50 ± 0.58; $t = 2.53$, $p < 0.05$); therefore, values in both sexes were pooled for subsequent analysis. Compared to Sβ^+-thalassemia, Sβ°-thalassemia manifested significantly higher Hb A_2, Hb F, and reticulocytes, and significantly lower Hb, MCHC, RBC, and MCV. Striking differences were also apparent in ISC counts, levels varying from 0–7% (median ISC count 3%) in Sβ°-thalassemia whereas in Sβ^+-thalassemia no ISCs were visible in 69 patients, and levels of 0.2–3.0 occurred in the remaining 7 patients.

DISCUSSION

These observations require cautious interpretation because of the greater median age of patients with Sβ^+-thalassemia. This has been seen to have diminished the apparent difference in painful crises; severe episodes being markedly more common in Sβ°-thalassemia when expressed in relation to the number of observation years. Qualitative differences in painful crises were also apparent—patients with Sβ^+-thalassemia often admitting to mild episodes of bone pain only on direct questioning and then only in childhood or during pregnancy. The increased prevalence of leg ulceration in Sβ°-thalassemia may also be more marked than apparent in Table 2, although some attempt was made to correct for age differences in the groups by expressing prevalence in patients aged 10 years and over. Similarly, the greater proportion of older patients in the Sβ^+-thalassemia group may have contributed to the apparent increase in this genotype of age-related features such as proliferative retinopathy and the number of pregnancies.

TABLE 4. Comparison of Some Hematologic Indices in Sickle Cell-β° Thalassemia and in Sickle Cell β^+-Thalassemia

	Sβ°-Thalassemia (59)		Sβ^+-Thalassemia (76)		Significance	
	Mean ± SD		Mean ± SD		t	p
Hb A_2 (%)	5.02	0.56	4.66	0.57	3.59	<0.001
Hb F ($\log_e$(%Hb F+4))	2.40(1)*	0.42	2.21(2)*	0.42	2.62	<0.01
Hb (g/dl)	8.85	1.13	11.55	1.27	12.54	<0.001
MCHC (g/dl)	0.318	0.018	0.336	0.013	6.55	<0.001
RBC (X10^{12}/l)	4.03	0.51	4.85	0.49	9.40	<0.001
MCV (fl)	69.3	5.1	73.3	5.2	4.37	<0.001
Retics ($\log_e$(% retics + 1))	2.10(3)*	0.50	1.27(4)*	0.37	11.0	<0.001

*Transformed variables reexpressed as percentages (1) 7.0, (2) 5.1, (3) 7.2, (4) 2.6.

These problems could be avoided by taking an age-stratified sample, but the small numbers of patients available did not generally allow this. Attempts were made to perform valid comparisons on the number of pregnancies in the 2 genotypes, but these reached conflicting conclusions. When observations were restricted to the number of pregnancies to female patients in the 20–29 year age group, there appeared to be no difference, 8 pregnancies occurring in 7 patients with $S\beta^{\circ}$-thalassemia and 10 pregnancies in 9 patients with $S\beta^{+}$-thalassemia. However, when pregnancies were expressed in relation to the number of fertile years observed, there were 18 pregnancies in 172 years (1/9.6 years) in $S\beta^{\circ}$-thalassemia compared to 75 pregnancies in 446 years (1/5.9 years) in $S\beta^{+}$-thalassemia, suggesting that pregnancy was less common in $S\beta^{\circ}$-thalassemia.

Despite these problems in interpretation of results, it is clear that there are highly significant hematologic and clinical differences between the 2 types of $S\beta$-thalassemia, $S\beta^{\circ}$-thalassemia generally manifesting features more similar to those of homozygous sickle cell disease. This is apparent in the greater anemia, greater hemolytic rate reflected in higher reticulocyte counts, greater intravascular sickling reflected in the ISC count, increased prevalence of severe painful crises and leg ulceration, and delay in puberty. The more severe clinical course of $S\beta^{\circ}$-thalassemia is also reflected in the earlier and more frequently symptomatic presentation.

Greater numbers of patients would have allowed more sophisticated statistical procedures and more confident definition of clinical differences, but both these genotypes are uncommon. In Jamaica, $S\beta^{+}$-thalassemia occurs once in every 3,000 births and $S\beta^{\circ}$-thalassemia once in every 6,000 births. The prevalence in adult populations would be further lowered by any excess mortality in childhood. The available results, however, indicate clear hematologic and clinical differences between the 2 genotypes. It is suggested that whenever possible the unspecific term sickle cell β-thalassemia be avoided and replaced by the terms sickle cell β^{+}-thalassemia or sickle cell β°-thalassemia allowing greater clinical specificity.

REFERENCES

1. Serjeant GR, Serjeant BE, Milner PF: The irreversibly sickled cell: A determination of haemolysis in sickle cell anaemia. Br J Haematol 17:527–533, 1969.
2. Millard DP, Mason K, Serjeant BE, Serjeant GR: Comparison of haematological features of the β° and β^{+} thalassemia traits in Jamaican Negroes. Br J Haematol 36:161–170, 1977.
3. Betke K, Marti HR, Schlicht I: Estimation of small percentages of foetal haemoglobin. Nature 184:1877–1878, 1959.

Incorporation of Screening and Genetic Counseling for β-Thalassemia Trait Into Primary Health Care: Effects on Knowledge and Attitudes*

Peter T. Rowley, MD, Lawrence Fisher, PhD, AND Mack Lipkin, Jr., MD

INTRODUCTION

Screening for β-thalassemia trait has frequently been conducted outside the health care system. In the United States, religious, fraternal, or educational institutions have sponsored screening, frequently relying on volunteered professional services and operating on a one-time or episodic basis. In Italy, the government supports thalassemia screening clinics which offer free testing.

Suitable lay sponsors are not available in every community in the United States. Government support for thalassemia screening is not forthcoming in most countries. Therefore, a more general solution to providing appropriate thalassemia screening is needed.

In Rochester, New York, we have asked "Should screening and genetic counseling for β-thalassemia trait be incorporated into primary health care?" We have tried to answer this question by providing screening and genetic counseling for β-thalassemia trait in a large comprehensive health care agency, and by analyzing the effects of counseling on knowledge and attitudes.

We chose a primary health care setting for thalassemia trait screening for several reasons. First, many individuals in developed countries have a primary physician, or access to one. Second, screening by the primary physician may reduce the likelihood of breaching the confidentiality of test results; with results known only to the physician and to the patient, there is little risk of stigmatization or discrimination. Third, the thalassemia trait individual thus found may be more likely to correctly identify the information as having primarily health significance, rather than ethnic or political significance, if identification is by a

*This project was supported by NIH Grant ROI-HL-17465 and the New York State Health Research Council Grants 146 and 664.

Birth Defects: Original Article Series, Volume 18, Number 7, pages 231–241
© 1982 March of Dimes Birth Defects Foundation

health organization, rather than by an ethnic or political organization. Finally, identification by the primary health provider facilitates adequate follow-up.

The primary health care setting that we chose for this project was a health maintenance organization (HMO). An HMO is an organization offering comprehensive health services to a defined population of enrolled members at a cost fixed in advance [1]. Clearly the HMO has an interest in reducing expenditures for medical care. It therefore emphasizes preventive measures, such as multiphasic health screening.

An HMO had three advantages as the setting of this study. First, since in the United States a federally certified HMO must be offered by employers to employees as one choice among health care providers, the membership of an HMO is quite representative of the employed members of the community. Thus, conclusions based upon HMO members are likely to apply to a large segment of the general population. Second, since no test which can be offered on a large-scale basis will detect every heterozygote for thalassemia, it was advantageous to transmit results only to positive subjects, and not to all subjects, as would have been necessary in a program in which subjects were asked whether or not they wished to be screened. Third, since an HMO offers prepaid care on a family basis, referral of other family members for screening could be used as a measure of the value the subject attaches to identification without the barrier represented by the cost of testing. Fourth, since the HMO provides comprehensive care, the total health impact of identification could be monitored.

Heterozygote identification may not be innocuous. Sickle-trait screening in the United States has provided illustrations of many undesirable outcomes. Hypochondriasis, discrimination for purposes of marriage, employment, or insurance, discovery of non-paternity, and overprotection of children by parents are a few examples.

Any medical intervention requires careful assessment of benefits and burdens before adoption as routine medical practice. In this study of thalassemia trait screening in an HMO, we therefore made a careful assessment of burdens as well as benefits by assessing, not only knowledge, but also attitudes of identified subjects.

METHODS

Figure 1 presents the design of the study, which has been described elsewhere [2–4].

Selection of Subjects

The population screened was that of the Genesee Valley Group Health Association which is located in Rochester, New York, and was the first federally certified HMO in New York State. Its subscribers, presently 36,000, are drawn prin-

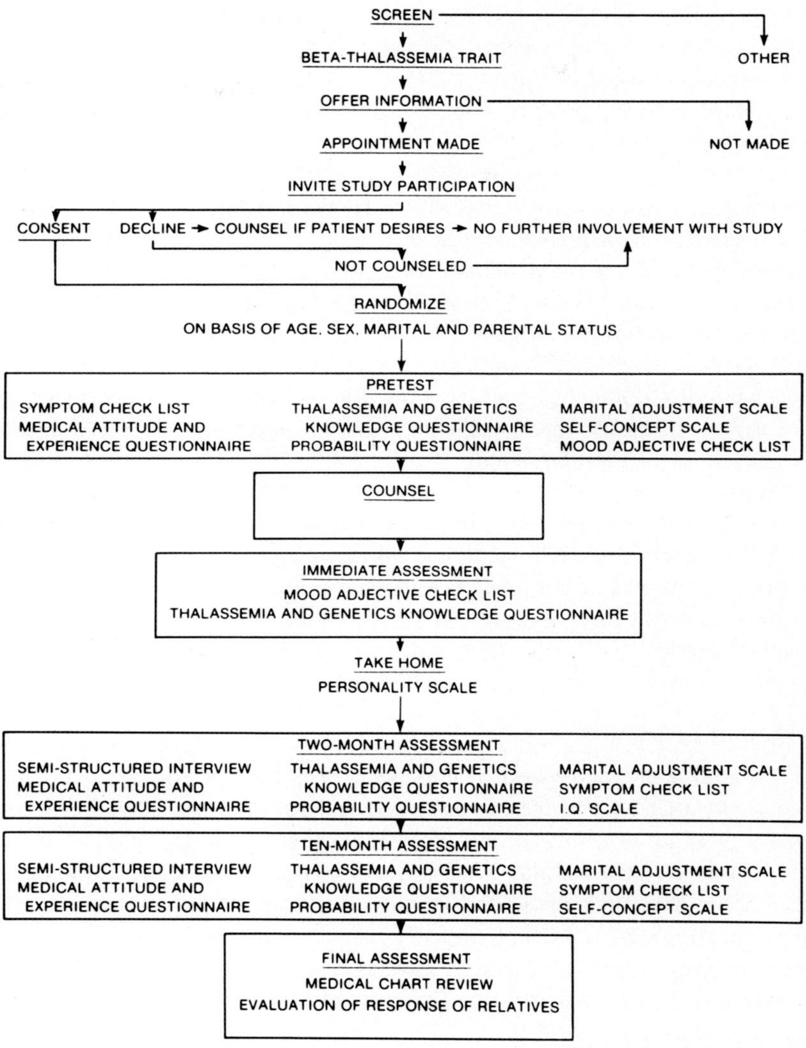

Fig. 1. Flow diagram of project to evaluate screening and genetic counseling for β-thalassemia trait. (From Rowley PT, Fisher L, Lipkin M Jr: Screening and genetic counseling for β-thalassemia trait in a population unselected for interest: Effects on knowledge and mood. Am J Hum Genet 31:718–730, 1979, with permission of the University of Chicago Press.)

cipally from Monroe county (population 711,917; 7.6% of Italian origin), and are representative of the employed population of the region except for an increased proportion of young adults and twice the birthrate of the general population.

All patients, aged 18-65, having phlebotomy for any reason including initial health assessment, were screened for β-thalassemia trait.

Screening consisted of a two-step procedure. In the first step, red cell mean corpuscular volume (MCV) was determined by an electronic cell sizer. On each sample with MCV ≤ 77 [5], Hb A_2 was determined chiefly by DEAE-cellulose microcolumn chromatography with stepwise elution [6].

Each patient with microcytosis and an elevated Hb A_2 (>3.5%) was sent a letter signed by his own HMO physician stating, "We would like you to receive an explanation of your hemoglobin laboratory results. Please contact (project coordinator) at (telephone no.) for an appointment." Most individuals responded promptly. Anyone not responding was sent a second letter and, if still not responding, was telephoned. Every trait patient identified was counseled if their physician did not object to our contacting the patient and the patient agreed to come in, regardless of whether they had been given information about thalassemia prior to our identifying them.

Just prior to counseling, the individual identified was asked to participate in a study of how physicians can best present medical information to patients. In order that subject selection not be biased for interest, neither the name of the condition nor its genetic nature was mentioned in requesting informed consent. It was explained that participation would involve time to complete questionnaires and several return visits. Each was told that, should he decline, he would still be offered the same information.

Selection of Controls

A control population was selected to establish that any changes occurring in counseled subjects were due to counseling and not the psychologic testing, the passage of time, or information from other sources. Control subjects were selected from subjects simultaneously screened from the same population, but found not to have thalassemia trait. Control and trait subjects were matched on the basis of age, sex, marital status, parental status, and education. For the control subject, a film dealing with general health maintenance was substituted for counseling about thalassemia. The same battery of pre- and postcounseling evaluations was performed.

Testing and Counseling

The experimental design involved approximately 2 hours of precounseling assessment, 40 minutes of genetic counseling, 10 minutes of postcounseling assessment, and 2- and 10-month follow-up visits. On the initial visit, following subject consent, baseline information was collected. The 6 questionnaires administered assessed symptoms, medical experience, and knowledge of thalassemia, of genetics, and of probability, marital adjustment, self-concept, and mood.

The patient was then counseled by 1 of 3 methods. Immediately following counseling, mood and knowledge of thalassemia and of genetics were reassessed. The California Psychological Inventory was given to the patient to do at home. The Shipley-Hartford IQ test was administered at the 2-month follow-up visit.

The content of counseling is given in Table 1. This information was transmitted by one of three different methods to be described later.

Follow-Up

At 2 months and again at 10 months after counseling, the patient was contacted by letter and asked to return for assessment. In a semistructured interview he was asked what impact the new knowledge had had on his life. The thalassemia and genetics knowledge questionnaire, health check list, medical attitude and experience questionnaire, marital adjustment inventory, and self-concept scale were also administered.

RESULTS

Results of Screening

The results of screening are shown in Figure 2. Of 21,575 adults screened, 20,855 had a normal MCV. To make certain there were no individuals with an elevated Hb A_2 but an MCV>77, 720 samples with MCV>77 were chosen randomly and tested, all had normal Hb A_2 values. Thus, we have confirmed the result in a smaller previous study [5] that microcytosis is a satisfactory screening criterion for individuals with an elevated Hb A_2.

TABLE 1. Information Provided at Counseling

Names for the condition:	Thalassemia
	Mediterranean anemia
	Cooley anemia
Two forms of thalassemia:	
Trait:	Detected by a blood test
	Mild anemia common
	Usually without symptoms
	Inherited from one parent
Major:	Severe anemia
	Growth often slow
	Appearance often abnormal
	Transfusions required
	Life shortened
	Both parents have trait
Risk to each offspring of trait individual:	If mate is normal
	50% trait + 50% normal
	If mate has trait,
	25% normal + 50% trait + 25% MAJOR

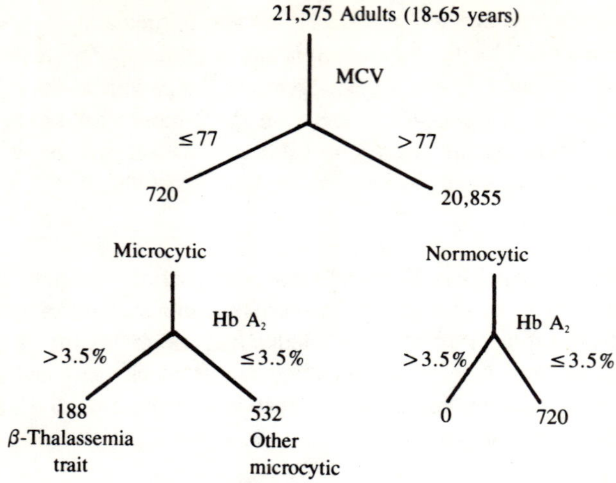

Fig. 2. Results of 2-step screening procedure for β-thalassemia trait among phlebotomy samples from patients of health maintenance organization.

Of the 720 who were microcytic, 188 had Hb A_2 values >3.5% and were considered to have β-thalassemia trait. Screening for MCV ≤ 77 reduced the average number of Hb A_2 determinations for each β-thalassemia individual identified from 115 to 3.8.

Of 154 subjects asked to participate in the study, 142 consented, representing a 92% consent rate.

Effects of Counseling on Knowledge

The effects of counseling on knowledge of thalassemia and genetics are shown in Figure 3. Results were similar for knowledge of both thalassemia and genetics. Knowledge of thalassemia for counselees significantly increased compared to controls immediately after counseling and declined only slightly after 2- and 10-month intervals. Individuals who previously knew that they had thalassemia trait had a greater knowledge of thalassemia than did naive subjects prior to counseling, but were not distinguishable by postcounseling scores from those who were previously unaware.

Comprehension following genetic counseling is often disappointing, as shown in many studies of retrospective counseling [7]. Comprehension may be even poorer in counseling following identification in a screening program, since the counselee generally has no affected family member to impress on him the seriousness of the disease. In our study, since screening was not requested by the subject, less interest in the subject matter might be anticipated than in the self-selected subject. In view of this, we tried to maximize learning by a number of

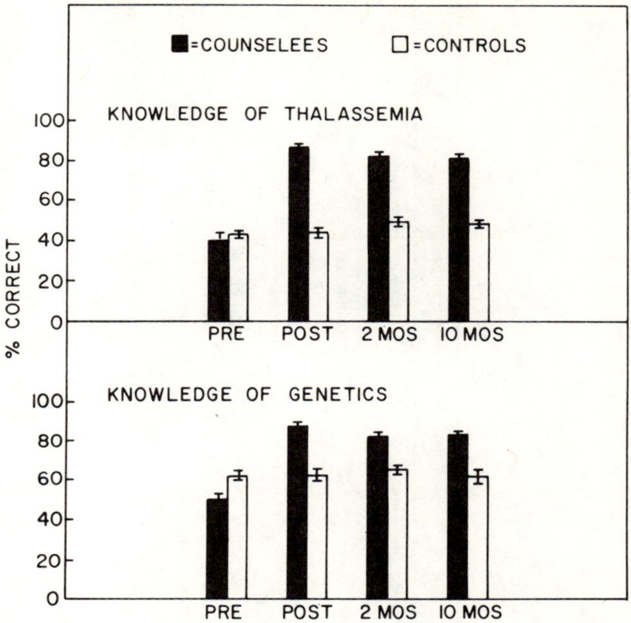

Fig. 3. Effects of genetic counseling for β-thalassemia trait on knowledge: Comparison of counselees and control subjects.

strategies including communicating only the essential information, repetition during presentation, encouragement of learning through questioning the subject, and providing illustrations of random events (eg coin tossing). It is thus gratifying that knowledge increased so markedly following counseling and was largely retained over a 10-month period.

Comparison of Effects of Different Counseling Methods

With emphasis today on containment of health costs, the best counseling method is the most economical one which achieves an acceptable result. We have compared three counseling methods, identical in information presented, viz programmed counseling, conventional counseling, and patient-structured counseling, which are compared in Table 2. *Programmed counseling* employed a specially produced color videotape depicting an actual counseling session by a physician in which the counselee readily understood the information presented, and indicated intent to use it, with interspersed comments by a narrator. Active learning was promoted by questions on the tape directed at the viewer, followed by intervals for recording answers. Following viewing, the patient had an opportunity to question the physician-counselor. In the *conventional counseling*

TABLE 2. Counseling Methods Compared

	Programmed	Conventional	Patient-structured
Structure	Self-instruction	Determined by interviewer	Determined by patient
Sequence	Fixed	Flexible	Flexible
Dealing with facts	Exclusively	Exclusively	Not exclusively
Dealing with feelings	Not done	Not done	Yes
Interview style	Programmed	Directed	Open-ended
Primary goal	Learning	Learning	Learning and adjustment
Discussion of alternatives	Without	Structured but complete	Determined by patient

method, the physicians were trained to present the same information in the same order as on the videotape. A physician's training included counseling surrogate patients until the audio recording of his counseling indicated that his performance was similar to the videotape in style, and identical to it in content. In the third method, called *patient-structured* counseling, the counselor followed the patient's lead in terms of the manner and order of presentation of the factual material. In this third method, in addition to relaying factual content, the counselor dealt with how the patient felt about the material and its implications. For this type, the counselors were specially trained physician members of a medical-psychiatric liaison group.

As shown in Figure 4, all three counseling methods gave similar results for thalassemia knowledge and for genetic knowledge.

Effects of Counseling on Attitudes

Genetic screening can have deleterious effects. Following sickle screening some identified individuals have developed hypochrondiacal complaints, marital problems, or an impaired self-image.

No such deleterious effects were observed in this study. As shown in Table 3, there was no increase in health complaints, no decrease in sexual frequency/satisfaction or in marital adjustment, and no change in perception of self.

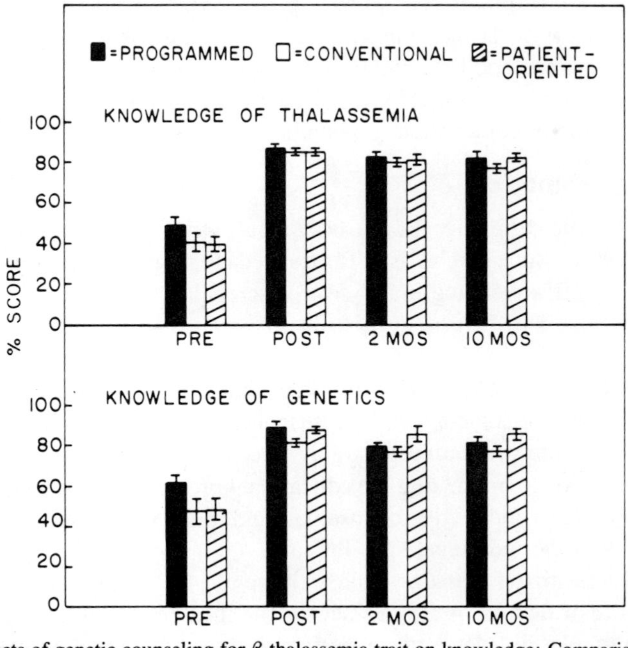

Fig. 4. Effects of genetic counseling for β-thalassemia trait on knowledge: Comparison of 3 counseling methods.

TABLE 3. Effects of Counseling on Attitudes

Parameter	Measure	Significant Change
Health complaints	Cornell Health Index	No increase
Sexual frequency/satisfaction	Special questionnaire	No decrease
Marital adjustment	Special questionnaire	No decrease
Perception of self	Tennessee Self-Concept Scale	No change

DISCUSSION

Screening Procedure

The two-step screening method originally proposed by Pearson et al [5] involving first a mean corpuscular volume determination and, second, a Hb A_2 determination if the MCV were low, is here validated on a much larger sample. In our population, an MCV cut-off value of 77 is satisfactory, does not miss any subjects with high Hb A_2, and reduces the number of Hb A_2 determinations necessary by 97%.

Learning

Learning was excellent. Mean postcounseling scores for nearly all subjects were satisfactorily high. Retention was prolonged. This finding is especially significant in view of the fact that individuals did not ask to be screened.

We attribute these good results to reducing the amount of information transmitted to the essentials, to making its presentation maximally clear, and to the use of visual aids to demonstrate probability and inheritance.

Counseling Method

We found little difference in the three counseling methods compared. The finding that a videotape can be used for the pedagogic part of carrier counseling promises a significant saving in the cost of screening.

Side Effects

Although other carrier screening programs have been plagued by undesirable side effects such as misunderstanding, misconceptions of ill health, discrimination and the like, our program was largely free of these problems. We think that this was due in part to optimizing the educational program, to ensuring confidentiality of results, to nondirective counseling, and to the integration of the screening process with the individual's health care.

Whether screening for thalassemia trait should be widely adopted depends upon a number of factors. A major factor is the incidence of thalassemia trait in the population. We did not find deleterious effects even though permission to screen was not solicited in advance. This may be due to the special character of the HMO in which individuals expect to be screened for conditions not individually specified.

Future

Since this program began, safe and accurate prenatal diagnosis for thalassemia major has become possible through DNA restriction fragment analysis [8]. This makes it possible for most trait individuals for whom termination of pregnancy is acceptable to have only healthy children. We are currently planning an analysis of the benefits and burdens of carrier screening during pregnancy.

REFERENCES

1. Saward EW, Fleming S: Health maintenance organizations. Sci Am 243:47–53, 1980.
2. Rowley PT, Fisher L, Lipkin M Jr: Screening and genetic counseling for β-thalassemia trait in a population unselected for interest: Effects on knowledge and mood. Am J Hum Genet 31:718–730, 1979.
3. Fisher L, Rowley PT, Lipkin M Jr: Predicting immediate outcomes of genetic counseling following genetic screening. Soc Biol 26:289–301, 1979.
4. Fisher L, Rowley PT, Lipkin M Jr: Genetic counseling for β-thalassemia trait following health screening in a health maintenance organization: Comparison of programmed and conventional counseling. Am J Hum Genet 33:987–994, 1981.
5. Pearson HA, O'Brien RT, McIntosh S: Screening for thalassemia trait by electronic measurement of mean corpuscular volume. N Engl J Med 288:351–353, 1973.
6. Huisman THJ, Schroeder WA, Brodie AN, Magneson SM, Jakway J: Microchromatography of hemoglobins, III. A simplified procedure for the determination of hemoglobin A_2. J Lab Clin Med 86:700–702, 1975.
7. Shaw MW: Review of published studies of genetic counseling: A critique. In Lubs HA, de la Cruz F (eds): "Genetic Counseling." New York: Raven Press, 1977, pp 35–52.
8. Kazazian HH, Phillips JA III, Boehm CD, Vik TA, Mahoney MJ, Ritchey AK: Prenatal diagnosis of β-thalassemia by amniocentesis. Blood 56:926–930, 1980.

The Control of Genetic Disease by Carrier Screening and Antenatal Diagnosis: Social, Ethical, and Medicolegal Issues*

Michael M. Kaback, MD

INTRODUCTION

The availability of a simple, accurate, and relatively inexpensive method for the detection of heterozygous carriers of a specific recessive trait, and the option of antenatal detection of the homozygous condition early in fetal gestation provide the foundations for one approach to "prospective control" of selected autosomal recessive conditions. Carrier screening among individuals of reproductive age should enable identification of at-risk couples (both partners: carriers) prior to the birth of index cases. Subsequent monitoring of all pregnancies to such couples could provide a method of "genetic disease prevention" and, simultaneously, enable at-risk families to have unaffected children selectively (assuming they would elect to terminate pregnancies in which the fetus is found to be affected). This possibility is further enhanced if the disorder in question tends to occur predominantly in a defined subpopulation. In practical terms, this greatly limits the extent of carrier screening which is required to gain optimal disease control.

In 1970, the first prospective disease control program of this type was initiated — directed to the prevention of Tay-Sachs disease (TSD), a fatal neurodegenerative disorder of infancy, occurring primarily in children of European Jewish ancestry [1,2]. The identification of heterozygous TSD carriers through serum hexosaminidase A quantification can be employed in a highly accurate, automated, and relatively inexpensive fashion [3-5]. Prenatal diagnosis of the homozygous condition is well established [6-8].

*Supported in part by a grant from the National Tay-Sachs Disease and Allied Diseases Association and by a contract from the Maternal and Child Health Branch of the Department of Health, State of California.

Birth Defects: Original Article Series, Volume 18, Number 7, pages 243–254
© 1982 March of Dimes Birth Defects Foundation

In 1970, a pilot program involving multiphasic education, voluntary screening, and follow-up counseling was initiated in the Baltimore, Maryland-Washington, D.C. communities. Extensive efforts were made to involve community, religious, and organizational leaders, as well as physicians in a saturation campaign of community education prior to the initiation of neighborhood-based screening sessions. The media similarly became involved in this genetic education effort. The first screening took place in 1971 [1]. The communities enthusiastically supported the screening, and similarly designed programs soon followed in Montreal and Toronto, as well as in many other North American cities. Within a few years, carrier screening programs had been initiated in more than 40 North American cities as well as in England, Israel, South Africa, Mexico, and Brazil [9].

As of June 1980, approximately 350,000 young Jewish adults have been screened voluntarily (Table 1). Nearly 15,000 heterozygotes have been identified, and more important, 298 couples have been identified as being at risk for this fatal condition in their offspring. None have had children with this disorder previously. A heterozygote frequency in the American Jewish population of 0.034 (1 in 29.7) has been determined. Of 844 pregnancies monitored by amniocentesis through June 1980, 184 fetuses were identified with TSD. All but 6 of these pregnancies were electively terminated, the others resulting in children with TSD, as predicted. There were 652 infants born unaffected with TSD. One child with TSD was misdiagnosed as being unaffected in utero.

The impact of this experience has been considerable. Data concerning new cases of TSD in the North American Jewish population during 1979-1980 indicate that the aforementioned efforts have contributed to a 70-85% decrease in the incidence of this fatal neurodegenerative disorder in the past decade. Whereas in 1970, approximately 50 cases of TSD were identified each year in Jewish infants

TABLE 1. Tay-Sachs Disease: Carrier Screening and Prenatal Diagnosis in 102 Worldwide Centers, 1969–1980

Total Persons Screened	348,117
Total Carriers Identified	14,368
"At-Risk" Couples Identified	298
Number Pregnancies Monitored	844
Tay-Sachs Fetuses Identified	184
Elective Abortions	177
Unaffected Offspring Born	652
Heterozygote Frequency in Jewish Population:*	0.034 1 in 29.7

*Based on California data only: >80,000 screened.

[10,11] only 13 new cases were reported in the North American Jewish population in 1979-80 [12].

SPECIAL ISSUES IN CARRIER SCREENING AND PRENATAL DIAGNOSIS

A number of critical similarities have been identified between issues involved in carrier screening and prenatal diagnosis for TSD with those associated with β-thalassemia prevention [13,14]. The purpose of this report is to further explore certain of those sensitive issues associated with this approach to prospective genetic disease control. Four major areas of consideration will be addressed: technical issues, psychosocial considerations, ethical issues, and medicolegal matters. Again, it is highly probable that considerations of this kind, as identified in TSD screening, will have direct relevance to similar efforts, targeted to different diseases in other populations.

Technical Considerations

Once a carrier detection method and prenatal diagnostic test have been established, it is essential that some *standardization of testing procedures* be established in laboratories carrying out these critical and sensitive determinations. The international experience with Tay-Sachs disease carrier screening has emphasized the need for establishing a specific laboratory facility which serves the major role of maintaining quality control, procedural standardization, and laboratory surveillance. Since methodologies may vary from one laboratory to another, it is of primary importance to establish that each laboratory can accurately identify carriers for the trait involved. This can be achieved through the communication of coded samples at regular intervals to all laboratories involved in such determinations. A central committee for quality control then is able to evaluate the results communicated by each laboratory on "blind" samples. This enables a critical assessment to be made of each laboratory involved and for rapid resolution and correction of problems where they are identified. Table 2 is a summary of results of the most recent quality control study for TSD carrier identification. This involved 41 laboratories including centers in the U.S., Canada, Israel, South Africa, Mexico, Brazil, and Australia. Further interaction of the 5 laboratories (where errors were made) with the International Quality Control Center in California has led to correction of specific methodologic problems in these centers [15].

Another critical technical matter in population screening is that of *manpower requirements*. Since carrier screening and prenatal diagnosis are targeted to sizeable subpopulations, it becomes essential that adequate personnel be available who are appropriately trained and capable of handling both the educational

TABLE 2. TSD Heterozygote Identification (Serum): Quality Control Assessment, 1981

Number laboratories participating	41
Noncarrier identification	
# samples analyzed	264
misidentified as carrier	2
# labs in error	2*
False-positive frequency	0.8%
Carrier identification	
# samples analyzed	205
misidentified as noncarrier	5
# labs in error	3*
False-negative frequency	2.4%
Number labs with no false + or –	36/41

*On retesting, 2 of these 5 laboratories have performed with 100% accuracy; 2 had repeated errors and have desisted from further testing; one dropped out until further methodologic modifications can be made.

phases of the genetic disease prevention program as well as the counseling needs it generates. This, of course, further emphasizes the importance of appropriate training programs and even licensure capability for both laboratory and counseling staff. In the U.S., an American Board of Medical Genetics recently has been established, which, through licensure examination, will certify individuals with appropriate training for genetic counseling positions. A similar structure exists in Canada. While this is, perhaps, a bit grandiose for all countries, it is an important first step in trying to establish a quality control mechanism for the adequacy of community education and carrier-related and prenatal diagnosis-related genetic counseling.

Social Issues

At the outset, before a carrier screening-prenatal diagnosis program is initiated, it is essential that the *goals of such an effort be clearly defined,* both by the professionals and within the community where it is targeted. One could envision several potential goals of such an effort. First, one could invoke a carrier screening and prenatal diagnosis program for the purpose of reducing disease, and the health benefits it might provide for individuals and families. A second goal, although distinctly different in implication, is that associated with the conduct of research. A screening program within a population for the purpose of establishing gene frequencies or predicting disease incidence has a definite value as long as that goal is clearly defined for those people agreeing to participate. Third, some have suggested carrier screening and prenatal diagnosis as a way of reducing the "genetic load of deleterious genes" within a population. This unquestionably has a eugenic implication, and one which has not been advocated in any area. When one appreciates that all human beings carry several recessive deleterious genes, the notion of changing the human gene pool by carrier screening and prenatal diagnosis is hardly tenable. In theory, carrier screening and prenatal diagnosis should have little impact, if any, on the frequency of the specified recessive allele in the target population. What is most likely to be achieved is the reduction in the incidence of homozygous disease, with no significant change (or even a slight relative increase) in the frequency of the gene itself within that population [16].

Another major social issue deals with *the mechanism by which such a program should be delivered.* Some have advocated that legislation be passed mandating carrier screening in individuals of the defined subpopulation. Others, both ethically and practically oriented, have strongly advocated an education/voluntarism approach to such an endeavor. The concept of legislated genetic screening raises serious ethical and practical issues [17]. It has been the judgment of many that effective education and voluntary response to screening opportunities is a far better way to proceed. What may be the best solution is mandatory (legislated) programs *requiring* education about human genetics and human genetic disorders in the schools or at the time of marriage, with the option for testing being provided on a voluntary basis.

If voluntary screening is employed, *the community to whom such a program is targeted should play an active role in the planning, organization, and delivery of such an effort.* Certainly, expertise as to the social dynamics of a defined community is best found from within that community, rather than in the "academic center." Experiences with Tay-Sachs carrier screening in many parts of North America have suggested that the excellent response of individuals in these programs has been enhanced greatly by the active involvement of community leaders, who encouraged them to do so.

To whom should carrier testing be targeted? In some instances, carrier screening has been directed to teenagers or to children entering the school system. Of course, such information during early school years has little, if any, relevance to such individuals. Carrier identification only has implications either for mate selection or for reproduction. For this reason, it has been the experience in most of the Tay-Sachs screening efforts to target screening opportunities to individuals of childbearing age (18–50 years). In certain instances, where individuals above or below this age range have requested testing, it has been provided after appropriate counseling. Testing of young teenagers has been associated with some ill effects. In a Montreal, Canada program which tested high school students, there was some "loss of self-esteem" indicated by 4 of 40 young carriers previously identified by that program [18]. Since carrier detection has implications for an individual's reproduction or mate selection, it is the author's opinion that such information should be provided only to that person on their request. Even parental request for testing should not be regarded as sufficient reason to carry out such a test on a youngster. Until further studies have been conducted in this area, carrier screening among children less than 18 years of age (with the exception of those married and/or considering reproduction) should be approached most cautiously.

Whether any significant stigmatization occurs in an individual identified as a carrier of a lethal recessive trait remains open to question. Possible stigmatization may occur within that individual's family or perhaps within the entire subpopulation where screening is conducted. Several follow-up studies among carriers of the TSD gene have not borne evidence of significant stigmatization in any sizeable number of individuals. While initially concerned or upset after learning of their carrier status, follow-up counseling appears to be an effective means of alleviating ongoing anxieties or possible stigmata. In fact, nearly every carrier evaluated 2-3 years after their designation has advocated continuation of the program, and indicated that he/she would choose to be tested again if given that choice [19,20]. In these follow-up carrier evaluations, individuals were not hesitant to speak of their carrier status with relatives or friends. In fact, in many instances, they become the strongest advocates for continued testing within their community.

A different experience was identified with sickle cell trait screening in its early stages [21,22]. Here, many young individuals (tested prior to reproductive years) became confused as to the meaning of being a carrier because of the possible medical significance of sickle cell trait. Certain employers and insurance companies felt that employment might be dangerous for individuals with sickle trait or that increased premiums for health or life insurance were appropriate. Critical education programs and careful follow-up counseling were not, however, strongly emphasized in the early sickle cell screening experience in North America. At least in great part, it is felt that for this reason many of these problems may have resulted.

Ethical Issues

A widely held ethical precept is that *an individual should be appropriately informed* prior to complying to any medical procedure. In so doing, it is implicit that an individual be made aware of the potential hazards and risks (both medical and psychologic) of the performance and outcome of any procedure or test. With regard to carrier screening, this becomes a rather complex matter. Although no one would expect each person screened to have a full knowledge of genetics and its subtle psychologic implications prior to a carrier screening test, it is felt that *a reasonable level of knowledge should be evident* prior to testing an individual. In the Tay-Sachs programs, intensive education always precedes the screening opportunity. Even then, clients are requested to read educational material which designates potential hazard areas, prior to testing. Then an informed consent statement with signature is required from all individuals prior to performance of the test itself. Although some may argue that this does not achieve a truly informed consent, in the fullest sense of the word, it is at least a reasonable effort.

Genetic screening and the resultant information it provides have important potential implications for an individual, his/her family, and other individuals in the community. It is paramount that the *privacy of each individual be protected* and not be intruded upon through inappropriate release of results of carrier screening tests. No release of such information should be made without the clear consent and approval of the tested individual. This issue becomes somewhat complicated when one considers *the familial implications of a positive carrier screening result.* Should the medical facility be responsible for informing other close family members when an individual is identified as a carrier? This potentially creates a conflict between the invasion of privacy of relatives and confidentiality of the tested person. In TSD testing programs, this issue is dealt with by simply providing written information to each identified carrier to give or send to close relatives. This material informs them of their increased risk of being a carrier and instructs them how to proceed to be tested, if they so choose.

From an ethical perspective, it is reasonable that *an individual have the right not to know information about himself.* While this may appear "anti-intellectual," it is clear that one must protect against subtle or even overt coercion forcing people to submit to a carrier screening test. It may be that some individuals would choose not to have this information about themselves for fear of potential anxiety or restrictions of their freedom. This becomes a rather difficult issue when one is presenting a very strong educational campaign to a community and strongly encouraging individuals within that community to submit to the screening test. Subtle and not-so-subtle coercions may develop within families or among friends by which individuals who would choose not to have such information become forced to participate in the screening program.

A basic concern with much of the "new genetics" is that our technologies are giving us enormous capabilities to assess the human organism early in its development. In the instance of carrier screening, we are able to assess the "potential" organism even before it exists. Because of the imperfection of our knowledge, and our inability to effectively treat or cure many of these disorders, the option of prenatal diagnosis has become an acceptable, although imperfect, alternative. This leads us, of course, into the difficult problem of selective termination of pregnancy. Does our technology provide us with sufficient information to judge a pregnancy as not being of sufficient "quality" to go to completion? Who has the right to make such a decision? Does our increasing technical capability to evaluate more and more imperfections in the fetus lead us to a state of intolerance for any imperfection? What would be the implications of such a notion on a society-wide scale? Certain of these questions may be premature at this time, but with the explosive development in technical capability, vis-à-vis fetal diagnosis and screening, such considerations are not entirely unrealistic. Others have raised the question of whether individuals, afflicted with disorders which could have been prevented through prenatal diagnosis and selective abortion, will come to be considered as less-than-equal members of society. Would there be prejudices against those born with conditions which could have been prevented, and what would be the social implications of such attitudes?

An obvious and major concern with this approach is that it is a *secondary form of prevention.* The conception of affected individuals is not prevented in this way, at least in most cases. Rather, it is the use of selective abortion that enables the prevention of births of affected individuals to be accomplished. Some would argue that the fetus has full and equal rights with other individuals in society and, therefore, abortion in itself is ethically unacceptable. In this context, it is not inappropriate to raise the issue of what choices the fetus might make, if, in fact, it were aware of its condition and the impact this condition would have on its own life and on the lives of its loved ones. Although this may seem absurd, it does have merit in an ethical discussion about freedom of choice and fetal rights.

Ultimately, it is hoped that effective therapies or even cures for many of these disorders will be discovered. Such achievements would obviate greatly the use of abortion as a means of disease control. Until that time, however, this alternative remains an important and positive option for those who find this choice acceptable.

Legal Issues

A number of legal actions have been initiated in conjunction with TSD carrier screening and prenatal diagnosis in the U.S. These are listed in Table 3. Although it is clear that legal precepts and practices may vary from one country to another, as well as between regions of the same country, such experiences may have important applications to similar programs in other areas. In a medicolegal

TABLE 3. Reasons for Litigation Associated With Tay-Sachs Disease Carrier Screening and Prenatal Diagnosis

Carrier Screening	
Failure to recommend testing	
Advice not to be tested	
Mislabeling of blood samples:	
Incorrect counseling	
Laboratory error in carrier identification	
Private lab: no assurance of communication of results	
Prenatal Diagnosis	
Laboratory error:	Affected child born
Insufficient controls:	Affected child born
Incorrect interpretation:	Affected child born

context, a *physician has a duty to disclose* hazards, risks, etc to the patient. Accordingly, it has been judged by several U.S. courts that a physician's duty is to inform his Jewish patients of the potential hazards of offspring affected with Tay-Sachs disease in light of their genetic heritage. This has led to several litigations in which physicians were alleged either to have omitted giving such information to their patients or advised them against carrier testing (because of their own misinformation or desire not to make their patient anxious). In both such instances, the patients went on to have children afflicted with Tay-Sachs disease. It may be implied from such judicial decisions that physicians have a responsibility to inform patients in reproductive years, who are of specified ethnic backgrounds, and in which defined hereditary conditions are more common, that they may be carriers of such recessive traits and therefore at risk for such conditions in their children. This would most likely be the case where carrier screening and prenatal diagnostic options were available for the disorder in question.

A second legal issue relates to the *standard of care expected of a physician.* In Western medicine a physician, particularly a specialist, is expected to remain current with advances in his field of practice. Recently, several U.S. courts have ruled that the standard of practice is no longer defined by the immediate community in which the physician functions. Rather, in light of modern communication and transportation, the physician is expected to make services which are available in the "greater community" (ie the state, country) available to his or her patients. Accordingly, it has been found unacceptable, in several judgments, that because amniocentesis, for example, is not available in a small rural community, a physician is not expected to inform his patients of the possible applications of this procedure in an at-risk pregnancy. Needless to say, such a decision has far-reaching implications for genetic medicine, as well as other fields. The local definition of quality-of-care would appear to be no longer acceptable.

As previously mentioned, the notion of *informed consent* has direct relevance to the area of carrier screening and prenatal diagnosis. This notion is of primary importance, not only from a social and ethical perspective, but also from a legal point of view. While the specific definition and requirement of "informed consent" remains enigmatic, it has generally been held in U.S. courts that all information that any "reasonable person" would expect to have before deciding whether or not to undergo a procedure or test should be made available prior to undergoing such a procedure. As mentioned previously, this raises certain dilemmas, particularly for carrier screening. To what extent must one inform an individual volunteering for carrier screening to establish that an informed consent has been obtained? How many potential complications of a procedure, both medical and psychologic, must be identified to achieve a "reasonable level" of understanding? Although this issue is gaining wider and wider attention in Western medicine, it remains obscure at this time as to how this matter will be handled in the courts.

Some of the most complex and difficult issues in this new field relate to the birth of a child with hereditary disease or congenital defect whose birth might have been prevented if appropriate advice, counseling, testing, and/or intervention had been introduced either prior to conception, or during pregnancy. Because of the important predictive power of genetic knowledge, and the available technologies of carrier screening and prenatal diagnosis, there have been several litigations in which an individual, born with a defect or disease, has brought suit *against physicians and others for having wrongfully brought them into life.* The courts initially regarded this concept as an imponderable one and not an appropriate basis for legal action. Recently, however, the California Supreme Court has upheld the legitimacy of a "wrongful life" action brought by a child born with Tay-Sachs disease whose parents were screened in a private laboratory and given incorrect results regarding their carrier status. As yet, this case has not been heard, but the courts have ruled that a wrongful life action is an acceptable basis for litigation in this instance. Needless to say, enormously far-reaching implications can be drawn from such a decision. All individuals involved in interacting with reproductive or prereproductive couples may have responsibilities for the advice and counsel they provide, particularly if insufficient or inaccurate information is conveyed. This may expose them to possible litigation by afflicted offspring for negligence or malpractice which wrongfully leads to their birth. While this is a complex and almost impossible notion, there is definitely a trend in the U.S. courts in the direction of allowing such actions to be taken.

The question of *communicating information to relatives of tested individuals who have been found to be carriers* of a recessive lethal trait previously has been mentioned. Although to date there has not been any specific legal action which has resulted from failure to communicate with such relatives, it is clear that the potential for litigation exists in this area. If an individual, identified as a carrier, fails to communicate the information regarding increased risk to his or her close blood relatives — who then go on to have children afflicted with serious and untreatable disease — it may be held that the physicians involved in screening the initial relative may be found negligent and culpable for not having communicated this high-risk status to the extended family of the original screenee. Whether or not the physician will be held responsible for not having done so, or whether, having done so, he will be guilty of invading the privacy of the other individuals, creates a dilemma of sizeable proportion for the physician in genetic screening. As mentioned previously, the Tay-Sachs program has attempted to counsel each identified carrier to convey essential information to appropriate blood relatives. However, no action has been taken where the identified carrier has chosen not to do so. This could lead to complex legal issues should close relatives give birth to affected children (not having been informed by their carrier relative).

CONCLUSIONS

This report summarizes the experiences of the past decade with Tay-Sachs disease carrier screening and prenatal diagnosis. It looks at the experience from the perspective of important social, ethical, and medicolegal issues which have been identified and which could have clear relevance to other carrier screening programs in different populations. Unquestionably, the experience with Tay-Sachs disease has greatly increased our awareness of these important issues and hopefully has provided at least some modicum of data with which such issues can be appraised. Clearly, differences in other screening programs will exist. However, many similarities undoubtedly are evident. As genetic technology continues to develop, and as new methodologies become available for expanded carrier screening and prenatal diagnostic capabilities, it is likely that other genetic disorders will be approached in the same fashion. In this context, the prototypic aspects of the Tay-Sachs disease carrier screening and prenatal diagnosis experience should prove of continued value.

REFERENCES

1. Kaback MM, Zeiger RS: Heterozygote detection in Tay-Sachs disease: A prototype community screening program for the prevention of recessive genetic disorders. In Yolk BW, Aronson SM (eds): "Sphingolipids, Sphingolipidosis, and Allied Disorders," Advances in Experimental Medicine and Biology. New York: Plenum Press, 1972, vol 19, p 613.
2. Kaback MM, Zeiger RS, Reynolds LW, Sonneborn M: Approaches to the control and prevention of Tay-Sachs disease. In Steinberg AG, Bearn A (eds): "Progress in Medical Genetics." New York: Grune & Stratton, 1974, vol 10, p 103.
3. O'Brien JS, Okada S, Chen A, Fillerup DL: Tay-Sachs disease: Detection of heterozygotes and homozygotes by serum hexosaminidase assay. N Engl J Med 283:15, 1970.
4. Kaback MM: Thermal fractionation of serum hexosaminidases: Applications to heterozygote detection and diagnosis of Tay-Sachs disease. In Ginsburg V (ed): "Methods of Enzymology." New York: Academic Press, 1973, vol 28, p 862.
5. Lowden JA, Skomorowski MA, Henderson F, Kaback MM: The automated assay of hexosaminidases in serum. Clin Chem 19:1345, 1973.
6. Schneck L, Friedland J, Valenti C, Adachi M, Amsterdam D, Volk BW: Prenatal diagnosis of Tay-Sachs disease. Lancet 1:582, 1970.
7. O'Brien JS, Okada S, Fillerup DL, Veat ML, Adornato B, Brenner PH, Leroy JG: Tay-Sachs disease: Prenatal diagnosis. Science 172:61, 1971.
8. Navon R, Padeh B: Prenatal diagnosis of Tay-Sachs genotypes. Br Med J 4:17, 1971.
9. Kaback MM (ed): "Tay-Sachs Disease: Screening and Prevention." New York: Alan R Liss, 1977.
10. Myrianthopoulos NC, Aronson SM: Population dynamics of Tay-Sachs disease. Am J Hum Genet 18:313, 1966.
11. O'Brien JS: Tay-Sachs disease: From enzyme to prevention. Fed Proc 32:191, 1973.
12. Kaback MM, Greenwald S, Brossman R: Carrier detection and prenatal diagnosis in Tay-Sachs disease: Summary experience of the first decade. Pediatr Res 15:1138A, 1981.

13. Kaback MM: Prospective control of genetic disease: Achievements and psychosocial considerations. In Bianco I (ed): "La Prevenzione delle Malattie Microcitemiche." Rome: Minerva Medica, 1981.
14. Modell B, Ward R, Fairweather D: Effect of introducing antenatal diagnosis on reproductive behavior of families at-risk for thalassemia major. Br Med J 1:1347, 1980.
15. Kaback MM, Roy C, Lim J, Greenberg D: The quality of Tay-Sachs disease carrier identification: A worldwide assessment. (Abstract) Proc Am Soc Hum Genet no 197, p 65A, 1981.
16. Motulsky AG, Fraser GR, Felsenstein J: Public health and long-term genetic implications of intrauterine diagnosis and selective abortion. In Bergsma D (ed): "Intrauterine Diagnosis." White Plains: The National Foundation-March of Dimes, BD:OAS VII(5):22, 1971.
17. Lappé M, Gustafson V, Roblin R: Ethical and social issues in screening for genetic disease. N Engl J Med 286:107, 1972.
18. Clow CL, Scriver CR: Knowledge about and attitudes toward genetic screening among high-school students: The Tay-Sachs experience. Pediatrics 59:86, 1977.
19. Childs B, Gordis L, Kaback MM, Kazazian HH Jr: Tay-Sachs screening: Social and psychological impact. Am J Hum Genet 28:550, 1976.
20. Massarik F, Kaback MM: "Genetic Disease Control: A Social Psychological Approach." Los Angeles: Sage Publishers, 1981.
21. Bowman JE: Mass screening programs for sickle cell hemoglobins: A sickle cell crisis. JAMA 222:1650, 1972.
22. Fost N, Kaback MM: Why do sickle screening in children? The trait is the issue. Pediatrics 51:742, 1973.

Fetal Blood Sampling*

Charles H. Rodeck, MD

In the early 1970s, experimental fetoscopy was being performed [1,2] using fairly large endoscopes at laparotomy. A purse-string suture was placed in the uterus and the myometrium was incised down to the fetal membranes. The success rate was not high enough to justify the risks to mother and fetus, and the technique did not find a place in clinical practice. In the mid-1970s, the need to obtain fetal blood became more pressing as the biochemical methods for the prenatal diagnosis of hemoglobinopathies became available. Placentesis [3] and fetoscopic chorionic plate sampling [4] were evolved to obtain fetal reticulocytes for the study of globin-chain synthesis. Another fetoscopic method for obtaining pure fetal blood from umbilical cord vessels was developed [5,6], which greatly simplified the laboratory work. I shall briefly discuss these three techniques and their advantages and disadvantages, and present our results using the third; Dr. Alter will describe the world experience in prenatal diagnosis of hemoglobinopathies.

TECHNIQUES OF FETAL BLOOD SAMPLING

Placentesis

This method [3], also called "blind needling," was widely used at first, but with the advent of fetoscopic methods most centers now use it only occasionally, if at all. The placental site is located by ultrasound, a 20-gauge needle is introduced through the abdominal wall, and a fetal vessel on the chorionic plate is punctured. It can be used for anterior or posterior placentae but has considerable disadvantages. The samples are nearly always heavily contaminated with maternal blood or amniotic fluid or both. A diagnosis can be made on samples containing as few as 3% fetal erythrocytes by enriching methods and/or prior blood transfusion of the mother, but not even this is possible in some 10–15% of pa-

*This work has been generously supported by Action Research for the Crippled Child.

Birth Defects: Original Article Series, Volume 18, Number 7, pages 255–261
© 1982 March of Dimes Birth Defects Foundation

tients in whom the sample may contain no fetal erythrocytes; in these patients the procedure has to be repeated. The other problem is fetal hemorrhage, the main cause of the appreciable fetal mortality. This, initially around 15% can, with experience, be brought down to 9% [7].

Puncture of Chorionic Plate Vessels by Fetoscopy

This technique was reported in 1974 [4]. The Needlescope® (Dyonics, Inc.) was narrow enough to be inserted transabdominally with local anesthesia, and had an acceptably low complication rate. The same vessels are punctured as in placentesis, but the samples are better and the fetal mortality is lower, because 27- or 26-gauge needles are used under direct vision. Pure blood is rarely acquired, but samples often consist of fetal cells in amniotic fluid; frequently, there is also feto-maternal hemorrhage because the needle tip easily passes through the fetal vessel into the intervillous space.

Initially, this technique was used for posterior placentae, and placentesis for anterior placentae. The chorionic plate of the latter is difficult to sample, and it may be damaged on insertion of the trocar and cannula, but experience showed that success was possible in the majority of cases.

Puncture of Umbilical Cord Vessels by Fetoscopy

In our view, a successful method for fetal blood sampling should reliably yield pure fetal blood, and it was clear that a new target was needed. Despite earlier warnings that the cord should be avoided, puncture of its vessels has proved to be most successful, preferably at the relatively fixed points at the cord insertion or the umbilicus. There are a number of advantages in the use of these two sites.

A) Puncture is easier because mobility is less than that of the rest of the cord or the chorionic plate [8].

B) Pure fetal blood can be aspirated from within the lumen of these large vessels. Therefore,

   1) Plasma assays are more accurate [9].
   2) Prenatal diagnosis of hemophilia A and B by coagulant assay of factors VIIIC and IXC is possible, and avoids the need for the more complex immunoassays [10,11].
   3) Methods for enriching fetal erythrocytes, or maternal blood transfusion prior to prenatal diagnosis of hemoglobinopathies can be avoided.
   4) Simpler, more rapid methods such as isoelectric focusing or the Biorex technique [12] can be used for the prenatal diagnosis of hemoglobinopathies.

C) Penetration of the intervillous space is very unlikely, hence there is no contamination with maternal blood, or feto-maternal hemorrhage.

D) Hemostasis is more efficient than at the chorionic plate vessels, and fetal blood loss is minimal.
E) Sampling the cord insertion of an anterior placenta is much easier than the chorionic plate.
F) Direct access to the fetal circulation permits transfusions or other therapeutic possibilities.

The technique of umbilical vessel puncture has been described in detail [6,13].

A Needlescope®, 1.7 mm in diameter is used with a cannula slightly wider than the standard Hobbins cannula to accommodate a 21-gauge blood sampling needle with 26-gauge tip [14]. The patient receives local anesthesia and sedation, and a linear array real-time scanner is used under sterile conditions immediately before and during fetoscopy. The importance of the preliminary scan in selecting the best entry point for trocar and cannula cannot be over-emphasized. The main aims are that cord insertion and/or umbilicus are accessible for sampling, and that the placenta is not perforated. A lateral or fundal introduction is therefore usually chosen.

The most conveniently approached vessel is punctured, whether it be umbilical artery or vein. Immediately beforehand, the dead space of the needle is flushed with normal saline, as amniotic fluid may initiate coagulation. After puncture, an assistant aspirates 1 ml of pure fetal blood, although more could be taken if needed. A particle size analyzer (Coulter Channelyzer) is at hand to confirm the absence of maternal erythrocytes and to estimate the hematocrit. Our criteria of purity of fetal blood have been described [5]. The safety of this technique was assessed by continuous fetal heart rate monitoring during umbilical vessel puncture, and by histologic examination of the cord after fetoscopy [15]. The results were reassuring and have been confirmed by experience with over 400 diagnostic procedures.

RESULTS

Two hundred and fourteen patients were referred for prenatal diagnosis of a hemoglobinopathy, 7 of whom had twin pregnancies. The indications are shown in Table 1. A diagnosis was made in 213 patients (Table 2) by fetoscopy; placentesis has not been used. In one patient a sample was not obtained; the fetus died soon after the procedure due to retroplacental hemorrhage (see below). It was aborted one week later and postmortem blood could not be taken.

In Table 3, the results in the first 100 patients (early series) are presented. An adequate sample was obtained in all but the patient mentioned above, and in 89, the sample was pure fetal blood. One repeat fetoscopy was necessary in 6 patients because of borderline results or laboratory problems.

TABLE 1. Prenatal Diagnosis of Hemoglobinopathies by Fetoscopic Blood Sampling

Fetus At Risk for		No. of Patients
β-Thalassemia		195
Sickle Cell Disease		12
Sickle/Thalassemia		6
β-Thalassemia/Hb Pylos		1
	Total	214
		(Includes 7 twin pregnancies)

TABLE 2. Prenatal Diagnosis of Hemoglobinopathies by Fetoscopic Blood Sampling

Diagnosis made in 213 out of 214 patients	
Homozygous affected	49
Heterozygous	111
Homozygous normal	53

TABLE 3. Results in the First 100 Patients

No. of patients	100	
Procedure repeated once	6	
Adequate sample	99	
Pure fetal blood	89	
Failure to obtain sample	1	
Fetal loss before result available[1]	2	
Termination of pregnancy	21	
Continuing pregnancies		77
Abortions[2]		2
Late fetal losses[3]		2
Amniotic fluid leakage		5
Induced delivery < 37 weeks		2
Spontaneous delivery < 37 weeks[4]		9
Delivery > 37 weeks		61
Neonatal deaths		0
No information		1

[1] 1 IUD; 1 amnionitis
[2] 1 week after repeat fetoscopy; 26 weeks
[3] severe preeclampsia, abruptio and IUD at 34 weeks; unexplained IUD at term
[4] 1 twin pregnancy; 1 delivery at 32 weeks, the rest at 34-36 weeks; all babies alive and well

Two fetal losses occurred before the results were available: one has been mentioned above, and the other developed amnionitis and aborted 36 hours after fetoscopy. This fetus was heterozygous.

Of the 77 continuing pregnancies, 2 aborted spontaneously. One occurred a week after a repeat fetoscopy, and the other was 6 weeks after an uncomplicated

TABLE 4. Results in the Next 114 Patients

No. of patients	114	
Procedure repeated once	1	
Adequate sample	114	
Pure fetal blood	113	
Failure to obtain sample	0	
Fetal loss before result available	0	
Termination of pregnancy	27	
Continuing pregnancies		87
Abortions[1]		1
Late fetal losses[2]		2
Amniotic fluid leakage		2
Induced delivery < 37 weeks		2
Spontaneous delivery < 37 weeks[3]		8
Delivery > 37 weeks		38
Neonatal death[4]		2
Undelivered		28
No information		8

[1] 2 weeks after fetoscopy
[2] 1 IUD at 30 weeks; 1 fresh IUD (40 weeks, cord around neck)
[3] 2 twins; 6 singletons delivered at 28, 31, and 34 to 36 weeks
[4] 1 28-week twin; 1 abruptio at 28 weeks

procedure. There were 2 late fetal deaths, which were probably unrelated to the fetoscopy. Nine patients delivered before, and 63 after, 37 weeks' gestation and all these babies did well. In one, however, the result was a false-negative: the β:γ ratio at 18 weeks was in the heterozygous range but the child developed β-thalassemia at 6 months of age.

Table 4 summarizes the results in the next 114 patients (late series). An adequate sample was obtained in all, and in 113 it consisted of pure fetal blood; a repeat fetoscopy was necessary in only one patient because of a borderline β:γ ratio.

No fetal losses occurred before the results were available, and of the 87 continuing pregnancies, one aborted spontaneously 2 weeks after fetoscopy. There were 2 late fetal losses: an intrauterine death at 30 weeks' gestation which might have been related to the fetoscopy, but was otherwise unexplained, and a fresh stillbirth at term which was delivered with the umbilical cord wound tightly several times round the neck. Two babies died in the neonatal period: one was a twin delivered at 28 weeks, and the other was also delivered at 28 weeks' gestation following abruptio placentae. The other preterm deliveries, as well as those at term, have resulted in healthy babies. Some are as yet undelivered and follow-up at present is incomplete; no further diagnostic errors have come to light. A

TABLE 5. Comparison of Early and Late Series

	First 100 Patients		Next 114 Patients	
	No.	%	No.	%
Diagnosis made	99	99	114	100
Procedure repeated	6	6	1	1
Pure fetal blood	89	89	113	99
Failure to obtain sample	1	1	0	0
Total fetal/neonatal deaths (% of all patients)	6	6	5	4
Deaths probably related to fetoscopy (% of continuing pregnancies)	4	5	2	2
Preterm labor (Singleton pregnancies < 37 weeks as % of continuing pregnancies)	8	10	6	7
Amniotic fluid leakage (% of continuing pregnancies)	5	6	2	3

small but significant proportion of patients leak amniotic fluid per vaginam; they are more prone to deliver early, but some may go to term without harm to the baby.

In Table 5, the early and late series are compared, although the latter is incomplete in that not all patients have yet delivered. Procedure-related deaths and preterm deliveries are therefore expressed as a percentage of continuing pregnancies. A category of total fetal and neonatal loss is included and is shown as a percentage of all patients, since 2 of the deaths due to fetoscopy occurred before diagnostic information was available. In all the points compared, the later series shows some improvement over the earlier.

CONCLUSION

Fetoscopic puncture of umbilical cord vessels is the method of choice for obtaining fetal blood, particularly if a pure sample is needed for fetal plasma or serum assays. This technique can be used for prenatal diagnosis of thalassemia with a high degree of success and a relatively low complication rate. It will need to be available in the future, even though an increasing proportion of such diagnoses will be made from amniocyte DNA. Access to the umbilical vessels also makes therapeutic intervention possible [14].

ACKNOWLEDGMENTS

The laboratory work was carried out in the Department of Hematology, King's College Hospital, under the direction of Professor J.M. White; initially, generous help had been given by Dr. Bernadette Modell, University College Hospital, and Professor Rosa and Drs. Y. Beuzard and M. Goosens, Paris.

REFERENCES

1. Valenti C: Antenatal detection of hemoglobinopathies. Am J Obstet Gynecol 115:851, 1973.
2. Scrimgeour JB: Clinical experience with fetoscopy. In Kaback MM, Valenti C (eds): "Intrauterine Fetal Visualization. A Multidisciplinary Approach." Amsterdam: Excerpta Medica, 1976, p 150.
3. Kan YW, Valenti C, Carnazza V, Guidotti R, Rieder RF: Fetal blood sampling in utero. Lancet 1:79, 1974.
4. Hobbins JC, Mahoney MJ: In utero diagnosis of hemoglobinopathies: Technic for obtaining fetal blood. N Engl J Med 290:1065, 1974.
5. Rodeck CH, Campbell S: Sampling pure fetal blood by fetoscopy in second trimester of pregnancy. Br Med J 2:728, 1978.
6. Rodeck CH: Fetoscopy guided by real-time ultrasound for pure fetal blood samples, fetal skin samples, and examination of the fetus in utero. Br J Obstet Gynaecol 87:449, 1980.
7. Fairweather DVI, Ward RHT, Modell B: Obstetric aspects of midtrimester fetal blood sampling by needling and fetoscopy. Br J Obstet Gynaecol 87:87, 1980.
8. Rodeck CH, Campbell S: Umbilical cord insertion as source of pure fetal blood for prenatal diagnosis. Lancet 1:1244, 1979.
9. Rodeck CH, Mibashan RS, Peake IR, Bloom AL: Prenatal diagnosis of severe von Willebrand's disease. Lancet 2:637, 1979.
10. Mibashan RS, Rodeck CH, Thumpston JK, Edwards RJ, Singer JD, White JM, Campbell S: Plasma assay of fetal factors VIIIC and IX for prenatal diagnosis of haemophilia. Lancet 2:1309, 1979.
11. Mibashan RS, Peake IR, Rodeck CH, Thumpston JK, Furlong RA, Gorer R, Bains L, Bloom AL: Dual diagnosis of prenatal haemophilia A by measurement of fetal factor VIIIC and VIIIC antigen (VIII CAg). Lancet 2:994, 1980.
12. Blouquit R, Beuzard Y, Varnavides L, Chabret C, Dumez Y, John PN, Rodeck CH, White JM: Antenatal diagnosis of haemoglobinopathies by Biorex chromatography of haemoglobin. Br J Haematol 50:7–15, 1982.
13. Rodeck CH: Fetoscopy at King's College Hospital. In Rocker I, Laurence KM (eds): "Fetoscopy." Amsterdam: Elsevier/North-Holland Biomedical Press, 1981, pp 233–259.
14. Rodeck CH, Kemp JR, Holman CA, Whitmore DN, Karnicki J, Austin MA: Direct intravascular fetal blood transfusion by fetoscopy in severe rhesus isoimmunisation. Lancet 1:625, 1981.

Prenatal Diagnosis of Hemoglobinopathies: Worldwide Experience*

Blanche P. Alter, MD

Prenatal testing for hemoglobinopathies using fetal blood began in July, 1974, in the laboratories of DG Nathan and YW Kan and their respective colleagues. An unofficial International Registry of cases has been maintained for the past 3 years, and the data have been published [1-3]. This report will summarize the most recent Registry update, and also outline new approaches to techniques for testing fetal samples. The techniques for obtaining fetal blood or amniotic fibroblasts, and for analysis of globin chain synthesis or globin gene structure have been described elsewhere [4-9]. So far, almost 2,000 cases have been tested for thalassemia or sickle cell disorders. The birthrate of children with homozygous thalassemia is beginning to decline in parts of Italy, Greece, England, and Cyprus, because of the impact of the combination of population screening, genetic counseling, and prenatal testing. What began as a laboratory research procedure in 1974 has now been transferred successfully to clinical application. Technical improvements are still needed, however, in order to make these tests simpler and less expensive.

FETAL BLOOD REGISTRY

As of March 1981, there were 21 centers using fetal blood for prenatal testing. These are listed in Table 1. Five centers had examined more than 100 cases each, while 4 more had tested from 50 to 100 samples. Of the remaining 12 centers, only 3 or 4 might anticipate studying more than 50 cases each year.

The diagnoses for which samples were obtained are listed in Table 2. A total of 1,856 cases were examined. There were 1,705 at risk for thalassemia (92%). Of these, 1,688 were for β-thalassemia, while the rest were for $\delta\beta$, E/β, α, $\alpha\beta$, and Lepore/β-thalassemia. There were 151 cases at risk for sickle disorders (8%). Of these, 115 were for sickle cell anemia, 33 for sickle/β-thalassemia, 2 for

*Supported by NIH grant HL 26132, and by an Irma T. Hirschl Career Scientist Award.

Birth Defects: Original Article Series, Volume 18, Number 7, pages 263–274
© 1982 March of Dimes Birth Defects Foundation

TABLE 1. Centers for Prenatal Diagnosis of Hemoglobinopathies

>100 cases	<50 cases
Athens	Melbourne, Queen Victoria Medical Center
Sardinia	Sydney, Royal Women's Hospital
London, University College Hospital	Sydney, Prince of Wales Hospital
London, King's College Hospital	Sydney, Crown Street Women's Hospital
New Haven	Montreal
	Toronto–Hamilton
50–100 cases	Jerusalem
	Ferrara
Paris	Milan
Munich	Boston
Rome	Baltimore
San Francisco	New York

(Tables 1, 4, 6, 8, and 11 from Alter BP: Prenatal diagnosis of hemoglobinopathies. A status report. Lancet 2:1152, 1981, with permission.)

SC and 1 for S/O_{Arab}. The preponderance of cases at risk for thalassemia reflects the fact that most of the patients studied came from the Mediterranean area.

Fetal blood was obtained by fetoscopy in 1,252, or 67% of cases, and by placental aspiration in 604 (33%). Most samples were obtained between 18 and 20 weeks gestation, and ultrasound guidance was always employed. Each center defined the adequacy of a sample according to its own criteria (Table 3). The range of the proportion of fetal red cells in an acceptable sample was from 5–40%. A Coulter cell size distribution analyzer was used for immediate analyses by almost all centers; the percent of fetal cells was subsequently confirmed with the acid elution technique of Kleihauer and Betke.

The proportion of adequate samples, as defined by each center, is summarized in Table 4. An adequate sample was obtained on the first attempt in 86% of the cases studied by fetoscopy, and 77% of those by placental aspiration. Two or more attempts were made in most of the unsuccessful cases, and eventually useful specimens were obtained in 97% of cases. In total, 1,791 of the 1,856 cases did provide a sample which could be analyzed.

The proportion of erythrocytes in the sample was higher when fetoscopy was used (Fig. 1). The overall mean was 92% fetal by fetoscopy, and only 57% by placental aspiration. The range of the means for each center was from 68–100% by fetoscopy, and 24–60% by aspiration. Thus, the problem of maternal contamination of samples was much less if fetoscopy were used. The percent of fetal blood also improved significantly as each obstetrician gained experience with fetoscopy. In the first 125 cases previously reported in the literature, fetoscopy

TABLE 2. Fetal Risk

Diagnosis	Number	Per Cent
Thalassemia:	1705	92
β	1688 (99%)	
$\delta\beta$	3	
E/β	3	
α	3	
$\alpha\beta$	5	
Lepore/β	3	
Sickle:	151	8
SS	115 (76%)	
S/β-Thal	33	
SC	2	
S/0-Arab	1	
Total	1856	100

Adapted from reference [3].

TABLE 3. Definition of Adequate Sample

% Fetal	No. of Centers
5	8
10	1
15	1
20	3
40	2

TABLE 4. Adequacy of Sample

Attempts	Fetoscopy (%)	Aspiration (%)	Total (%)
One	1,072 (86)	468 (77)	1,540 (83)
Two or more	115 (9)	136 (23)	251 (14)
Total adequate	1,214 (97)	577 (96)	1,791 (97)
Total cases	1,252 (100)	604 (100)	1,856 (100)

had yielded a mean of 76% fetal cells, and aspiration 53% [4]. Placental aspiration did not improve with experience, perhaps because most obstetricians no longer use that technique.

In those cases where maternal contamination is still a problem, 12 centers reported using selective hemolysis of the maternal cells to purify the fetal sam-

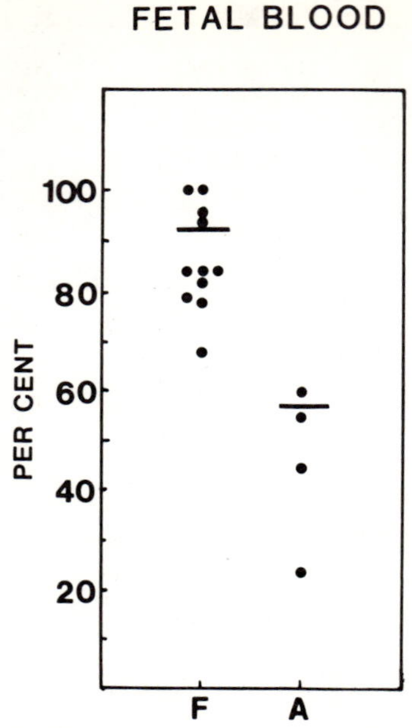

Fig. 1. Percent fetal blood obtained by fetoscopy (F) and placental aspiration (A). The mean for each was obtained by multiplying the means reported by each center (●) by the number of cases studied at that center. Data are incomplete, because not all centers reported their mean values.

ples [10], while 3 used agglutination of fetal cells with anti-i [11], and only one center still suppresses maternal reticulocyte production by transfusion of the mother 1–2 weeks before the fetal blood sampling [6].

The risks of the procedure are outlined in Table 5. Fetal loss rates were initially as high as 15% [6,7], and declined progressively to 9.3% of the first 522 cases, 4.4% of the next 609, and 3.9% of the most recent 725 cases. In addition, the loss rate for all cases studied by fetoscopy was 5.2%, while it was 6.5% by placental aspiration. Thus, the single rapid puncture under direct vision through the fetoscope is slightly less traumatic than the multiple placental aspirations guided only indirectly by ultrasound, but the differences are not statistically significant. Most losses were due to fetal death in utero or spontaneous abortion, with the majority occurring within a week of the procedure.

Additional complications of the procedure included 29 cases of maternal problems, usually benign amniotic fluid leakage. Data on the rate of prematurity are incomplete, because the denominator of total births is not known. The reported premature rate was 5.6% of cases which were not lost or terminated

TABLE 5. Outcome of Pregnancies

Outcome	Fetoscopy (%)	Aspiration (%)	Total (%)
Total cases	1,252 (67)	604 (67)	1,856 (100)
Fetal losses[a]	65 (5.2)	39 (6.5)	104 (5.6)
Cases corrected for terminations and losses	902 (66)	473 (44)	1,375 (100)
Premature births[b]	54 (6.0)	23 (4.9)	77 (5.6)

[a] Losses were 49 of first 522 (9.3%), 27 of next 609 (4.4%), and 28 of last 725 (3.9%).

[b] Premature births not corrected for undelivered cases, because data incomplete.

Adapted from reference [3].

(6.0% following fetoscopy and 4.9% after placental aspiration). In addition, follow-up on the children is clearly both short and incomplete, but no significant birth defects or long-term effects have been reported. Acquisition of this sort of information will require intensive effort by the local centers.

Currently, all 21 centers incubate the small samples of fetal blood with radioactive leucine, prepare globin, and separate the globin chains by chromatography on carboxymethyl cellulose columns in urea. Examples of this technique are shown on the right in Figure 2, and are compared with another method which will be discussed subsequently. Diagnoses are based on the biosynthetic ratio of β/γ globin. These ratios depend on the quality of the β and γ separation on the column, how the baseline is drawn for the determination of the radioactivity in each peak, and whether the pre-γ radioactivity is included in the γ (which we do not do). In our own experience, the mean β/γ in normal fetuses was 0.11, and in fetuses proven after birth to have thalassemia trait, 0.06. We proposed that the cutoff below which β^{o}- or β^{+}-thalassemia major would be most likely was a β/γ ratio of 0.025. In the Registry, 17 centers reported their cutoff: 2 use 0.01, 7 use 0.02, 4 use 0.025, and 4 use 0.03. The lower ratios are in regions where β^{o} thalassemia is prevalent.

The rate of known mistaken diagnoses is less than 1% (Table 6). For thalassemia, there were 11 homozygotes who were not diagnosed prenatally, and 4 fetuses terminated for homozygosity but shown subsequently to be heterozygotes. Most of the false-negative diagnoses in the thalassemia group turned out to have β^{+}-thalassemia. Only one error was made in the sickle group, due to technical problems with the assay [6].

Homozygous thalassemia was in fact predicted in 387 of the 1,671 adequate samples, or 23%, which is close to the 25% expected for an autosomal recessive condition (Table 7). Addition of the 11 false-negatives brings the total proportion of cases of thalassemia major to 24%. In the group at risk for sickle disorders,

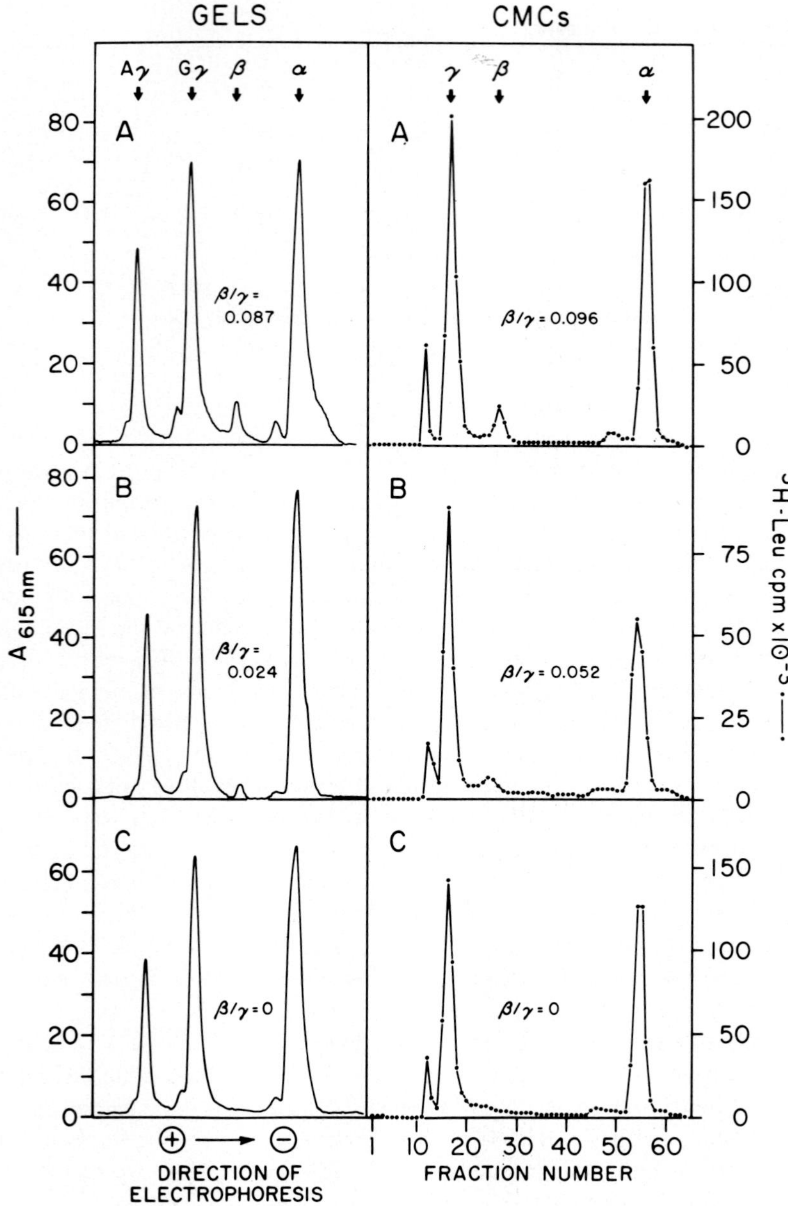

Fig. 2. Comparison of analysis of fetal globin chain synthesis by polyacrylamide gel electrophoresis (left) with carboxymethyl cellulose chromatography (right). A) Normal. B) Thalassemia heterozygote. C) Thalassemia homozygote. (Figs. 2 and 3 from Alter BP et al: Globin chain electrophoresis for prenatal diagnosis of β thalassemia. Hemoglobin 5:357, 1981, with permission of Marcel Dekker, Inc.)

TABLE 6. Errors

Diagnosis	False-Negative (%)	False-Positive (%)	Total/Adequate Samples (%)
Thalassemia	11 (0.66)	4 (0.24)	15/1671 (0.90)
Sickle	1 (0.84)	0 (0)	1/120 (0.83)
Total	12 (0.67)	4 (0.22)	16/1791 (0.89)

TABLE 7. Affected Fetuses

Diagnosis	Number/Adequate	(%)
Thalassemia	387/1,671	(23)
Sickle	18/120	(15)
Total	405/1,791	(23)

TABLE 8. Summary, Fetal Blood (June, 1974 – March, 1981)

	Number	%
Cases: total	1,856	
thalassemia	1,705	92
sickle	151	8
Adequate samples	1,791	97
Affected fetuses	405	23
Errors: false-negatives	12	0.67
false-positives	4	0.22
total	16	0.89
Fetal losses	104	5.6
Premature infants	77	5.6*

* Corrected for terminations and losses.

only 18 of 120 adequate samples, or 15% were predicted to have the disease for which they were tested.

Table 8 summarizes all of the fetal blood data for the current Registry. Of the 1,856 cases tested, 92% were at risk for thalassemia. Overall, 97% of the cases yielded an adequate sample, although the number of multiple attempts required was greater with placental aspiration than with fetal blood sampling by fetoscopy. The fetal loss rate was 5.6% overall, again less by fetoscopy than aspiration. Twenty-three percent of adequate samples were found to demonstrate the disease for which that fetus was at risk. The prematurity rate was approximately 6%, although this is an underestimate.

Analysis of globin chain synthesis by CMC chromatography is expensive, cumbersome, and time-consuming. Several alternative approaches have been proposed (Table 9), although none are currently used to the exclusion of CMC columns. Globin-chain separations may be performed by electrophoresis on polyacrylamide gels [12], cellulose acetate membranes [13], isoelectric focusing [14], or high pressure liquid chromatography [15]. Hemoglobin tetramers can be analyzed by isoelectric focusing [16] or column chromatography [17,18]. Antibodies to fetal and adult Hbs can be used to analyze single cells by fluorescence microscopy or cell sorting [19].

One example of these recent methods is our own use of globin-chain electrophoresis on polyacrylamide gels [12]. ^{3}H-leucine-labeled lysates of fetal blood are electrophoresed, and the gels then processed for fluorography. The x-ray films can be examined visually (Fig. 3), and scanned in a densitometer (Fig. 2 left side). The β/γ ratios are determined by integration of the peak areas. We found that the results from this method correlated well with those from CMC columns. β/γ ratios were slightly lower by gel, and we proposed that samples which gave a β/γ ratio of 0.03 or below on gel should then be analyzed by CMC column chromatography. With sufficiently high specific radioactivity, 12 or more fetal samples can be processed daily, and results available within 3–5 days.

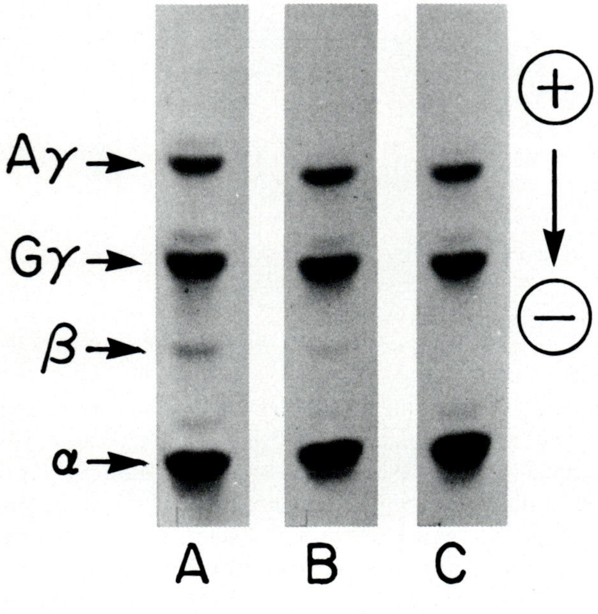

Fig. 3. Fluorograms of globin-chain synthesis analysis by gel electrophoresis. Samples as in Fig. 2.

The time is similar to that required for one set of our CMC columns, but the cost and effort involved for large numbers of samples is much less.

Many hemoglobinopathies may soon be diagnosed by mapping of fibroblast DNA, thus eliminating the need for fetal blood analyses for this purpose (see below). However, the methods for obtaining fetal blood in utero which were developed for the hemoglobinopathies have now been applied to other disorders as well. Some of these are listed in Table 10. They include nonhemoglobinopathic red cell disorders, as well as studies of white cells and plasma factors. Gene mapping techniques cannot yet be applied for those purposes. Thus, obstetricians skilled in obtaining pure fetal blood will not be totally displaced by the gene mappers.

FETAL FIBROBLAST DNA REGISTRY

Several of the hemoglobinopathies can now be diagnosed from studies of the globin genes in fibroblast DNA. For this purpose, an amniocentesis of 20 ml is performed at 16–18 weeks. The fetal fibroblasts are recovered by centrifugation,

TABLE 9. Laboratory Methods

Method		No. of Centers
Globin chain	- chromatography on CMC	21
	- electrophoresis—polyacrylamide gel	1
	—cellulose acetate	1
	- isoelectric focusing	1
	- high pressure liquid chromatography	1
Hemoglobin	- chromatography	2
	- isoelectric focusing	1
	- antibodies and single cells	1

TABLE 10. Applications of Fetal Blood Sampling

Red Cells —	hemoglobinopathies
	blood grouping
	galactosemia
	transfusion
White Cells —	chronic granulomatous disease
	chromosomes
Plasma —	coagulation (VIII, IX, VW)
	$alpha_1$-antitrypsin
	Tay-Sachs (hexosaminidase)

TABLE 11. Summary, Fetal Fibroblasts

Study	Number	%
Total	70	
SS	57	87
S/Other	4	
Thalassemia: α	2	
β	6	13
$\delta\beta$	1	
Affected	17	24
Diagnosis = exclusion	18	26
Fetal blood test	8	
Error = false-negative	1	1.4

and either cultured or analyzed directly. DNA is extracted and examined with restriction endonuclease mapping [4,8,9]. Many cases of α-thalassemia and some of $\delta\beta$ are due to gene deletions, which are readily detected by these methods. More than half the cases of sickle cell disease, and some forms of β-thalassemia (particularly in Sardinia) can be detected from restriction enzyme polymorphisms linked to the β genes of interest [8,20]. Very recently, it was pointed out that the specific nucleic acid mutation in sickle cell disease could be detected because it was the site of action of a restriction enzyme [21]. Thus, the use of direct analyses of DNA will play an increasingly important role in prenatal diagnosis of hemoglobinopathies.

There were 70 cases which were analyzed by DNA methods and reported to the Registry (Table 11). Most of the cases were at risk for sickle disorders (87%). This probably reflects the introduction of studies of polymorphisms linked to β^s in the USA in the past 2 years. There has been at least one error, due to incomplete information regarding the specific linkage of the polymorphism to the sickle gene. The obstetric component of these methods is a simple amniocentesis, and thus can be done in many places. The laboratory component is more specialized, and is available in less than a half dozen of the 21 centers listed in Table 1. Because the fetal risk is less, use of this approach must be expanded, as more enzyme polymorphisms are described, and more specific gene defects detected in sickle and thalassemia.

SUMMARY

Prenatal testing for hemoglobinopathies is now a reality, using both fetal blood and fetal fibroblast DNA. New techniques are being developed in the laboratories, and new skills by the obstetricians. Until thalassemia and sickle cell anemia can be cured, they will remain costly public health problems in specific parts of the world. Prenatal testing has provided an additional consideration for the governments and the families in such places, providing an acceptable alternative in many cases.

ACKNOWLEDGMENTS

Prenatal testing for hemoglobinopathies has been realized because of the initial efforts of Drs. D.G. Nathan, Y.W. Kan, H.H. Kazazian, Jr., B. Modell, D.J. Weatherall, J.B. Clegg, and their colleagues in the laboratories, and C. Valenti, J.C. Hobbins, M.J. Mahoney, and C.H. Rodeck in the obstetric operating room. The following have reported their annual data to the Registry and coordinated their programs: Athens: D. Loukopoulos. Sardinia: A. Cao. London, University College Hospital: B. Modell and E. Huehns. London, King's College Hospital: C.H. Rodeck, J. White. New Haven: M.J. Mahoney, J.C. Hobbins, B.G. Forget. Paris: Y. Beuzard, M. Goossens. Munich: M. Jensen. Rome: A. Pachi, L. Tentori. San Francisco: Y.W. Kan, M.S. Golbus. Melbourne, Queen Victoria Medical Center: R. Matthews. Melbourne, Royal Women's Hospital: M.N. Cauchi. Sydney, Prince of Wales Children's Hospital: V. Berdoukas. Sydney, Crown Street Women's Hospital: Y. Holcombe. Montreal: T. Perry. Toronto-Hamilton: R. Benzie. Jerusalem: E.A. Rachmilewitz, G. Civadelli. Ferrara: C. Vullo. Milan: M. Ferrari. Boston: D.G. Nathan. Baltimore: H. Kazazian. New York: B.P. Alter.

REFERENCES

1. Alter BP: Prenatal diagnosis of hemoglobinopathies and other hematologic diseases. J Pediatr 95:501, 1979.
2. Alter BP: Pre- and postnatal diagnosis of the hemoglobinopathies. In Bloom AD, James LS (eds): "The Fetus and the Newborn." New York: Alan R Liss for the March of Dimes Birth Defects Foundation, BD:OAS XVII(1):181-199, 1981.
3. Alter BP: Prenatal diagnosis of hemoglobinopathies: A status report. Lancet 2:1152, 1981.
4. Alter BP, Orkin SH, Nathan DG: Prenatal diagnosis of hemoglobinopathies. In Barson AJ (ed): "Laboratory Investigation of Fetal Disease." Bristol: John Wright and Sons Ltd, 1981, p 337.
5. Benzie RJ: Fetoscopy and fetal blood sampling. Ibid, p 320.
6. Alter BP, Modell CB, Fairweather D, Hobbins JC, Mahoney MJ, Frigoletto FD, Sherman AS, Nathan DG: Prenatal diagnosis of hemoglobinopathies. A review of 15 cases. N Engl J Med 295:1437, 1976.
7. Kan YW, Golbus MS, Trecartin RF, Filly RA, Valenti C, Furbetta M, Cao A: Prenatal diagnosis of β-thalassemia and sickle cell anaemia. Experience with 24 cases. Lancet 2:269, 1979.
8. Kan YW, Dozy AM: Antenatal diagnosis of sickle cell anaemia by DNA analysis of amniotic fluid cells. Lancet 2:910, 1978.
9. Orkin SH, Alter BP, Altay C, Mahoney MJ, Lazarus H, Hobbins JC, Nathan DG: Application of endonuclease mapping to the analysis and prenatal diagnosis of thalassemias caused by globin-gene deletion. N Engl J Med 299:166, 1978.

10. Alter BP, Metzger JB, Yock PG, Rothchild SB, Dover GJ: Selective hemolysis of adult red blood cells: An aid to prenatal diagnosis of hemoglobinopathies. Blood 53:279, 1979.
11. Kan YW, Nathan DG, Cividalli G, Crookston MC: Concentration of fetal red blood cells from a mixture of maternal and fetal blood by anti-i serum - An aid to prenatal diagnosis of hemoglobinopathies. Blood 43:411, 1974.
12. Alter BP, Coupal E, Forget BG: Globin chain electrophoresis for prenatal diagnosis of β thalassemia. Hemoglobin 5:357, 1981.
13. Boccacci M, Massa A, Tentori L: Application of cellulose acetate electrophoresis to globin chain separation for antenatal diagnosis of beta thalassemia. Clin Chim Acta (In press).
14. Gianni AM, Polli E, Giglioni B, Comi P, Ottolenghi S, Ferrari M, Furbetta M, Angius A, Cao A: Isoelectric focusing of globin chains for antenatal diagnosis of β^{o}-thalassemia. Hemoglobin 5:349, 1981.
15. Congote LF: Rapid procedure for globin chain analysis in blood samples of normal and β-thalassemic fetuses. Blood 57:353, 1981.
16. Dubart A, Goossens M, Beuzard Y, Monplaisir N, Testa U, Basset P, Rosa J: Prenatal diagnosis of hemoglobinopathies: Comparison of the results obtained by isoelectric focusing of hemoglobins and by chromatography of radioactive globin chains. Blood 56:1092, 1980.
17. Hollenberg MD, Kaback MM, Kazazian HH Jr: Adult hemoglobin synthesis by reticulocytes from the human fetus at midtrimester. Science 174:698, 1971.
18. Gloquit Y, Beuzard Y, Varnavides L, Chabret C, Dumez Y, John PN, Rodeck C, White JM: Antenatal diagnosis of haemoglobinopathies by Biorex chromatography of haemoglobins. (Submitted for publication).
19. Thorpe SJ, Huehns ER: A double labelling immunofluorescence microscopy technique for the antenatal diagnosis of β-thalassemia major. (Submitted for publication).
20. Kan YW, Lee KY, Furbetta M, Angius A, Cao A: Polymorphism of DNA sequence in the β-globin gene region. N Engl J Med 302:185, 1980.
21. Geever RF, Wilson LB, Nallaseth FS, Milner PF, Bittner M, Wilson JT: Direct identification of sickle cell anemia by blot hybridization. Proc Natl Acad Sci USA 78:5081, 1981.

Prenatal Diagnosis by DNA Analysis*

Yuet Wai Kan⁺ MD, Judy C. Chang, MS, and Andrée M. Dozy, MT

INTRODUCTION

Since first introduced in 1974, prenatal diagnosis of sickle cell anemia and thalassemia has been performed in medical centers throughout the USA, Europe, and Australia [1]. Initially, the method of diagnosis depended on analyzing fetal blood obtained either by placental aspiration or fetoscopy. Advances in nucleic acid technology have paved the way for prenatal diagnosis by analysis of amniotic fluid DNA obtained by amniocentesis. An increasing number of disorders are being diagnosed by this method. Amniocentesis, a well-established and widely available procedure, is safer than fetal blood sampling, which carries a small but definite fetal risk, and is available only in a few medical centers.

The conversion from fetal blood sampling to amniocentesis was made possible by applying the Southern blot technique [2] for DNA analysis to the globin genes [3–5]. In this method, DNA is first digested with a restriction enzyme which cleaves DNA at specific nucleotide sequences. The fragments generated are separated according to size by electrophoresis on agarose gels. The DNA is then transferred to, and immobilized on, nitrocellulose filters and the fragments that contain the globin genes are then identified by hybridization with a globin-specific ^{32}P-labeled probe. The technique is extremely sensitive; in most cases, sufficient DNA for analysis can be isolated from the cells obtained from 20 ml of uncultured amniotic fluid at the 16th–18th week of gestation [6].

Normal DNA yields distinct and reproducible patterns with each restriction enzyme. A mutation on the human genome can be detected either directly or indirectly (Table 1). Direct analysis localizes the mutation, while indirect analysis uses sequence polymorphisms in surrounding regions of DNA for linkage analysis of the lesion.

*Supported in part by NIH grant AM 16666, a grant from the March of Dimes Birth Defects Foundation, and a contract from the State of California, Department of Health Services, Maternal & Child Health Branch.

⁺ Y.W.K. is a Howard Hughes Medical Institute Investigator.

Birth Defects: Original Article Series, Volume 18, Number 7, pages 275–283
© 1982 March of Dimes Birth Defects Foundation

TABLE 1. Prenatal Diagnosis by DNA Analysis

Direct Analysis of the Mutation
a) Deletion defects: α-thalassemia, $\delta\beta$-thalassemia
b) Point mutations: Hb O^{Arab}, Hb S
Indirect Analysis with Restriction Endonuclease Polymorphism
a) *Hpa* I polymorphism for Hb S and Hb C
b) *Hin* dIII polymorphism for Hb S and β-thalassemia
c) *Bam* HI polymorphism for β-thalassemia

DIRECT ANALYSIS

A mutation can alter the normal restriction pattern of the globin genes in two different ways. When a long stretch of nucleotide sequences is deleted, the patterns that restriction enzymes normally generate in this region change. Similarly, if a small lesion, such as deletion of a few nucleotides, or a single nucleotide substitution, happens to involve a restriction endonuclease recognition site, the restriction patterns of that particular enzyme will be affected. These small changes can abolish a normal recognition site, or create a new one in the normal DNA.

The first hereditary disorder detected prenatally by direct DNA analysis was α-thalassemia. The severe form of the disease, which occurs predominantly in Southeast Asia, is most frequently caused by deletion of the duplicated α-globin loci [7,8]. The homozygous disorder, hydrops fetalis associated with Hb Barts, causes fetal death either during the last trimester of pregnancy, or shortly after birth [9]. Terminating an affected pregnancy reduces the gestation period by approximately 20 weeks and forestalls two common complications of hydropic pregnancies, maternal toxemia and postpartum hemorrhage. Prenatal diagnosis for this condition was initially performed using cDNA-DNA hybridization in solution [10]. The amount of α-globin-specific ^{32}P-labeled probe that hybridizes to DNA prepared from amniotic fluid cells is quantitated. The large quantity of DNA required for this method of analysis necessitates cell culture. Solution hybridization has now been replaced by restriction analysis. In this assay, the fragments that contain the α-globin genes are absent on Southern analysis. The assay can be applied to uncultured amniotic fluid cells and has been used to test many pregnancies at risk for α-thalassemia [11] (Fig. 1).

Some β-thalassemia syndromes are due to deletions that involve the β-globin gene. One form of β^0-thalassemia found in India is caused by deletion of the 3′ portion of the β-globin structural gene [12,13]. Several of the $\delta^0\beta^0$-thalassemias involve deletion of varying lengths of DNA. In one, the entire β-globin gene and the 3′ portion of the δ-globin gene are deleted [14,15]. In another, a more extensive deletion involves the $^A\gamma$-, δ-, and β-globin genes [16]. In theory, these dele-

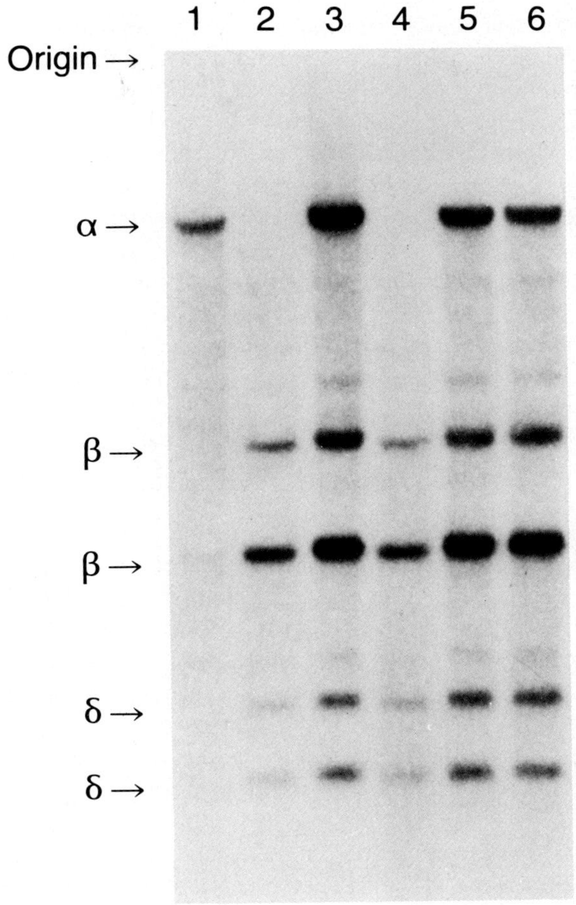

Fig. 1. Prenatal diagnosis of α-thalassemia. DNA was cleaved with *Eco* RI and hybridized with a globin cDNA probe. DNA are from 1) HPFH, 2) homozygous α-thalassemia, 3) normal, 4) amniocytes from a pregnancy at risk for α-thalassemia, and 5,6) parents of fetus. the DNA fragments containing the α-, β-, and δ-globin genes are indicated (adapted from reference 11).

tions are detectable prenatally by direct DNA analysis. In practice, however, this approach is seldom applied since gene deletion rarely causes β-thalassemia, and homozygosity for $\delta^0\beta^0$-thalassemia is usually mild.

An example of a point mutation that abolishes a restriction endonuclease recognition site is the β-globin mutant, Hb O^{Arab} [17]. A GAA to AAA (Glu→Lys) mutation at amino acid number 121 abolishes the *Eco* RI recognition site (GAATTC) normally present in this position. A case of Hb S-O^{Arab} has been tested prenatally by restriction endonuclease analysis with this enzyme [18].

The most important hemoglobinopathy caused by a point mutation is sickle cell anemia. The sickle mutation occurs in a region of the β-globin gene that contains recognition sites for several enzymes. The first enzyme described, *Mnl* I [19], could not be used because it cleaves the DNA in this region into very small fragments which are difficult to detect. Recently, Geever et al showed that *Dde* I generates fragments that are large enough for analysis [20]. This enzyme cleaves the sequence CTNAG (C = cytosine, T = thymine, A = adenine, G = guanine, N = any of the four bases), and normally cuts at the nucleotide sequences (CCT, GAG) which encode for amino acid numbers 5 and 6 (Pro, Glu) of the β-globin chain. The Glu→Val change at β6 in the sickle mutation abolishes this cleavage site. When sickle DNA is digested with *Dde* I, a single DNA fragment of 381 nucleotides replaces the two fragments of 180 and 201 nucleotides that are normally present in this region [21] (Fig. 2). Such small DNA fragments generally produce weak hybridization signals, and 10-20 μg of DNA is required to detect them; hence, the amniotic fluid cells must be cultured to obtain enough DNA.

Recently another restriction enzyme was shown to be even more sensitive than *Dde* I. *Mst* II recognizes the nucleotide sequence CCTNAG. In the normal β-globin gene, this sequence occurs in the region corresponding to amino acids 5, 6, and 7 (Pro,Glu,Glu: CCT GAG GAG). When normal DNA is digested with this enzyme, two fragments of 1.15 and 0.2 kb are produced 5′ and 3′ to this position. The sickle mutation abolishes the cleavage site and the resultant fragment is 1.35 kb long. Since larger DNA fragments produce stronger hybridization signals, less DNA is required, and the amniocytes do not have to be cultured. We successfully used this assay to test pregnancies at risk for sickle cell anemia [22].

One type of β^0-thalassemia is caused by a single nucleotide mutation which affects mRNA processing. The coding sequences of most eukaryotic structural genes are interrupted by noncoding intervening sequences which are transcribed, but are excised as the mRNA matures. The invariant nucleotide sequences at the 5′ and 3′ splice junctions of the intervening sequences are GT and AG, respectively. In this form of β^0-thalassemia, which is found in the Mediterranean area, the dinucleotide sequence GT at the splice junction of the second intervening sequence is mutated to AT (T. Maniatis, personal communication). The mRNA is improperly spliced at this junction and degrades rapidly in the nucleus. As a result, no β-globin mRNA emerges into the cytoplasm, and hence no β-globin chain synthesis occurs. This lesion abolishes an *Hph* I recognition site (GGTGA) which normally is present in this region. The restriction patterns produced by *Hph* I digestion of this DNA show only one 1.39 kb fragment, instead of the two normal fragments of 0.13 and 1.26 kb (A. Bank, personal communication).

INDIRECT DNA ANALYSIS

When a lesion does not involve a restriction endonuclease recognition site it can be detected by linkage analysis of sequence polymorphisms in regions of

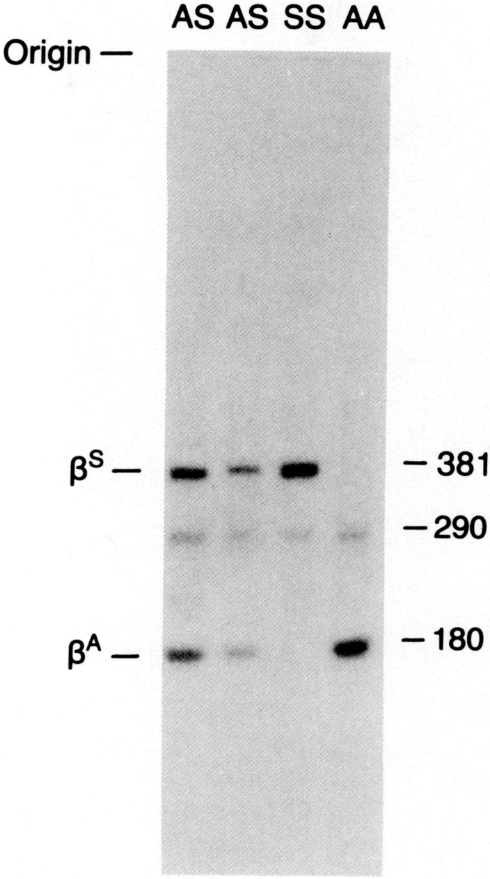

Fig. 2. Prenatal diagnosis of sickle cell anemia by *Dde* I analysis [21]. DNA samples are from parents at risk (AS, AS), a previous child with sickle cell anemia (SS), and amniotic fluid cells from which the AA diagnosis was made. The fragments specific for the β^S- and β^A-genotypes are 381 and 180 basepairs (bp) long, respectively. A faint 290 bp band, present in both genotypes, originates from a DNA fragment in the 5′ flanking region.

DNA surrounding the mutant gene. Traditional linkage analysis relies on protein polymorphism. Recent studies indicate that DNA sequence polymorphisms are more common since they may occur in regions that do not encode for proteins and are therefore not subjected to the functional constraints that restrict mutations in the coding regions. They provide a new class of markers for genetic analysis and can be used for linkage analysis of both normal and mutant genes [23].

Indirect DNA analysis was first used for prenatal diagnosis of sickle cell anemia [6]. When normal human DNA is digested with the restriction enzyme *Hpa* I, the β-globin gene lies in a 7.6 kb DNA fragment (Fig. 3). In people of West African and Mediterranean origin, a single nucleotide mutation abolishes

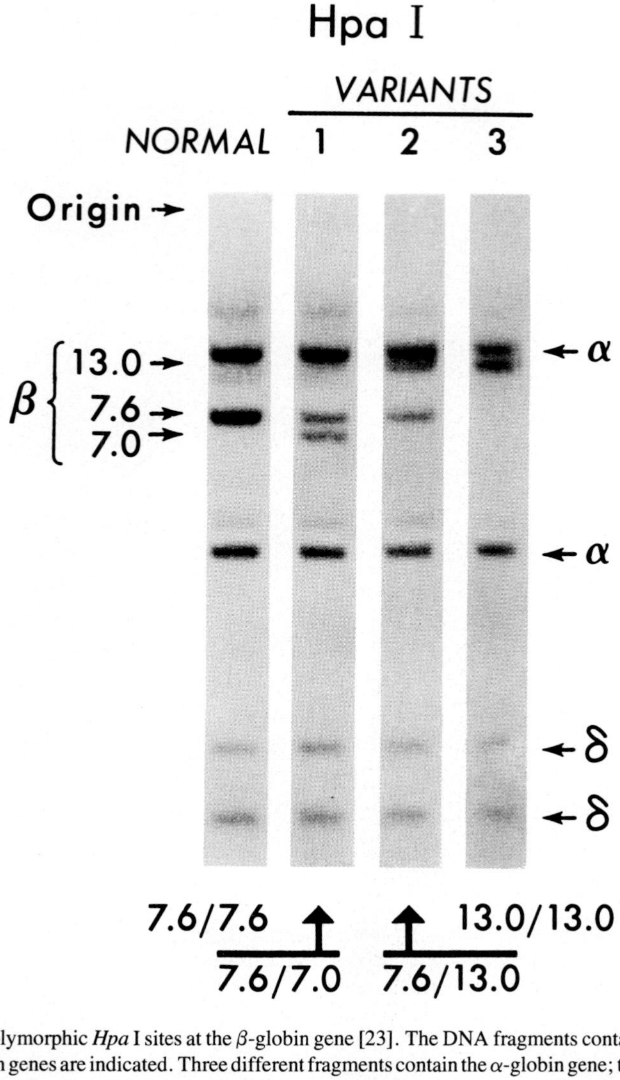

Fig. 3. Polymorphic *Hpa* I sites at the β-globin gene [23]. The DNA fragments containing the α-, β-, and δ-globin genes are indicated. Three different fragments contain the α-globin gene; the normal 7.6 kb fragment, and the variant 7.0 kb and 13.0 kb fragments. The 13.0 kb *Hpa* I fragment is frequently associated with the sickle mutation that originates from West Africa.

the recognition site on the 3′ flanking region of the β-globin gene, and the length of the DNA fragment that contains the gene increases to 13 kb. The sickle mutation in these areas is frequently associated with the 13 kb *Hpa* I fragment. In the American black population, about 70% of the sickle genes are linked to the 13 kb fragment [24]; when the linkage can be established through family studies, the size of the *Hpa* I β-globin gene-containing fragment in the amniotic fluid cell DNA indicates the presence or absence of the sickle gene in the fetus.

A polymorphic *Bam* HI site on the 3′ side of the β-globin gene is useful for prenatal diagnosis of β-thalassemia in certain populations [25]. This enzyme cleaves the coding region of the normal β-globin gene into two fragments, each containing a portion of the gene: a 1.8 kb fragment contains the 5′ portion, and a polymorphic 9.3 or 22 kb fragment contains the 3′ portion. This is an old polymorphism which exists in many different races, including European, African, and Asian. As the mutations that affect the β-globin gene probably occurred after these races diverged, they can be associated with either of the polymorphic *Bam* HI fragments. β^0-thalassemia in Sardinians, and β^0- and β^+-thalassemia in Chinese are always associated with the chromosome that contains the 9.3 kb fragment. Therefore in these two populations, finding a 22 kb fragment in DNA from a pregnancy at risk would exclude the existence of the β-thalassemia gene on that chromosome.

There is a polymorphic *Hin* dIII recognition site in each of the major intervening sequences of the $^G\gamma$- and $^A\gamma$-globin genes [26,27]. Three genotypes have been identified: *Hin* dIII sites present in both intervening sequences (G+A+), only in the $^G\gamma$-gene (G+A−), and absent from both genes (G−A−). When informative family members are available, these genotypes can be linked to the normal or abnormal β-globin gene and used for linkage analysis. This technique has been used successfully for prenatal diagnosis of sickle cell anemia and β-thalassemia [28,29].

Several other polymorphic restriction sites surrounding the β-globin gene have been described [30,31]. When studied in combination, these sites serve as useful markers for determining the normal and mutant states of the gene.

CONCLUSION

Direct DNA analysis can be applied to all pregnancies at risk for homozygous α-thalassemia. Until recently, sickle cell anemia was diagnosed by linkage analysis using the *Hpa* I polymorphism, supplemented with the *Hin* dIII polymorphism. Direct analysis with *Dde* I and *Mst* II will replace this approach in most cases. Currently, β-thalassemia is seldom diagnosed by DNA analysis, and fetal blood sampling remains the primary method of diagnosis.

When feasible, direct DNA analysis is preferable to indirect analysis which entails family studies to establish the linkage phase, ie which restriction fragment is linked to which genotype. Furthermore, since the restriction site under analysis is located some distance away from the actual mutation, the possibility of cross-over always exists. However, the chance of cross-over is lower with restriction analysis than with the classic linkage analysis because the distances between the recognition sites and the mutant gene are much shorter than those between the protein products. For example, the chance of cross-over between the *Hpa* I site and the sickle gene is estimated at 1/20,000 [32].

Linkage analysis will probably be applied to more genetic disorders than direct analysis. It can be performed without knowing the precise nature or the location of the lesion. As illustrated by the β-thalassemias, the same phenotype can be produced by many different mutations, most of which do not affect a restriction endonuclease recognition site. The molecular defects in many other genetic disorders are also probably heterogeneous. Thus, using DNA sequence polymorphisms for linkage analysis will be feasible in many situations where direct DNA analysis is impossible.

ACKNOWLEDGMENT

The author thanks Jennifer Gampell for editorial comments.

REFERENCES

1. Alter BP: Prenatal diagnosis of haemoglobinopathies: A status report. Lancet 2:1152–1155, 1981.
2. Southern EM: Detection of specific sequences among DNA fragments separated by gel electrophoresis. J Mol Biol 98:503–517, 1975.
3. Jeffreys AJ, Flavell RA: The rabbit β-globin gene contains a larger insert in the coding sequence. Cell 12:1097–1098, 1977.
4. Mears JG, Ramirez F, Liebowitz D, Nakaura F, Bloom A, Konotey-Ahulu FID, Bank A: Changes in restricted human cellular DNA fragments containing globin gene sequences in thalassemias and related disorders. Proc Natl Acad Sci USA 75:1222–1226, 1978.
5. Orkin SH, Alter BP, Altay C, Mahoney MJ, Lazarus H, Hobbins JC, Nathan DG: Application of endonuclease mapping to the analysis and prenatal diagnosis of thalassemias caused by globin-gene deletion. N Engl J Med 299:166–172, 1978.
6. Kan YW, Dozy AM: Antenatal diagnosis of sickle cell anemia by DNA analysis of amniotic fluid cells. Lancet 2:910–912, 1978.
7. Ottolenghi S, Lanyon WG, Paul J, Williamson R, Weatherall DJ, Clegg JB, Pritchard J, Pootrakul S, Wong HB: The severe form of α thalassemia is caused by a haemoglobin gene deletion. Nature 251:389–391, 1974.
8. Taylor JM, Dozy A, Kan YW, Varmus HE, Lie-Injo LE, Ganesan J, Todd D: Genetic lesion in homozygous α thalassemia (hydrops foetalis). Nature 251:392–393, 1974.
9. Lie-Injo LE, Lie-Hong G, Ager JAM, Lehmann H: α Thalassaemia as a cause of hydrops foetalis. Br J Haematol 8:1–4, 1962.
10. Kan YW, Golbus MS, Dozy AM: Prenatal diagnosis of α-thalassemia: Clinical application of molecular hybridization. N Engl J Med 295:1165–1167, 1976.
11. Dozy AM, Forman EN, Abuelo DN, Barsel-Bowers G, Mahoney MJ, Forget BG, Kan YW: Prenatal diagnosis of homozygous α thalassemia. JAMA 24:1610–1612, 1979.
12. Flavell RA, Bernards R, Kooters JB, de Boer E: The structure of the human β-globin gene in β-thalassemia. Nucleic Acids Res 6:2749–2760, 1979.
13. Orkin SH, Kolodner R, Michelson A, Husson R: Cloning and direct examination of a structurally abnormal human β^0-thalassemia globin gene. Proc Natl Acad Sci USA 77:3558–3562, 1980.
14. Fritsch EF, Lawn RM, Maniatis T: Characterization of deletions which affect the expression of fetal globin genes in man. Nature 279:598–603, 1979.

15. Ottolenghi S, Giglioni B, Comi P, Gianni AM, Polli E, Acquaye CTA, Oldham JH, Masera GG: Globin gene deletion in HPFH, $\delta^0\beta^0$ thalassaemia and Hb Lepore disease. Nature 278:654–656, 1979.
16. Orkin SH, Alter BP, Altay C: Deletion of the $^A\gamma$-globin gene in $^G\gamma$-δ β-thalassemia. J Clin Invest 64:866–869, 1979.
17. Flavell RA, Kooter JM, de Boer E, Little PFR, Williamson R: Analysis of the β-δ-globin gene loci in normal and Hb Lepore DNA: Direct determination of gene linkage and intergene distance. Cell 15:25–41, 1978.
18. Phillips JA, Scott AF, Kazazian HH Jr, Smith KD, Stetten G, Thomas GH: Prenatal diagnosis of hemoglobinopathies by restriction analysis: Pregnancies at risk for sickle cell anemia and S-O^{Arab} disease. Johns Hopkins Med J 145:57–60, 1979.
19. Nienhuis AJ: Mapping the human genome. N Engl J Med 299:195–196, 1978.
20. Geever RF, Wilson LB, Nallaseth FS, Milner PF, Bittner M, Wilson JJ: Direct identification of sickle cell anemia (SS) by blot hybridization. Proc Natl Acad Sci USA 78:5081–5085, 1981.
21. Chang JC, Kan YW: Antenatal diagnosis of sickle cell anaemia by direct analysis of the sickle mutation. Lancet 2:1127–1129, 1981.
22. Chang JC, Kan YW: A sensitive new prenatal test for sickle cell anemia. N Engl J Med (In press)
23. Kan YW, Dozy AM: Polymorphism of DNA sequence adjacent to human β-globin structural gene: Relationship to sickle mutation. Proc Natl Acad Sci USA 75:5631–5635, 1978.
24. Kan YW, Dozy AM: Evolution of the hemoglobin S and C genes in world populations. Science 209:388–391, 1980.
25. Kan YW, Lee KY, Furbetta M, Anguis A, Cao A: Polymorphism of DNA sequence in the β-globin gene region: Application to prenatal diagnosis of β^0 thalassemia in Sardinia. N Engl J Med 302:185–188, 1980.
26. Jeffreys AJ: DNA sequence variants in the $^G\gamma$-$^A\gamma$- and β-globin genes of man. Cell 18:1–10, 1979.
27. Tuan D, Biro PA, de Riel JK, Lazarus H, Forget BG: Restriction endonuclease mapping of the human gamma globin gene loci. Nucleic Acids Res 6:2519–2544, 1979.
28. Little PFR, Annison G, Darling S, Williamson R, Camba L, Modell B: Model for antenatal diagnosis of β-thalassaemia and other monogenic disorders by molecular analysis of linked DNA polymorphisms. Nature 285:144–147, 1980.
29. Phillips JA III, Panny SR, Kazazian HH Jr, Boehm CD, Scott AF, Smith KD: Prenatal diagnosis of sickle cell anemia by restriction endonuclease analysis: Hin dIII polymorphism in γ-globin genes extend test applicability. Proc Natl Acad Sci USA 77:2853–2856, 1980.
30. Driscoll MC, Baird M, Bank A, Rachmilewitz EA: A new polymorphism in the human β-globin gene useful in antenatal diagnosis. J Clin Invest 68:915–919, 1981.
31. Antonarakis SE, Boehm CD, Giardinia PJV, Kazazian HH Jr: Nonrandom association of polymorphic restriction sites in the β-globin cluster. Proc Natl Acad Sci USA 79:137–141, 1982.
32. Kurnit DM, Hoehn H: Prenatal diagnosis of human genome variation. Ann Rev Genet 13:235–258, 1979.

Social Consequences of Introducing Antenatal Diagnosis for Thalassemia

Bernadette Modell, MD, PhD, and Mary Mouzouras, BSc

Since 1955, thalassemia has been brought to Britain by two main ethnic groups. Greek and Turkish Cypriots, who have a 17% prevalence of β-thalassemia trait, have mainly settled in North London so that there is now a population of about 150,000 in the region of University College Hospital. Asians, originally from the northwestern part of the Indian subcontinent, with a lower prevalence of β-thalassemia trait (from 4–15%) have settled mainly in the industrial towns of the north.

For thalassemia, as for all other forms of antenatal diagnosis as practiced at present, diagnosis is possible only in midtrimester, and the only help we can offer following diagnosis of an affected fetus is termination of pregnancy at 18–20 weeks. This is a very traumatic intervention, and it may seem difficult to balance its disadvantages against the disadvantages of having a child with thalassemia major. It is only by observing the actions of at-risk couples actually faced with the decision of whether or not to request antenatal diagnosis, and whether or not to terminate an affected pregnancy, that we can obtain guidance about the kind of help that is useful to people at risk for genetic disease.

In 1979, with the intention of measuring the usefulness of antenatal diagnosis for thalassemia, we evaluated the reactions in Britain of at-risk couples to counseling and the offer of antenatal diagnosis; the results are presented here. All of our subsequent experience is consistent with these findings.

Between 1975 and 1979, 95% of pregnant at-risk Cypriot couples chose to have antenatal diagnosis (Table 1). Two of the three who refused requested an abortion instead, because of general anxiety and uncertainties about the accuracy and safety of the procedure in the early days. However, both of these couples have since come to us for antenatal diagnosis. In short, 98% of all pregnant at-risk Cypriot couples determined the fate of their pregnancy as a result of genetic counseling. Asians behaved rather differently, with just over 50% of counseled couples requesting antenatal diagnosis, and the others continuing their pregnancies undiagnosed. However, this is a very large and complex group, and requires

Birth Defects: Original Article Series, Volume 18, Number 7, pages 285–291
© 1982 March of Dimes Birth Defects Foundation

TABLE 1. Choices of Counseled Couples at Risk for Thalassemia Major Offspring, and Ethnic Origin

Ethnic origin	No. counseled	No. (%) Choosing AND*	No. (%) Rejecting AND
Cypriot	50	47 (94)	3 (6)
Indian and Pakistani	22	13 (59)	9 (41)
Italian	3	1 (33)	2 (67)
Total	75	61 (81)	14 (19)

*AND = antenatal diagnosis. (Tables 1, 2, and 3 from Modell B, Word RHT, Fairweather DVI: Effect of introducing antenatal diagnosis on reproductive behaviour of families at risk for thalassaemia major. Br Med J 280:1347–1350, 1980, with permission.)

further study. For the sake of simplicity we will concentrate here only on results among Cypriots. The data have been given in full by Modell and co-workers [1].

A similarly high acceptance of the offer of antenatal diagnosis has been found in Sardinia [2], the Ferrara region of Italy [3], Greece [4], and Cyprus [5].

Since the uptake rate of antenatal diagnosis by Cypriots is almost 100%, we are in essence examining the reaction of an entire community to a severe inherited disease. Among Cypriots, marriages are stable and the incidence of nonpaternity is low. Therefore, we are in the fortunate position of being able to follow the same set of families through the evolution of their knowledge about thalassemia: from ignorance, to the effect of genetic counseling, to the arrival of antenatal diagnosis. The obstetric history has proved a very useful tool for measuring their reactions, as shown in Table 2.

The reproductive lives of these couples could be divided into three phases; first was a "phase of innocence" from the time of marriage to the time they learned they were at risk, which usually (but not always) happened only when they had an affected child. The second phase was from the time they knew their risk, to the time that antenatal diagnosis became available; thus, there was nothing positive to be done; the third phase, following the introduction of antenatal diagnosis in 1975, was a period in which they knew both their risk, and the availability of antenatal diagnosis. In each of these three phases we counted the number of pregnancies undertaken, and their outcome.

In the first phase, the number of pregnancies generated was 1 per 3 married years, since Cypriots tend to reproduce soon after marriage, though the final family size is small. There was a very low rate of termination for social reasons; of the children born, only 43% (instead of 75%) were healthy, because at that time couples usually discovered their risk only by producing an affected child. The last column, the rate of production of healthy children, is in one sense the most important. It expresses the biologic viability of the group, and at 1 per 7 married years was about half what they had initially been aiming at.

TABLE 2. Reproductive Behavior of Families Choosing Antenatal Diagnosis for Thalassemia. Whole Group (59 Couples)

	No. couples	Married years	Married yr per pregnancy	% AND	% TOP*	% Children healthy	Married yrs per healthy child
Pregnancies started and completed not knowing risk	40	145	2.6	0	1.4	43	6.3
Pregnancies started knowing risk but no AND available	26	95	4.8	0	70	33	48.0
Pregnancies started not knowing risk, but counseled with offer of AND	24	49	2.0	95	27	100	3.1
Pregnancies started knowing risk and that AND is available	47	137	2.4	98	35	97	3.9

*TOP - termination of pregnancy

Once they knew of their risk of having a thalassemic child, the pregnancy rate fell by half, indicating that they were trying not to reproduce. There was a relatively high rate of accidental pregnancy, which probably reflects the ambivalence of a group of people on the one hand wanting children, but on the other, afraid to have them. No less than 70% of these pregnancies were terminated for fear of thalassemia. Unfortunately, of those that continued, some still produced children with thalassemia major, so the final rate of production of healthy children was one per 50 married years. This amounts to biologic suicide on the part of the group as a whole, as a result of their knowledge of the disease itself and its mode of inheritance. Their reaction could be expressed in this unambiguous way only because they live in a community which permits open access to contraception and to termination of pregnancy. In a society which does not permit the options of divorce, contraception, or termination of pregnancy, it would be impossible for genetic counseling to have any similar measurable effect, and this may explain why it was not observed by Barrai and Vullo [3] or Stamatoyannopoulos [6]. The figures are a clear indicator of the degree of distress within families already caring for one affected child and aware of the risk of having a second, but barred from any socially acceptable solution. It is under such circumstances that the disease can prove most tragically destructive to family life.

Since the introduction of antenatal diagnosis, the number of pregnancies undertaken by the same families rose to the previous level; 98% had antenatal diagnosis and 33% were terminated (29% had a diagnosis of thalassemia major and 5% fetal losses due to the procedure in this group). Of the continuing preg-

TABLE 3. Reproductive Behavior of Families Choosing Antenatal Diagnosis for Thalassemia. 24 Couples Without an Affected Child, Detected During Pregnancy

	No. couples	Married years	Married yr per pregnancy	% AND	% TOP	% Children healthy	Married yrs per healthy child
Pregnancies started and completed not knowing risk	6	39	3.5	0	18	100	4.3
Pregnancies started not knowing risk but counseled and offered AND	24	49	2.2	95	27	100	3.1
Pregnancies started knowing both risk and that AND is available	12	19	1.9	100	30	100	2.7

nancies, 97% produced healthy children (there was one misdiagnosis in 1977 which fortunately has not yet been repeated). The final rate of production of healthy children was 1/4.6 married years. The conclusion is clear. This community is using antenatal diagnosis to preserve family life and to obtain the healthy families they want.

One might think that this very clear-cut reaction depended on firsthand experience of the disease; therefore, we extracted the group of couples who had been identified prospectively in the antenatal clinic. Table 3 shows that their behavior does not differ from that of "experienced" couples. Table 3 also shows two additional interesting figures. One might expect that when couples had once been through this very distressing procedure it would be a long time before they undertook another pregnancy, but the figure of 1 pregnancy per 2 married years for pregnancies freely undertaken in the knowledge of risk and of what antenatal diagnosis involves proves the opposite for this particular set of families. The high figure is largely the result of second pregnancies undertaken by couples who terminated one pregnancy because of an affected fetus. There seem to be two reasons for the speed with which they undertake another pregnancy. First, it is impossible to go through a midtrimester termination of pregnancy without guilt feelings, which were expressed particularly well by one young couple (who incidentally chose to continue the pregnancy though they knew the fetus was affected). "Whichever way we look there is no right answer. To have the child is wrong, but to kill it is wrong . . . . If we have the baby we must make that the right solution. We must be strong enough to help him, and we must try to get him the very best treatment." Couples who terminate their pregnancies feel the same, but they make termination the right decision by undertaking another pregnancy very quickly, so that the termination becomes a constructive step towards obtaining the wanted normal child. A second reason seems to be that when a couple realizes that they have the capacity to produce an abnormal child they feel to some extent damaged themselves, and that they have unwittingly damaged each other. However, they feel they can repair themselves (and each other) by producing a normal child. This also explains the exceptional satisfaction of at-risk couples who produce a child that does not even carry the thalassemia trait.

Additional factors in the high acceptability of antenatal diagnosis among Cypriots are the high incidence of the disease (1 in 170 births) combined with the readiness of families to talk about it, which produce a high level of subliminal awareness in the community, and the attitude of the Greek Orthodox Church, which though disapproving termination of pregnancy allows the individual's conscience to be the final arbiter of right and wrong.

The second interesting figure in Table 3 in this group of young couples is the relatively high incidence of social termination of pregnancy in the early married years when they were ignorant of their risk of thalassemia. This contrasts with the low rate among the set of couples first presenting for diagnosis and reflects a social change. Traditionally in Cyprus, the parents of the bride provide the marital home at the time of marriage, so there is no reason to postpone reproduction. In Britain this pattern is changing of course, and the first task of the newly married Cypriot couple, and of the young English couple, is to establish their home, so there is an increasing tendency to terminate pregnancies accidentally started too soon. The numbers in Table 3 reflect this approximation of the young Cypriot to the English marriage pattern. However, once couples know they are at risk for thalassemia major they very rarely request termination of pregnancy on social grounds. All pregnancies become precious and all are tested, because, as they say, "This may be the normal one. If we terminate this, we may not be able to get a normal one when we try." In summary, the general effect of people knowing their genetic risks is improved attention to careful family planning.

The group of prospectively counseled at-risk couples is exceptionally interesting in other ways. We usually asked them two questions. 1) What would they have done if they had known they were both heterozygotes before they married? Those who had not known each other well beforehand but had been introduced with a view to marriage in the traditional Cypriot fashion usually said that, had they known at that early stage, they might not have married. However, when the marriage was a love match, the knowledge would not have affected their decision. 2) What would they have done had they discovered their risk after marriage but before the presenting pregnancy, and antenatal diagnosis was not available? Once again they split into two groups. Most of those with a thalassemic child in the extended family said they would not have had children under any circumstances (a typical remark is . . . "I couldn't possibly see my wife go through what my mother went through"), and some would have aborted the presenting pregnancy, but most of those without such imprinting would have taken the risk and tried to have at least one child. From his wider experience, Professor Vullo states that couples may marry with the intention of not having children, but generally after a few years, and in the absence of antenatal diagnosis, most do try to have a child. However, since antenatal diagnosis is in fact available, practically no couple is now prepared to undertake an undiagnosed pregnancy, because they would feel responsible if they produced a child with thalassemia major. Practically all Cypriot counseled couples say, "We have no choice. We could not knowingly bring a child into the world to suffer." In short, once antenatal diagnosis became available, it was strongly self-reinforcing, and this kind of dynamic effect makes it very difficult to introduce a preventive program in a phased or partial way.

Finally, the attitude of the older patients themselves is interesting. In our thalassemia society we have an articulate group of young men and women aged 17–24 available for consultation. All of the 15 young women we have asked approve of antenatal diagnosis and would make use of it themselves if it were indicated. They made comments such as, "It's bad enough going to hospital yourself never mind dragging the children along"; "I think it would be irresponsible"; "I couldn't go through all that again." The 8 young men were more ambivalent: 4 thought they would take advantage of antenatal diagnosis and 4 thought they would not. In a sense, these reactions give "permission" for an antenatal diagnosis program, but they are also a poignant reflection of the feelings of unworthiness that a severe disease of this kind can generate. The behavior of at-risk couples has also not changed with our increasing confidence in the effectiveness of treatment for thalassemia.

Paradoxically, in many ways antenatal diagnosis and treatment prove to be mutually reinforcing rather than antagonistic approaches to the same problem. The existence of treatment in itself increases the demand for antenatal diagnosis, because the feature of the disease that is most feared is the need to subject a vulnerable child to the harsh discipline of a demanding treatment. In addition, where patients must pay for treatment, parents cannot take the responsibility of committing the family to such a crushing financial load; in communities where the disease is very common, the prevention of further cases is an absolute necessity if the existing patients are to receive adequate treatment.

The existence of antenatal diagnosis also produces a reciprocal effect on treatment. From the time that a preventive method becomes available a new element of medical responsibility appears, since each new birth must now be a consequence of ignorance or error, or of a positive decision not to test a pregnancy, or not to abort an affected fetus. Clearly, new births should occur only for one of the last two reasons, as a result of parental choice. When we started our program the possibilities of diagnostic error and of fetal losses due to the procedure caused some anxiety that we could be subjected to legal action, but this has never occurred. The only people who have wanted to take legal action have been couples who were "missed" in antenatal clinics, and first became aware of their risk by producing an affected child; subsequently, they realized that this could have been avoided. For such couples, the existence of antenatal diagnosis makes it more difficult than before to accept the disease with all of its treatment implications; they see themselves together with their child as the victims of an avoidable disaster. Such parents, as well as those who decide to keep a fetus diagnosed as abnormal, are likely to press for an improved standard of treatment. Doctors with an increased awareness of responsibility for these cases share this desire for the highest possible standard of treatment; we now have a situation where antenatal diagnosis and treatment tend to push each other continuously to an improved level of performance.

The social effects described here seem to hold true for most European and Mediterranean communities. The next question to ask is, how would the pattern differ in the Middle Eastern and Oriental societies where thalassemia is an even greater public health problem?

ACKNOWLEDGMENTS

This data was derived from antenatal diagnoses for thalassemia done at University College Hospital with the help of many people, including the following: Professor D.V.I. Fairweather, Mr. H. Ward, Dr. V. Berdoukas, Dr. M. Matsakis, Ms. M. Mouzouras, Dr. M. Angastiniotis, Dr. P. Ioannou, Dr. B. Brambati, Dr. M. Ferrari, Miss M. Boussiou, Dr. M. Lucci, Dr. L. Camba, Mr. Vedat Azmi, Dr. L. Varnavides, and Dr. G. de Olim. We thank them all for their help in providing a wanted service to our patients. We are all deeply grateful to His Royal Highness Prince Sultan bin Abdulaziz of Saudi Arabia for the personal financial assistance that made this work possible.

REFERENCES

1. Modell B, Word RHT, Fairweather DVI: Effect of introducing antenatal diagnosis on reproductive behaviour of families at risk for thalassaemia major. Br Med J 280:1347–1350, 1980.
2. Cao A, Furbetta M, Galanello R: Screening for thalassaemia. Lancet 2:1189, 1980.
3. Barrai I, Vullo C: Screening for beta-thalassaemia heterozygotes. Lancet 2:1257, 1980.
4. Loukopoulos D, Tassiopoulos A, Fessas P: Screening for thalassaemia. Lancet 2:1188–1189, 1980.
5. Angastiniotis MA, Hadjiminas MG: Prevention of thalassaemia in Cyprus. Lancet 1:369–370, 1981.
6. Stamatoyannopoulos G: Problems of screening in the hemoglobinopathies. In Motulsky AG, Lenz W (eds): "Birth Defects." Amsterdam: Excerpta Medica, 1974, pp 268–276.

Prenatal Diagnosis of β-Thalassemia; The Greek Experience*

Dimitris Loukopoulos, MD, Aris Antsaklis, MD, Vassiliki Aleporou-Marinou, PhD, John Panourgias, BsC, Photini Karababa, BsC, and Phaedon Fessas, MD

Prenatal diagnosis of thalassemia and the hemoglobinopathies has now been adopted as the most realistic measure to reduce the incidence of these conditions in Greece. The project is expanding rapidly in conjunction with the program for premarital examination carried out by the Ministry of Social Services, and has already served a considerable number of couples at risk. Preliminary results have been published or presented elsewhere [1,2]. The present report summarizes the experience to date and comments on the feasibility of the program on a large scale, as well as on the expenses and expected benefits. The mean incidence of heterozygous β-thalassemia in this country is about 8%; the distribution is uneven and varies from near 0 to 15% and even as much as 20% [3,4]. In addition, there are some areas with an extremely high incidence of Hb S [4], the inhabitants of which nowadays seek their partners from regions all over the country, and give birth to babies with sickle cell thalassemia. The latter condition is severe in most Greek patients and constitutes a clear indication for prenatal diagnosis. β^+- and β^0-genes are encountered in almost equal proportion; their identification is possible through their interaction with Hb S, but in most cases, is difficult since the β^+-thalassemic genes contribute only traces of β^A-chains to the total cellular hemoglobin.

On the basis of the above data, the total number of newborns with thalassemia major is estimated at approximately 200/year plus a few cases of various thalassemia interactions. It is therefore evident that 1,000 prenatal examinations are adequate to reduce the load of thalassemic patients to numbers which can be managed satisfactorily today.

*This study was made possible by research contract 1926/R1/RB of the International Atomic Energy Agency to D.L. and support from the Greek Ministry of Social Services.

Birth Defects: Original Article Series, Volume 18, Number 7, pages 293–301
© 1982 March of Dimes Birth Defects Foundation

The pilot work for prenatal diagnosis of thalassemia in this country has been carried out through a research contract with the International Atomic Energy Agency; today the program is fully supported by the Greek Ministry of Social Services. It is still being developed and various technical and administrative problems remain unresolved. Presently, our Unit does 7-10 tests/week; however, this number must soon increase to meet the rapidly increasing demand.

Acceptance of the procedure by heterozygous prospective parents and the overall population is good and, to our knowledge, no couple at risk has ever been refused prenatal examination. Information regarding prenatal diagnosis is spreading by women who have undergone the procedure, obstetricians who are willing to collaborate, and the media which report on thalassemia from time to time. In addition, the Unit has prepared a simple leaflet with relevant information which is available free to all interested persons.

At the beginning, most of the women examined had a child with thalassemia major and sought assistance in the hope that they might have a normal child. The pattern is changing gradually. At the onset of pregnancy, many women at risk are now referred by their obstetricians when, on routine laboratory evaluation they are found to have "anemia." The number of prospective parents who consider prenatal diagnosis *prior* to starting pregnancy is still very limited, but will surely increase in the near future, as more and more young people become aware and seek the appropriate blood tests. The number of cases evaluated in the present report is 500. Of these, 482 were at risk for thalassemia major, 17 for various sickle cell syndromes, and one for α-thalassemia (Table 1). In all instances, counseling on methodology and on risks was given to pregnant women seeking the test. One hundred twenty-two families already had an affected child. Furthermore, the pregnant women reported at least 650 abortions, most of which were undergone for fear of having another child with thalassemia major. Placental blood sampling was carried out by fetoscopy in almost all recent cases and was successful on the first attempt in 88%. Placental "blind" aspiration, which was widely used initially, is now reserved for repeats following failures by fetoscopy (Fig. 1, Table 2). The procedure is monitored by ultrasound.

TABLE 1. Case Analysis. June 1977-May 1981

Total number of cases 500; at risk for:	
β^{th}/β^{th}	468
$\beta^{th}/\delta\beta^{th}$	14
β^{S}/β^{S}	5
β^{S}/β^{thal}	12
$(\alpha\alpha)^{th}/(\alpha\alpha)^{th}$	1
Ten pregnancies were twin.	

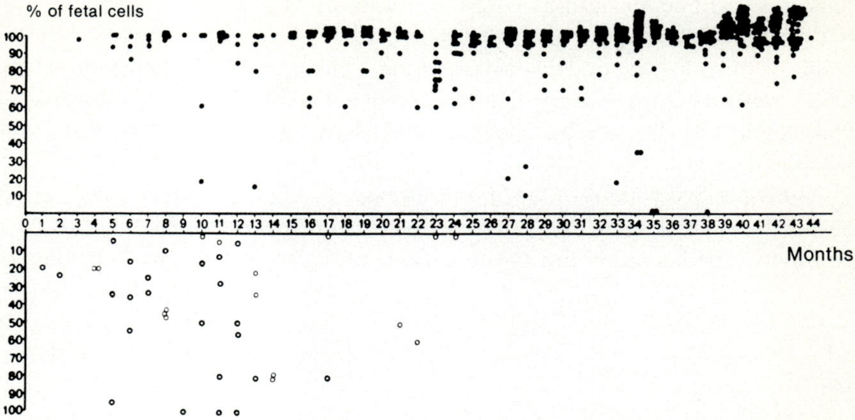

Fig. 1. Percentage of fetal cells obtained by "blind" aspiration (open circles, lower part) compared to those obtained by fetoscopy (black dots, upper part) throughout the progress of the study.

To avoid maternal red cell contribution to the in vitro globin biosynthesis, the first 100 cases were transfused with 4 units of packed red cells 15 days prior to the procedure. This resulted in complete suppression of erythropoiesis in the mothers, and thus all radioactivity in the (mixed) placental sample was considered to be of fetal origin. The subsequent cases were not transfused; maternal contamination was dealt with either by subtraction or by elimination of the maternal red cells by the Orskov technique [5]. However, with increasing experience the proportion of fetal cells is now 100% in most fetoscopies (Fig. 1). Study of the placental blood sample is still carried out by the standard method, ie

TABLE 2. Acquisition of Placental Blood Sample

	By Fetoscopy	By "Blind" Aspiration
On first attempt	427	12
On second attempt	27	19
On third attempt	–	5
On fourth attempt	–	2
Failure to obtain sample	4*	4*
Samples analyzed		492
472 from single pregnancies and		
10 from twin pregnancies (10×2)		

*Of these, 4 cases were followed by IUFD and 1 by premature rupture of membranes (26th week). The other 3 women elected to continue pregnancy and were lost to follow-up (2 from Cyprus).

biosynthesis of hemoglobin in vitro in presence of ^{3}H-leucine, separation of globin chains dissolved in urea-mercaptoethanol by chromatography on CM-cellulose columns [6], and evaluation of the β-chain/γ-chain radioactivity [1,2]. Other methods, such as electrophoresis in urea-Triton X gels [7] or hemoglobin chromatography [8], are being explored but have not yet been introduced routinely.

The β/pre-$\gamma + \gamma$ ratios of the 500 cases evaluated in this report are depicted in Figure 2 according to the week of gestation. In our laboratory, the ratio of 0.03 is considered the boundary line between cases of thalassemia major with some β-

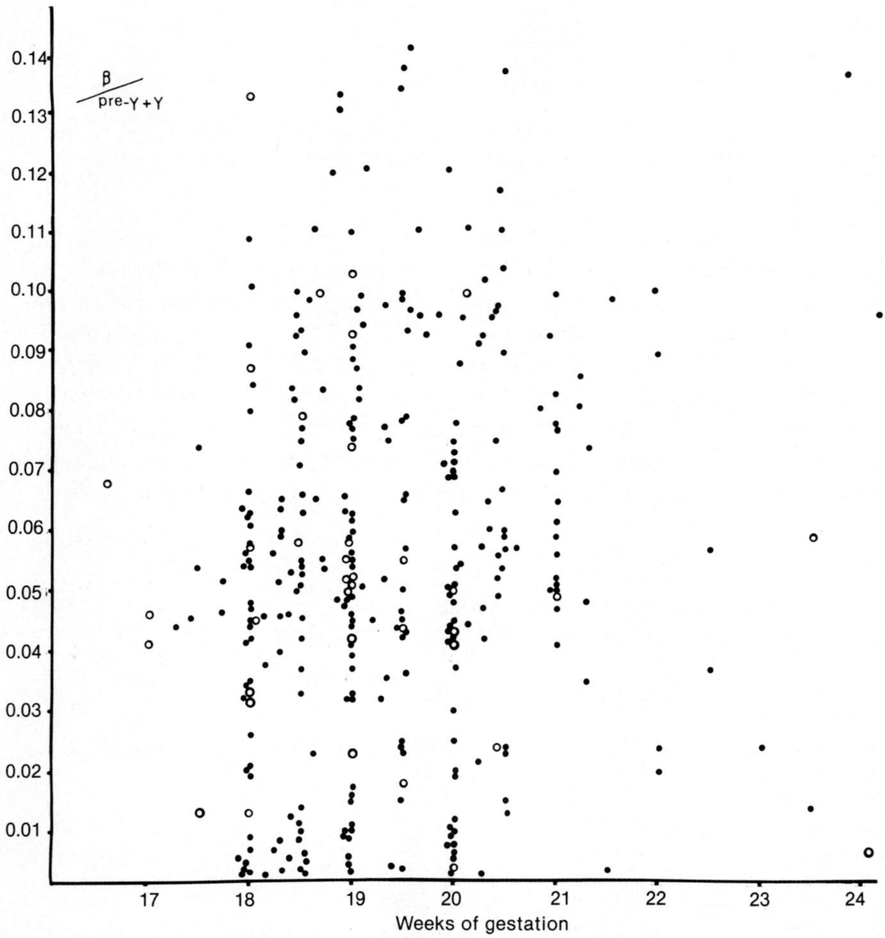

Fig. 2. Chart of the results obtained to date. Black dots denote cases studied by fetoscopy; open circles denote cases where the placental samples were obtained by "blind" aspiration.

chain production and cases with heterozygous β-thalassemia with very low β-chain production. This number has been decided by the experience from other Centers [9,10] and is realistic because 25% of the examined cases fall below this value. There is no doubt that a slight overlapping may occur; false-negative diagnoses have already occurred and will be difficult to avoid as a clear distinction between β^+-heterozygotes (hence, the β^+/β^+ combination) and β^0-heterozygotes is almost impossible in the Greek population [11]. False-positive diagnoses inadvertently aborted may also have occurred. A β/pre-$\gamma+\gamma$ ratio of 0.07 is taken to denote the lower normal level of β-chain synthesis. In fact, another 25% of cases exceed this level in our evaluation. Table 3 summarizes predictions and end results. It is estimated that by now about 420 children have been born. Confirmation is incomplete, since families are dispersed all over Greece and are somewhat reluctant to have their babies examined. Consequently, Table 3 includes confirmation obtained by blood examination of new-

TABLE 3. Predictions and Results Available to May 1981

Predictions					
Samples analyzed				492	
Fetuses predicted to be:					
β^A/β^A	125	(25.4%)			
β^A/β^{th}	234		359	373	(76.0%)
β^A/β^S			14		
β^{th}/β^{th}			115	118	(24.0%)
β^S/β^{th}			3		
No severe α-thalassemia				1	

Results available to May 1981

	Fetoscopy	Placental Aspiration	Total
Number of samples	454	38	492
Homozygotes predicted	111	7	118
confirmed	5 (5)	None	5
Heterozygotes predicted	227	22	249
confirmed	100 (85)	16 (13)	116 (98)
Normals predicted	116	9	125
confirmed	52 (46)	7 (7)	59 (53)
Numbers in brackets indicate confirmations by cord blood examinations (Hb biosynthesis or electrophoresis) *or* by hematologic evaluation at 6 months.			
False diagnoses			
Homozygotes not diagnosed in utero	4	1	5
Heterozygotes called homozygotes (laboratory error)	1	0	1
Inability to obtain results (laboratory problem; baby OK)	1	0	1

borns, as well as information given by the parents over the telephone that the baby is well. The same table presents an analysis of our false diagnoses. Of these, 3 negatives are due to wrong interpretation of marginal values (Fig. 3), another to an unexplained peak with β-chain mobility in a very satisfactory radiochromatogram, and 2 (1 false-negative and 1 false-positive) to interchange of samples during the procedure. To assure accuracy, whenever in doubt, our present policy is to repeat the whole procedure 2 weeks after the initial ambigu-

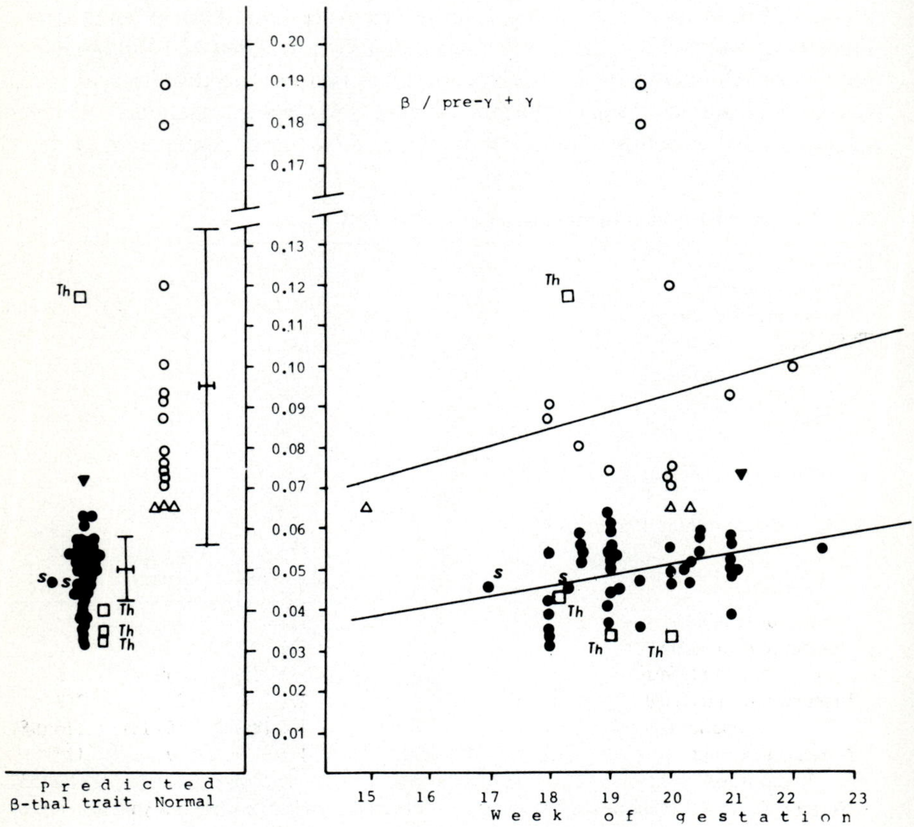

Fig. 3. Ratios β/pre-$\gamma+\gamma$ on fetuses predicted to have β-thalassemia trait (black dots), or no evidence of thalassemia (open circles), confirmed a few months after birth. Triangles pointing upward denote cases predicted to have heterozygous β-thalassemia but found entirely normal at birth. Triangles pointing downward denote cases predicted to be normal but found to have thalassemia trait. S denotes β^A synthesis on confirmed Hb A Hb S babies. Th corresponds to false-negative cases; 3 of them are close to the cutoff level. One remains unexplained. The means of (confirmed) normal vs heterozygous fetuses appear rather distinct; however, correlation of the ratios with gestational age is not significant.

ous diagnosis, to make sure that the β/pre-$\gamma+\gamma$ is at least increased or confirmed.

In conclusion, the overall picture is that prenatal diagnosis of thalassemia major is indeed an effective step toward control of the disease in Greece.

Reservations concerning the safety of placental aspiration cannot be a major obstacle, in our opinion. The total number of fetal losses (29) remains considerable (Table 4). However, analysis of these cases leaves no doubt that the occurrence of obstetric complications has decreased with increased experience, as the present rate of fetal losses directly associated with the procedure is less than 3%. On the other hand, it should be pointed out that not all cases of premature births can be ascribed with certainty to the procedure, as many of them may well represent a complication of pregnancy (Table 5).

Evaluation of the overall benefit from prevention versus treatment of thalassemia is summarized in Table 6. Under present conditions, the expense for treating a child with thalassemia major is estimated at $4,000/year. This sum represents cost of transfusion (blood processing, software, staff and hospitalization) and a mean cost of iron chelation therapy. This is expected to increase rather than decrease in the future because of various complications which endanger the patient's life when therapy is prolonged, and because of new therapeutic approaches which cannot be denied to the patients if they prove advantageous (neocyte transfusions mainly). The expense increases significantly when indirect expenses such as absence of parents from work, trips to specialized units, and nonproductivity of the patients are considered. An acceptable life, therefore,

TABLE 4. Obstetric Complications; Time Distribution

Obstetric complications	
Intrauterine fetal death	10
Including 4 cases which were followed by IUFD and 1 by premature rupture of membranes (26thw). The other 3 women elected to continue pregnancy and were lost to follow-up (2 from Cyprus).	
Intrauterine infections	2
Premature rupture of membranes	6
Premature birth (<28 weeks)	10
Total	28
Of these 14 are not necessarily related to the procedure (cf. Table 5).	

Time Distribution

	Number of cases	Complications definitely related	Total
June '77-May '78	59	4 (8.0%)	8 (16.0%)
June '78-May '79	98	7 (7.1%)	8 (8.2%)
June '79-July '80	202	3 (1.5%)	10 (5.0%)
August '80-May '81	141	0 (0.0%)	3 (2.1%)
TOTAL	500	14 (2.8%)	29 (5.8%)

TABLE 5. Fetal Losses Which Followed the Procedure but Are Not Considered Obligatory Complications

Intrauterine fetal deaths	
1.	At 8th month; colored amniotic fluid already present on day of amniocentesis
2.	At 9th month; umbilical cord knob
Premature rupture of membranes	
3.	Placental tap done on threatened abortion + cervical ligation
4.	One month later with no apparent cause
5.	Two days later but mother Wasserman (++++)
6.	One month later with no apparent cause
Premature births	
7.	30 days later following difficult trip
8.	60 days later; hydramnion; megacolon
9-14.	30-65 days later; no apparent cause
	The incidence of these complications in a normal pregnancy has not yet been established.

TABLE 6. Prevention Cost vs Benefit

Cost of Prevention:
Cost for identification of heterozygotes approximately $5/person when voluntary
Cost for examination of all couples marrying each year (100,000; one partner only) approximately $500,000
Cost of prenatal diagnosis with present methodology approximately $500/case
Cost of all estimated prenatal diagnoses to be necessary in Greece each year (1,000) approximately $500,000
Cost for total prevention per year approximately $1,000,000
Cost of Treatment:
Direct (hospital care, transfusions, iron chelation) by gross estimation $5,000/child year; significantly more when complications appear.
Indirect (parents out of work, traveling, no personal productivity) undefined but certainly very high.
Total expenses for treatment of children with thalassemia major alive today (2,000); by gross estimation $10,000,000/year
Total expenses for treatment of babies with thalassemia major born each year (200) about $1,000,000/year over the subsequent 20 years.

requires at least $5,000/patient/year; assuming a mean survival of 20 years and estimating that each year 200 newborns have thalassemia major, the conclusion is that each year the Greek Public Health Services are engaged in spending one million US dollars/year for the following 20 years for the treatment of new cases of thalassemia. Adding these increasing expenses to the huge cost of treatment now provided to patients already affected makes it clear that effective treatment soon will be impossible.

Prevention by screening, identification of the couples at risk, and prenatal diagnosis seem more realistic and less expensive. It is realistic because young people are now "sensitized" and demand premarital examination in many instances; antenatal clinics and private obstetricians are also helpful since they often advise pregnant women to have the appropriate tests. The national policy is to make identification of carriers readily available countrywide. The cost is no more than \$5/person examined, hence \$500,000 are adequate to cover all couples marrying each year (100,000/year; examination of one partner only). The cost of prenatal diagnosis with the present methodology is estimated at \$500/case; this means that another \$500,000 may cover the 1,000 examinations which become necessary in Greece annually. It ensues therefore, that with a cost of one million US dollars yearly, thalassemia can be controlled completely in this country; this relieves the Public Health Services from spending many millions over subsequent years as shown above, and is a convincing argument that the benefit of prevention is significantly greater than its cost.

REFERENCES

1. Aleporou-Marinou V, Sakarelou-Papapetrou N, Antsaklis A, Fessas Ph, Loukopoulos D: Prenatal diagnosis of thalassemia major in Greece; evaluation of the first large series of attempts. Ann NY Acad Sci 344:181, 1980.
2. Loukopoulos D: Prenatal diagnosis of thalassemia in Greece. In "la prevenzione delle malattie microcithemiche", Proc. 5th International Congress of the National Association for Control of Microcythemia. Rome 1980. Minerva Medica, 1980, p 255.
3. Malamos B, Fessas Ph, Stamatoyannopoulos G: Types of thalassemia trait carriers as revealed by their incidence in Greece. Br J Haematol 8:5, 1962.
4. Schizas N, Tegos K, Voutsadakis A, Arabatzis G, Angelopoulou P, Chrysanthopoulos K, Athanasiadou A, Bathrelou S, Rombos J, Skarlos D, Davakis M: The frequency and distribution of β-thalassemia and abnormal hemoglobins in Greece. A study of 15500 recruits. Hellenic Armed Forces Med Rev (Suppl 1) 11:197, 1977. (in Greek)
5. Alter BP, Metzger JB, Yock G, Rothchild S, Dawes GJ: Selective hemolysis of adult red cells: An aid to prenatal diagnosis of hemoglobinopathies. Blood 55:279, 1979.
6. Clegg JB, Naughton MA, Weatherall DJ: An improved method for the characterization of human hemoglobin mutants: Identification of $\alpha_2\beta_2{}^{95Glu}$ haemoglobin N (Baltimore). Nature 207:945, 1965.
7. Alter BP, Coupal E, Forget BG: Globin chain electrophoresis for prenatal diagnosis of β-thalassemia. Hemoglobin 5:357, 1981.
8. Blouquit Y, Beuzard Y, Varnavides L, Chabret C, Dumez Y, John PN, Rodeck C, White JM: Antenatal diagnosis of haemoglobinopathies by Biotex chromatography of haemoglobins. Br J Haematol 50:7, 1982.
9. Alter BP, Modell CB, Fairweather DVI, Hobbins JC, Mahoney MJ, Frigoletto FD, Sherman AS, Nathan DG: Prenatal diagnosis of hemoglobinopathies. A review of 15 cases. N Engl J Med 295:1437, 1976.
10. Matsakis M, Berdoukas VA, Angastiniotis M, Mouzouras M, Ioannou P, Ferrari M, Modell B, Fairweather DVI, Ward RHT, Loukopoulos D, Sakarelou N: Haematological aspects of antenatal diagnosis for thalassemia in Britain. Br J Haematol 46:185, 1980.
11. Fessas Ph, Agraphiotis A, Loukopoulos D: Hematological, biochemical and biosynthetic differences between β^0 and β^+ thalassemia heterozygotes. 17th Cong. International Soc. Hematology, Paris 1978, Abstracts.

Control of Homozygous β-Thalassemia by Carrier Screening and Antenatal Diagnosis in Sardinia*

A. Cao, MD, M. Furbetta, MD, R. Galanello, MD, M.A. Melis, A. Angius, C. Rosatelli, R. Ruggeri, M. Addis, T. Tuveri, A.M. Falchi, L. Maccioni, E. Paglietti, and M.T. Scalas

β-Thalassemia in Sardinia meets the prerequisites suggested for a prospective control of a recessive genetic disease through heterozygote screening and antenatal diagnosis [1]: A) the disease occurs in a defined population of 1.4 million inhabitants having a β-thalassemia carrier rate of 13%; B) there are simple and accurate methods for carrier identification [2]; and C) the homozygous condition can be detected in utero early in pregnancy [3,4].

In September 1977, on the basis of these considerations we started a pilot, voluntary genetic screening program directed at the prospective prevention of homozygous β-thalassemia in Southern Sardinia. Herein we are reporting the results of this program as of May 1981.‡

MATERIALS AND METHODS

Screening Program and Diagnostic Schema

The screening program directed at the adult population, primarily to couples of child-bearing age, was carried out in Southern Sardinia (Cagliari and Oristano provinces) on a voluntary basis. The program took 2 different approaches: 1) outreach community testing, and 2) hospital testing for an individual requesting the test.

Education, information, counseling, and sampling were carried out as previously described [5]. The diagnostic schema used is outlined in Figure 1 [6].

Screening Methods

Blood samples were drawn and stored in EDTA. Hematologic indices were obtained using the Coulter Counter model ZBI and Coulter Hemoglobinometer or Coulter Counter model "S." Hemoglobin electrophoresis was carried out on cellulose acetate plates (Helena Laboratories, Beaumont, Texas) in Tris-EDTA

*Supported in part by grants of Assessorato Igiene e Sanità Regione Autonoma della Sardegna; grant number 80.02252.83, Program of Preventive Medicine, CNR (Rome, Italy) Project M.E.E., and NIH grant number 5R01 HL-24173-02.

‡Preliminary results of this program have been published in Am J Hum Genet [5].

Birth Defects: Original Article Series, Volume 18, Number 7, pages 303–311
© 1982 March of Dimes Birth Defects Foundation

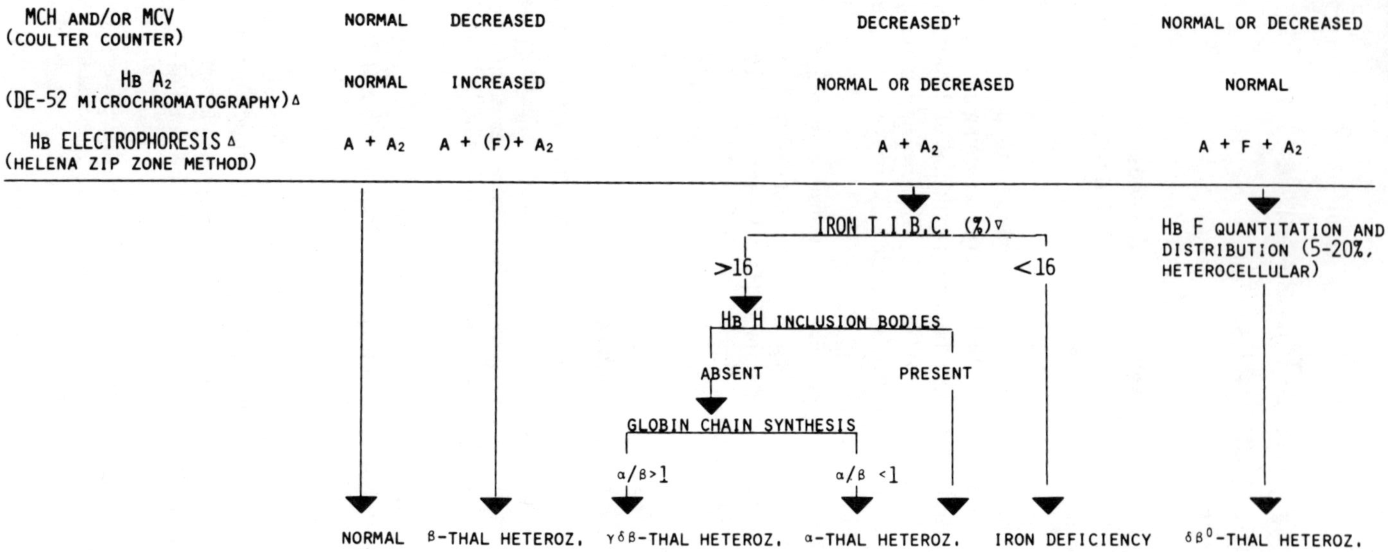

† VALUES LOWER THAN NORMAL MEAN -2 STANDARD DEVIATIONS

Δ HEMOLYSATES PREPARED ADDING FEW DROPS OF DISTILLED WATER TO PACKED RED CELL

▽ T.I.B.C. TOTAL IRON BINDING CAPACITY

Fig. 1. Scheme for mass screening for thalassemia syndromes.

borate buffer pH 8.6. Hemoglobin A_2 was quantified by DE-52 microchromatography [7]. Hemoglobin F was measured by alkali denaturation [8]. Erythrocyte Hb F distribution studies were performed with the Betke-Kleihauer stain [9] using commercial kits (Boehringer, Mannheim) or with the immunofluorescence method with anti-γ antiserum (kindly provided by Doctor Bernini, Leiden, Holland). Serum iron and iron-binding capacity were determined by the method of Lauber [10]. Hemoglobin H inclusion bodies were obtained by mixing equal volumes of whole blood and 1% brilliant cresyl blue in citrate saline solution and incubating at 37°C for 20 minutes to 1 hour.

Antenatal Diagnosis

Fetal blood was sampled by placental aspiration with a 20-gauge needle between the 18th and 20th week of pregnancy after placental localization with ultrasound (Picker Echoview model 80L) as described [11]. The placental samples obtained were checked immediately for the presence of fetal red blood cells with a Coulter particle size analyzer [3]; (^3H) leucine incubation, anti-i differential agglutination, NH_4Cl-NH_4HCO_3 differential lysis of maternal cells and globin chain synthesis analysis were performed according to previously described methods [3,11,12]. The diagnosis of homozygous state was based on a β/γ-globin chain synthesis ratio < 0.011. However, 95 of 98 homozygous fetuses identified to date had no β-chain synthesis [13]. The lowest β/γ ratio found in heterozygous fetuses was 0.022.

RESULTS

Outreach Community Testing

Testing was requested by 61% of the couples of child-bearing age living in the villages where the program was run. Twenty-five couples, in whom both husband and wife were found to be β-thalassemia carriers and hence at risk of producing thalassemia major offspring, were identified. Adding to this the number of couples who already had an affected child, the total number of at-risk couples in these villages was 45, which was very close to the expected figure of 61, with a carrier rate of 13.6% (Table 1).

Hospital Testing

The genetic service of the 2nd Pediatric Clinic, where the testing was carried out, takes care of the population of Cagliari and Oristano provinces. The villages, where the outreach testing was performed, are located in these provinces.

Of the total population of couples, 11.2% requested testing, and of 8,720 couples examined, 246 at-risk couples were identified (Table 2). Including 546 couples known to be at risk, as they already had affected children, 792 couples at risk were observed out of 1,300 expected. Pregnancy was in progress in 41.5%

TABLE 1. Outreach Community Testing: Demographic Characteristics and Overall Results

	Pimentel*	Samassi*	Samatzai*	S. Andrea Frius*	Sarroch*	Serrenti*	Settimo S. Pietro*	Villacidro*	Total
Population	1,160	4,742	1,574	1,763	3,944	4,674	3,583	12,690	34,130
Population at child-bearing age (15–44 yrs)	410	1,683	473	632	1,622	1,653	1,398	4,790	12,661
Population examined	101	1,050	109	191	527	477	442	1,161	4,058
% Population examined	24.6	62.4	22.9	30.2	32.5	28.9	31.6	24.2	32.0
Couples at child-bearing age (15–44 yrs)	100	448	156	155	412	508	313	1,227	3,319
Couples at child-bearing age examined	60	301	77	30	215	194	263	885	2,025
% Couples at child-bearing age examined	60.0	67.2	49.4	19.4	52.2	38.2	84.0	72.1	61.0
β-Thalassemia carriers identified	12	180	20	30	91	76	43	170	622
β-Thalassemia carrier frequency	11.9	17.1	18.1	15.7	17.3	15.9	9.7	14.6	15.3
Adjusted carrier frequency	11.5	14.9	16.3	13.7	14.8	12.9	9.1	13.9	13.6
Couples at risk identified	1	8	2	1	1	1	0	11	25

*Sardinian villages.

of the couples, and 329 out of 792 couples identified at risk, included 160 with and 169 without affected children. After counseling couples without affected children, 136 out of 169 elected to have antenatal testing, 23 (13.6%) decided against having the test and continued the pregnancy, and 10 aborted spontaneously during the interval between counseling and the day scheduled for the placental tap (Table 3). In the group with affected children, 129 out of 160 decided to have antenatal diagnosis, 18 (11.2%) decided against, and 13 (8.1%) spontaneously terminated before fetal blood sampling was performed (Table 3). The refusal of prenatal testing in both groups of couples showed a steady decline from 1977 to 1981 (Fig. 2).

Prenatal Diagnosis

In 129 pregnancies occurring in couples with previous affected offspring, 29 (22.4%) homozygous β-thalassemia fetuses were identified. In all instances but one, which was spontaneously terminated a few days after fetal blood sampling, the parents requested elective termination (Table 4).

There were 7 (5.4%) fetal losses due to premature labor or fetal hemorrhage. To date, 87 nonhomozygous fetuses have been born. The other pregnancies are still in progress. In 136 monitored pregnancies occurring in couples with no previous offspring, 35 (25.7%) homozygous fetuses were identified; in all but 2 cases the parents requested elective abortion (Table 4).

In the 2 pregnancies with β-thalassemia homozygous fetuses that continued to term, the respective offspring developed thalassemia major. There were 2 fetal losses due to premature labor and 81 nonhomozygous fetuses have been born to date. The other pregnancies are still in progress.

A survey of all in- and outpatient admissions to the hospitals of the provinces showed a steady decline of thalassemia major incidence at birth from 1976 to 1979 (Table 5).

TABLE 2. Hospital Testing: Demographic Characteristics and Overall Results

	Number
Population	802,888
Population at child-bearing age (15–44 yrs)	339,121
Population examined	16,279 (4.8%)
Total couples at child-bearing age (15–44 yrs)	77,490
Couples at child-bearing age examined	8,720 (11.2%)
Total carriers identified	3,215
Adjusted carriers	2,500
Heterozygote frequency	0.154
Couples at risk identified	246

TABLE 3. Outcome of the Couples at Risk Identified Who Had Had a Previous Pregnancy

	With Previous Affected Offspring	Without Previous Affected Offspring	Total
Couples at risk identified	546[a]	246	792
Couples who had had pregnancy	160[b]	169	329
Couples refusing antenatal diagnosis	18 (11.2%)	23 (13.6%)	41 (12.4%)
Pregnancies terminated before fetal blood sampling	13 (8.1%)	10 (5.9%)	23 (6.9%)

[a]Only couples identified in the hospital testing who had had a previous pregnancy.
[b]The total number of couples calculated from the heterozygote frequency is ~1,300.

DISCUSSION

In spite of the relatively low number of people tested, the results of this program, which was designed with the ultimate aim of controlling β-thalassemia major in the southern Sardinian population, are encouraging.

The outreach testing was very effective. Including the couples with a previously affected child, the total number of couples identified at risk was 45, which

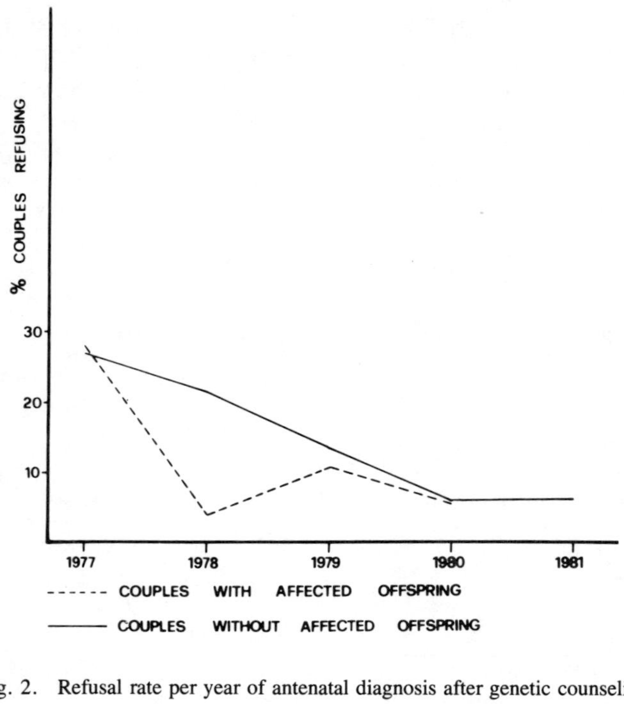

Fig. 2. Refusal rate per year of antenatal diagnosis after genetic counseling.

TABLE 4. Results of Antenatal Diagnosis of Thalassemia Major (Cagliari Center: May 1977 – April 1981)

	With Previous Affected Offspring	Without Previous Affected Offspring	Total
Pregnancies monitored	129	136[a]	265
Homozygous fetuses	29 (22.4%)	35 (25.7%)	64 (24.1%)
Electively terminated	28[b]	33[c]	61
Unaffected offspring born	87	81	168
Complications	7 (5.4%)	2 (1.4%)	9 (3.3%)
In progress	7	20	27

[a]One was a complication.
[b]Pregnancies of 2 homozygous fetuses were continued to term.
[c]One twin pregnancy, one unsuccessful fetal blood sampling attempt.

is very close to the expected figure of 61 with a carrier rate of 13.6%. Notwithstanding the low percentage tested (11.9% of the couples), and although less effective, the hospital testing gave promising results. In fact, considering couples, both with and without affected children, the total number of at-risk couples detected was 57% of the expected figure.

This highly apparent effectiveness of the screening and counseling could be due to the fact that many people requesting testing were relatives of homozygotes or heterozygotes, or went to the hospital for confirmatory testing but did not reveal prior positive results obtained in previous programs carried out in the schools. In order to increase the effectiveness of the program, we are now planning a more intensive screening which will be based on the activity of mobile units, each composed of a nurse and a social worker. According to the above described outreach approach, the main tasks of the units will be education, blood sampling, and counseling of the population of the district.

The consistent number of pregnant women requesting testing, particularly in the hospital, probably results from the educational publicity and counseling that stresses the availability of the prenatal diagnosis service.

TABLE 5. Newborn Incidence of Thal Major in Cagliari and Oristano Counties

Year	Number Thal Major Newborns[a]	Number Live Births	Incidence
1976	71	15,138	1:213
1977	58	14,850	1:256
1978	51	14,204	1:279
1979	21	13,398	1:638
1980	14		

[a]Number patients diagnosed in the different hospitals of the counties up to July, 1980.

After nondirective genetic counseling, most of the couples at risk (87.6%) who had a pregnancy requested testing. Similar attitudes were noted in the Cypriot community living in Britain [14].

The absence of statistically significant differences between the number of couples with and without previously affected offspring requesting antenatal testing is again encouraging, since it shows that even couples without the personal dramatic experience of the homozygous state were well informed and accepted antenatal testing as a method of having healthy offspring.

The refusal of antenatal testing after genetic counseling in 12.4% of the at-risk couples may be due to fear of complications or to ethical reasons. The steady decline of the refusal rate from the beginning (approximately 27%) to the actual figure (approximately 6%), without differences between couples with and without affected children, suggests that fear was the most prevalent reason against antenatal testing. The high number of pregnancies (approximately 7%) spontaneously terminated between counseling and fetal blood sampling sessions may be due to anxiety, to a decision to interrupt the pregnancy before attending counseling, or the misunderstanding of the counseling.

The steady decline from 1976 to 1979 in the incidence of Cooley anemia at birth seems to be extremely accurate since ours is a referral center and all Cooley anemia patients present at our hospital at least once. This decline is probably due partially to antenatal diagnosis, partially to the rational decision not to have other children, and to wider knowledge of family planning techniques.

The success of our program contrasts with previous experience in Greece concerning the sickle cell trait [15] and in Ferrara [16] concerning β-thalassemia, where the effects of genetic screening and counseling, carried out without the option of prenatal diagnosis, were negative. This was shown by the lack of difference in the observed and expected (in the case of random mating) figures of mating between carriers.

According to our previous experience [5,13], fetal blood sampling with needling was highly successful with a success rate of 98.8%, and the biochemical analysis of fetal blood by globin-chain synthesis seemed to be very accurate. In fact, no affected children have been born to date, and the homozygous incidence figure of 24.7% is very close to that expected for a recessively inherited disorder.

The 3.3% fetal loss is an acceptable figure as it is very close to the 3.2% and 3.5% values found in a prospective study concerning normal and amniocentesis midtrimester pregnancies, respectively [17].

In conclusion, this experience in the control of thalassemia major through carrier screening and prenatal diagnosis is promising; but a prospective controlled study, now in progress, is necessary to evaluate the long-term effects of screening and counseling of the target population.

ACKNOWLEDGMENTS

We thank Drs. Y.W. Kan and M.M. Kaback for their continuing advice, and Rita Loi and Kathleen Stark for their excellent editorial assistance.

REFERENCES

1. Kaback MM, Zeiger RS, Reynold LW, Sonnerborn M: Approaches to the control and prevention of Tay-Sachs disease. Prog Med Genet 10:103, 1974.
2. Weatherall DJ, Clegg JB: "The Thalassaemia Syndromes," 2nd Ed. Oxford: Blackwell Scientific Publication, 1972.
3. Kan YW, Golbus MS, Klein P, Dozy AM: Successful application of prenatal diagnosis in a pregnancy at risk for homozygous β-thalassemia. N Engl J Med 292:1096, 1975.
4. Alter BP, Nathan DG: Antenatal diagnosis of hematological disorders-1978. Clin Hematol 7:195, 1978.
5. Cao, A, Furbetta M, Galanello R, Melis MA, Angius A, Ximenes A, Rosatelli C, Ruggeri R, Addis M, Tuveri T, Falchi AM, Paglietti E, Scalas MT: Prevention of homozygous β-thalassemia by carrier screening and prenatal diagnosis in Sardinia. Am J Hum Genet 33:592, 1981.
6. Galanello R, Melis MA, Ruggeri R, Addis M, Scalas MT, Maccioni L, Furbetta M, Angius A, Tuveri T, Cao A: β°-thalassemia trait in Sardinia. Hemoglobin 3:33, 1979.
7. Huisman THJ, Schroeder W, Brodie AN, Mayson SM, Jakway J: Microchromatography of hemoglobins. III. A simplified procedure for determination of hemoglobin A_2. J Lab Clin Med 86:700, 1975.
8. Pembrey ME, McWade P, Weatherall DJ: Reliable routine estimation of small amount of foetal hemoglobin by alkali denaturation. J Clin Pathol 25:738, 1972.
9. Kleihauer E, Braun H, Betke K: Demonstration von fetalem Hämoglobin in den Erythrocyten eines Blutansstrichs. Klin Wochenschr 35:637, 1957.
10. Lauber K: Demonstration of serum iron and iron binding capacity without deproteinization. Z Klin Chem 3:96, 1965.
11. Kan YW, Golbus MS, Trecartin RF, Filly RA, Valenti C, Furbetta M, Cao A: Prenatal diagnosis of β-thalassemia and sickle cell anemia. Experience with 24 cases. Lancet 1:269, 1977.
12. Furbetta M, Angius A, Ximenes A, Tuveri T, Rosatelli C, Scalas MT, Fais R, Cao A, Angioni G, Caminiti F: Prenatal diagnosis of β-thalassemia with red cell enrichment with NH_4Cl-NH_4HCO_3 differential lysis of maternal cells. Br J Haematol 44:441, 1980.
13. Cao A, Furbetta M, Angius A, Ximenes A, Rosatelli C, Tuveri T, Scalas MT, Falchi AM, Angioni G, Caminitti F: Hematological and obstetric aspects of antenatal diagnosis of β-thalassemia. Experience with 200 cases. J Med Genet (In press).
14. Fairweather DVI, Ward RHJ, Modell B: Obstetric aspects of midtrimester fetal blood sampling or fetoscopy. Br J Obstet Gynecol 87:87, 1980.
15. Stamatoyannopoulos G: Problems of screening and counseling in the hemoglobinopathies. In Motulsky AG, Lenz W (eds): "Birth Defects. Proceedings of the Fourth International Conference." Amsterdam: Excerpta Medica, 1974, pp 268–276.
16. Barrai I, Vullo C: Genetic counselling in β-thalassemia in Ferrara. J Genet Hum 28:97, 1980.
17. NICHD Study Group: Midtrimester amniocentesis for prenatal diagnosis. Safety and accuracy. JAMA 236:1471, 1976.

Prenatal Diagnosis of β-Thalassemia: The Experience of the Center of Rome*

Leonardo Tentori, MD, Antonio Pachì, MD, Maurizio Bresadola, MD, Fabrizio De Gado, MD, Pasquale Bilotta, MD, Ester Alvino, PhD, Rosalba Paesano, MD, Adriana Massa, PhD, Marino Marinucci, PhD, Marco Vignetti, MD, Nadia M. Sposi, PhD, and Bruno Dallapiccola, MD

The Center of Rome operates in the II Obstetric Clinic, University of Rome, and the biochemical analyses are performed in the Hematology Laboratory of the Istituto Superiore di Sanità.

The diagnostic activity began in October 1979; as of June 1981 we had tested 102 couples at risk for different hemoglobinopathies:

— 95 couples at risk for β-thalassemia homozygosity
— 5 couples at risk for Hb S/β-thalassemia
— 1 couple at risk for Hb Lepore homozygosity
— 1 couple at risk for Hb Lepore/β-thalassemia

Fifty-one of the couples examined already had an affected child. The couples came from 10 different Italian regions, but mainly (75) from southern Italy.

Fetal blood sampling was obtained either by placental aspiration or by fetoscopy; in total, 62 placental aspirations and 40 fetoscopies were performed (Table 1). An adequate fetal blood sample, sufficient to carry out biochemical analyses, was obtained in all cases, usually on the first attempt. Fetal blood sampling was repeated in 3 cases because biochemical results were not definitive. Fetal losses were 7, more numerous in the beginning of our work; only one of the lost fetuses was homozygous.

Biochemical analyses were carried out on double samples, when feasible, according to the methods previously described [1], after enrichment of fetal erythrocytes, when necessary, by the Orskov selective lysis [2].

*This work has been partially supported by a CNR grant, Progetto Finalizzato Medicina Preventiva, contr. no. 81.00332.23.

Birth Defects: Original Article Series, Volume 18, Number 7, pages 313–315
© 1982 March of Dimes Birth Defects Foundation

The evaluation of β/γ-biosynthetic ratio has allowed us to predict 26 homozygous fetuses, 52 heterozygotes, and 24 normals. But the limit values for each group are not yet well established, as we have few controls at 6 months of age.

We have tried to express graphically in a histogram the β/γ-ratios, with a range of 0.005 (Fig. 1). It is clear that there are only two classes of higher frequency: the first for homozygotes (ranging from 0.005 to 0.01), and the second for heterozygotes (ranging from 0.04 to 0.045); there is no evidence for a higher frequency class for normals.

A problem not yet completely solved is the determination of cut-off point to distinguish between heterozygotes and homozygotes: on the basis of data resulting from a preliminary study on expression of β-thalassemia in southern Italy [3], and the Greek experience with β^+-thalassemia [4], we have fixed it at a value of β/γ below 0.03. The most important of several factors considered in the evaluation of the β/γ-ratios were the tested couples' regional origins, and the presence of previous, affected children.

The summary of the results is shown in Table 2.

Follow-up presents some difficulties due particularly to the fact that our couples live in different and distant areas. Twenty-four out of 26 homozygous fe-

TABLE 1. Fetal Blood Sampling

Number of Cases Attempted: 102	
a) Placental aspiration: 62	Mean percentage of fetal cells: 42
b) Fetoscopy: 40	Mean percentage of fetal cells: 86
Adequate Samples: 102	
a) Obtained at the 1st attempt: 87 (85.3%)	
b) Obtained at the 2nd attempt: 12 (11.8%)	
c) Obtained at the 3rd attempt: 3 (2.9%)	
Fetal Losses: 7 (6.9%)	

TABLE 2. Results of Prenatal Diagnosis for Hemoglobinopathies

Fetuses at risk: 102		Diagnoses performed: 102
	Homozygotes: 26 (24 for β-thalassemia; 1 for Hb S/β-thalassemia; 1 for Hb Lepore).	after abortion: homozygotes 24
		Tested: only at birth: 19
		at 6 months: 5 (3 heterozygotes and 2 normals)
Predicted:	Heterozygotes: 52	
	Normals: 24	
Diagnoses awaiting confirmation: 17		
Not yet born: 31		
Impossible to test: 6		

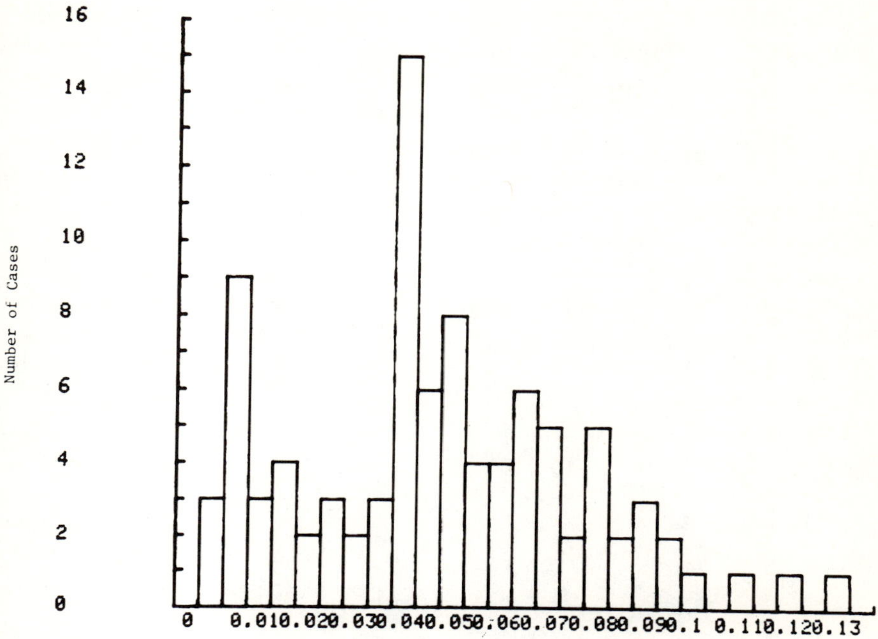

Fig. 1. Histogram of β/γ synthetic ratio distribution of 95 fetuses at risk for β-thalassemia (width: 0.005).

tuses have been tested after abortion; 24 babies have been tested, either at birth (19) or at 6 months (5), by biosynthesis and hematologic study. All the analyses were in agreement with the diagnoses made in utero. Seventeen newborns have not yet been tested.

REFERENCES

1. Massa A, Marinucci M, Tentori L, Alvino E, Pachi A: Diagnosi prenatale di beta-talassemia omoigote. In Pachi A, Dallapiccola B (eds): "Diagnosi Prenatale Precoce." Ed. Societia Editrice Universo (Roma), 1980, pp 241–251.
2. Boyer, SH, Noyes AN, Boyer ML: Enrichment of erythrocytes of fetal origin from adult-fetal blood mixtures via selective hemolysis of adult blood cells: An approach to prenatal diagnosis of thalassemia. Pediatr Res 8:883–897, 1976.
3. Tentori L, Marinucci M, Massa A, Mavilio F, Guerriero R, Gabbianelli M, Giampaolo A, Cianciulli P, Sposi NM, Masi M, Cecconi M, ANtimi M, Pratesi G: β-thalassemia in southern Italy: A preliminary approach. This volume.
4. Aleporou-Marinou V, Sakarelou-Papapetrou N, Antsaklis A, Fessas P, Loukopoulos D: Prenatal diagnosis of thalassemia major in Greece: Evaluation of the first large series of attempts. Ann NY Acad Sci 344:181–188, 1980.

Prenatal Diagnosis of Thalassemia by Fetoscopy: The Experience of the Milan Center

Bruno Brambati, MD, Maurizio Ferrari, Umberto Nicolini, and Angelo Cantù-Rajnoldi

The incidence of heterozygous β-thalassemia in Italy ranges between 2–20% [1]. The areas with the highest carrier rate are the Po Delta, the coast of southern Italy, Sicily, and Sardinia. After World War II an enormous migration from these regions to the industrial areas of northern Italy was observed, causing a marked growth in the thalassemia carrier rate, which, at present, ranges between 2.7% in Milan and 4.5% in Turin [1].

Surprisingly, in a country where the Roman Catholic Church resolutely opposes abortion, an increasing number of women, both from rural and industrial areas, are seeking prenatal diagnosis. Two important events concerning voluntary abortion were the decision of the Italian Supreme Court in 1975, and the popular referendum in 1978, both emphasizing a pregnant woman's freedom of choice. Until very recently there was no experience in antenatal diagnosis of thalassemia in mainland Italy, and hundreds of pregnant women at risk were obliged to attend different centers in foreign countries with considerable economic and obstetric burdens. For these reasons, the thalassemia prevention program of the Lombardy region has added prenatal diagnosis to public education, population screening, and genetic counseling [2].

In setting up antenatal diagnosis, fetoscopy was the method of choice for several reasons: 1) the rate of fetal loss is less than with placental aspiration; 2) the success rate in fetal blood sampling is not entirely dependent on the location of the placenta; 3) a 100% fetal sample is quite usual and the total number of fetal red cells is very large; and 4) this approach makes possible the acquisition of pure fetal blood allowing for prenatal diagnosis of other forms of genetic diseases [3–6].

When the obstetrician is introduced to fetoscopy without any prior experimental training, a substantially enhanced rate of fetal loss and unsuccessful sampling

Birth Defects: Original Article Series, Volume 18, Number 7, pages 317–321
© 1982 March of Dimes Birth Defects Foundation

characterizes the first series of cases. Moreover, the risk for the pregnancy is higher when a failed fetoscopy is followed by a second procedure [4]. The poor success rate of the first attempted procedure to obtain an adequate sample proves the value of increasing experience. Unfortunately, no experimental models have been devised to simulate the fetoplacental unit of human pregnancy for fetoscopy training. Nevertheless, for a center starting prenatal diagnosis the experimental training constitutes the only concrete reference to quantitate the risk of the diagnostic procedure. Consequently, we utilized late terminations of pregnancy to provide the experience necessary for diagnostic cases (Fig. 1).

The results of fetal blood sampling in 24 consecutive experimental fetoscopies performed by one of us (B.B.) are reported in Table 1. The analysis of the results clearly shows improved skill. In fact, in the second series of 12 procedures a success rate of 91% was attained and over 50% of the specimens were characterized by a 100% of fetal red cells. The placental site was not a serious problem

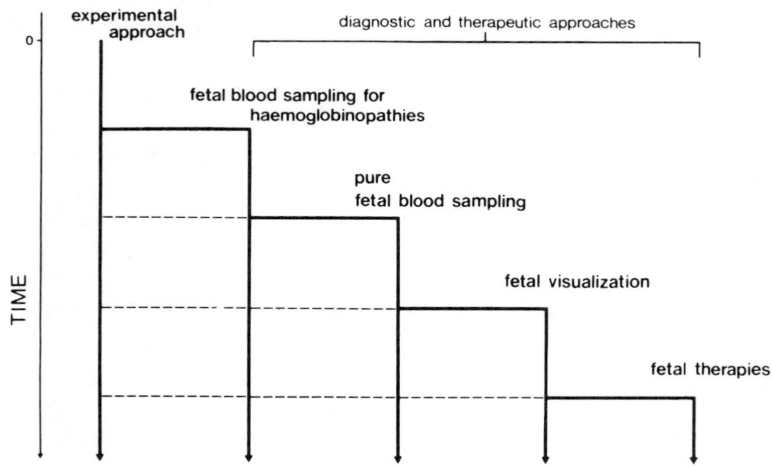

Fig. 1. Timetable in fetoscopy technique: priorities and potential use.

TABLE 1. Summary of Fetal Blood Sampling by Fetoscopy in 24 Experimental Cases

	No. of Cases	Successful Sampling (%)	No. of Specimens With 100% of FCs	Site of Placenta Ant.	Post.
1st Series	12	6 (50%)	3	4	8
2nd Series	12	11 (91%)	6	4	8
(Gestational Age: 15–23 Weeks)					

affecting the quality of the blood sampling. Hence, in December 1980 our team decided to start our prenatal diagnosis program.

The results of diagnostic fetoscopies up to May 1981 are reported in Table 2. A total of 23 procedures were performed on 22 patients. In one case at 17 weeks, we failed to obtain any fetal blood: the failure was due to stripping the membranes; 2 weeks later the sampling was successful. In 17 cases (77% of the total), a 100% fetal blood samples were obtained. In 5 cases, 97%, 87%, 80%, 67%, and 35% of fetal blood samples, respectively, were obtained. The last very low percentage characterized a sampling in a pregnancy at 22 weeks with an anterior placenta: in another center placental aspiration was attempted twice but no diagnosis was made. In this case, the amniotic fluid appeared extremely cloudy and the sampling was possible by means of a continuous flushing of the saline solution. In all but 2 cases the procedure took less than 20 minutes. In one case, an adequate blood sample was obtained only after 1 hour. The Hobbins cannula was introduced through the edge of a large anterior placenta: the maternal hemorrhage obscured the visual field, and the sampling was very difficult. There were some thousand million fetal red cells contained in the samples, the lowest value observed being 300 million cells. Fetal karyotype and AFP are always performed: in 14 cases the fetal karyotype was obtained in 4 days using fetal blood. Thalassemia major was diagnosed in 4 cases and selective abortion was performed by dilatation and evacuation technique within 24 hours. The diagnosis was confirmed in all cases. Fetal loss related to fetoscopy occurred in 1 case: the first case of our series, coming from the south at 22 weeks, aborted 2 weeks after an uncomplicated fetoscopy. In one of the 21 continuing pregnancies an ambiguous laboratory result on an adequate blood sample required a second procedure 2 weeks later, but the couple refused, deciding to continue the pregnancy regardless of test results.

When the test results suggested the presence of a thalassemia major fetus, the mode of termination was discussed with the patient and her husband. In communicating the diagnosis it seemed essential to try to identify the patient susceptible to significant emotional disturbances. For patients undergoing termination, careful reproductive counseling appeared very useful in reducing depression and obtaining a better emotional recovery. Considerable care and support was neces-

TABLE 2. Summary of β-Thalassemia Prenatal Diagnoses Attempted by Fetoscopy in 22 Cases

No. of Cases	No. of Procedures	Range of Gestational age (Weeks)	Quality of Specimens*	Fetal Losses
22	23	17–22	17	1

*Samples with 100% of fetal red cells; in 8 cases pure fetal blood was obtained.

sary for the case for which we failed to provide a test result: the pregnancy continues and the emotional state is being closely monitored.

Figure 2 shows how the increasing experience of the operator through the experimental phase improved both the success rate of obtaining a fetal blood sample and the percent of fetal red cells. It also clearly demonstrates the high success rate in obtaining 100% fetal red cells over the 5-month period of diagnostic activity.

In conclusion, we should keep in mind the following: 1) Experimental training is necessary in fetoscopy before starting with diagnostic procedures. We agree with the guidelines suggested by the most important centers [7] according to which adequate experience can be obtained with at least 20–25 midtrimester termination cases. Consequently, the training of fetoscopists can be accomplished only in the principal centers for late pregnancy terminations. 2) The

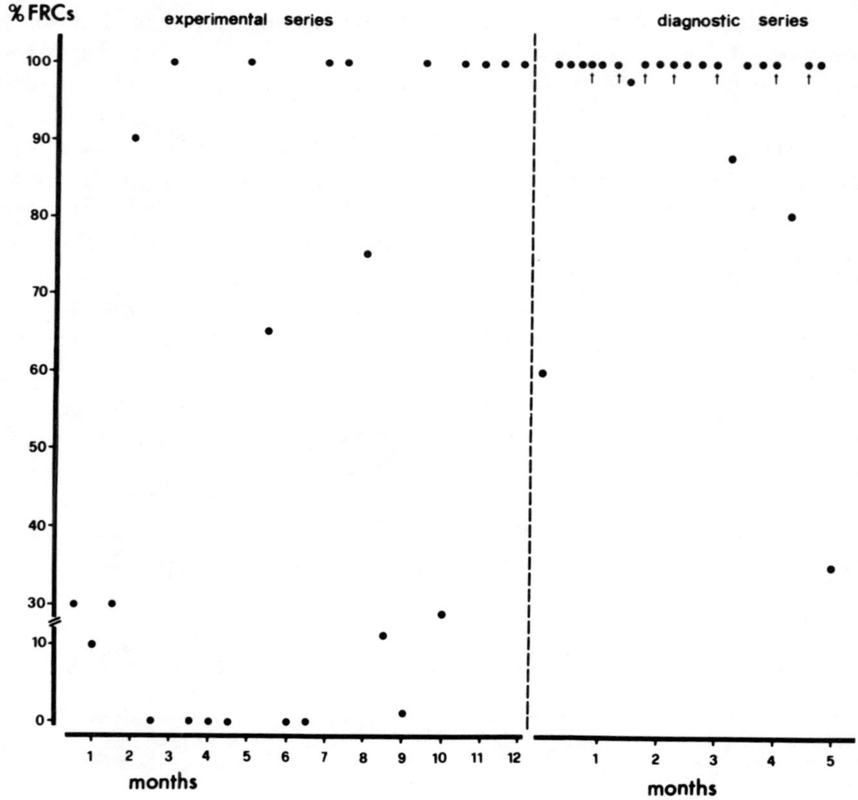

Fig. 2. Sequential time histogram of fetal blood samples (% of fetal red cells) in the experimental and diagnostic phases. The arrows point out samples of pure fetal blood.

dilatation and evacuation technique produces great technical and emotional involvement by the physician. However, the gains for women in speed, comfort, and acceptance are very great. Moreover, it is usually very easy to obtain a segment of umbilical cord to confirm the diagnostic results. 3) The evacuation of the uterus in less than 24 hours following the announcement of the fetus having thalassemia major appeared essential to reduce the distressing reactions. 4) After the termination of pregnancy, careful reproductive counseling and support should be insured as an essential means in preventing persistent adverse psychologic and behavioral reaction.

REFERENCES

1. Mazza U, Ciocca Vasino MA, Carena C, Colombero G: Diffusione e frequenza della microcitemia in Italia. In: Atti del VI Congresso Internazionale "La prevenzione della, malattia microcitemica." Ed. Minerva Medica, Roma, 1981, p 51.
2. Ferrari M, Cantù-Rajnoldi A, Brambati B, Nicolini U, Masera G: Il ruolo della diagnosi prenatale della talassemia in un program ma di prevenzione in Lombardia. In: Atti del V Corso Nazionale di aggiornamento in Medicina Perinatale, Milano, 2-4 giugno 1980. Ed. Cofese, Palermo, 1981, p 157.
3. De Vore GR, Mahoney MJ, Hobbins JC: Antenatal diagnosis of hemoglobinopathies, hemophilia, Von Willebrand's disease, Duchenne's muscular dystrophy, and chronic granulomatous disease by fetal blood analysis. Clin Obstet Gynaecol 7:41, 1980.
4. Fairweather DVI, Ward RHT, Modell B: Obstetric aspects of midtrimester fetal blood sampling by needling or fetoscopy. Br J Obstet Gynaecol 87:87, 1980.
5. Rodeck CH: Fetoscopy guided by real-time ultrasound for pure fetal blood samples, fetal skin samples, and examination of the fetus in utero. Br J Obstet Gynaecol 87:449, 1980.
6. Antsaklis A, Karayanopoulos C, Kaskarelis D: Clinical experience of 250 continuing fetoscopies for antenatal diagnosis. In Abstracts of 22nd British Congress of Obstetrics and Gynaecology, Edinburgh, July 8-11, 1980, p 86.
7. Hamerton JL, Simpson NF: Le diagnostic prénatal:hier, aujourd'hui et demain - Compte rendu d'un symposium international tenu à Val David, Québec, 4-8 novembre 1979. In: Le diagnostic prénatal. Cahiers de Bioéthique, Les Presses de l'Université Laval, Québec, 2:263, 1980.

TREATMENT OF THALASSEMIA

The Treatment of β-Thalassemia: Organization

Guiseppe Masera, MD

INTRODUCTION

Homozygous β-thalassemia is a genetically determined severe form of anemia, generally symptomatic early in life and, if not treated, leads to death in 2–3 years. Even though a cure for this disease has not yet been found, the life expectancy of a thalassemic child has been rising from 10–20 years in the 60s, to more than 20 years in the 70s, to reach an expected survival of more than 30 years in the 80s. These advances are essentially due to progress in transfusion and iron chelating therapy.

The good results achieved have enhanced our efforts to give total assistance (not only from a medical, but also from a psychologic and social point of view) aimed at ensuring the best quality of life for the thalassemic patient. Considering then the need for organized prevention programs, it becomes evident that thalassemia constitutes an important problem for many countries with a high incidence of the disease, not only insofar as medical care is concerned but also the social and economic aspects. The necessity to give these patients more qualified and rational assistance makes the planning of organized programs extremely important on a national or regional basis. Even if preventive and therapeutic policies must be strictly interlocked, we will deal only with the latter aspect.

In planning a therapeutic program for β-thalassemia we must consider several essential points: a) epidemiologic evaluation, b) analysis of needs and facilities, c) definition of aims, d) definition of all the points of the program and of the ways to fulfill them, and e) auditing. To make our discussion more concrete, we will discuss the program now in progress in the Region of Lombardy (RL), a northern Italian region of about 9 million inhabitants with an incidence of heterozygous β-thalassemia gene carriers of about 2–3%.*

*This program has been discussed and approved, at least in its general lines, by the Lombardy Section of Italian Association of Pediatric Haematology, by the Lombardy Association of Haemopatic Children's Parents, and by Regional Authorities.

Birth Defects: Original Article Series, Volume 18, Number 7, pages 325–328
© 1982 March of Dimes Birth Defects Foundation

EPIDEMIOLOGIC EVALUATION

In 1981, a census of all cases of β-thalassemia treated in the pediatric wards (up to about 15 yrs) in RL was taken. The 453 cases identified are distributed as follows: 1 hospital treats more than 100 patients, 2 hospitals treat from 51–70 patients, 5 hospitals from 11–50 patients, 10 hospitals from 6–10 patients, and 31 from 1–5 patients. In the coming years, a decrease in pediatric cases is expected, as births of thalassemic children are becoming progressively rarer (due to the prevention program, particularly prenatal diagnosis). We can assume that in 15 years thalassemia will become mainly an adult medical problem.

ANALYSIS OF NEEDS AND FACILITIES

At the present time, optimal treatment of thalassemia [1] requires periodic RBC transfusions and chelating therapy with microinfusors, which is done at home. Transfusions must be performed on an ambulatory basis in peripheral hospitals, as close as possible to the patient's home so as to minimize discomfort caused by traveling, and interference with school, play, and work. Transfer to a few specialized centers is not considered necessary as long as adequate training and updating of the operators are maintained.

Pediatric wards in RL have a low bed occupancy rate (about 50%); therefore, it would be feasible to exploit surplus room and working time for the creation of an ambulatory treatment service for thalassemic patients residing in the hospital area.

OBJECTIVES

A precise definition of the aims to be achieved is extremely important. Possible objectives might be: a) to ensure to all thalassemic patients living in RL the best total care (ie length and quality of life); b) to rapidly transfer research results into clinical practice; and c) to promote clinical and basic research.

LINES OF THE PROGRAM

Common Therapeutic Protocol

In 1981, the Italian National Research Council protocol [2], issued the main guidelines of the treatment to be followed: 1) minimum level of Hb of 11–12 gm/dl; 2) iron chelating therapy by subcutaneous route with personal portable infusors supplied directly by the hospitals; and 3) use of standardized clinical records.

Outpatient Clinic

In RL we have elected to create outpatient clinics as we consider them most acceptable by the patients; and we deem them suitable to permit the administering of the best therapeutic regimens. These units require: 1 bed for every 10 patients, 1 nurse for every 30 patients, and 1 physician every 50 patients. Operators work part time or full time according to local policy and needs.

Full Availability of Adequately Prepared Blood

In certain areas this could be a major problem requiring a special effort by the local health department. In RL there is no problem as far as fresh blood supplies are concerned, although the preparation of leukocyte-poor or -free derivatives requires better organization of blood banks. Transfusion of leukocyte-poor or -free RBCs is extremely important to avoid reactions in already immunized patients, and to prevent immunization in the others in order to give them the chance of receiving a bone marrow transplantation in the future.

The preparation of filtered red cells is quite simple and inexpensive, and thus is easily reproducible in all hospitals treating thalassemic patients [3].

Psychologic and Social Support

Other very important requirements are the presence of a psychologist and a social worker on the staff, and the elaboration of programs to provide a better social life for these patients. These programs include plans to help them at school, in looking for a job, and in play and sporting activities. In RL we are forming an operative link between psychologists and social workers dealing with thalassemic patients' problems at specialized centers, and those operators who deal infrequently with such cases. The final aim is to offer complete support to the child and to the family, to create a quality of life as normal as possible, including the opportunity of finding a job.

Continuous Education and Updating of all Personnel Operating in the Field

Every year, both medical schools of RL (University of Milan and University of Pavia), the Region itself, and the Association of Haemopatic Children's Parents organize an updating of physicians and nurses on the main hematologic topics. This part of the program is fundamental to ensure the best quality of care in all Region hospitals and to provide a rapid transfer of research results to clinical practice.

Research Programs

The follow-up of so large a series of patients under standardized conditions will permit the study of many problems: hepatitis B prevention, transfusion regimen's evaluation, iron chelating therapy, etc. Every subject will be thoroughly discussed by the staff to update participants. Another important point is the cooperation among different fields (medical practice, genetics, and biochemistry) to enhance basic research.

Data Bank

In RL we plan to collect information (vital statistics, social characteristics, and essential clinical data) and several standardized indicators (eg number of transfusions, minimum pretransfusional Hb levels, etc) for each patient to monitor the quality of care and evaluate future needs.

CONCLUSION

1) The planning of rational and organized assistance for thalassemic patients must first consider the socioeconomic and cultural situation in which health providers work; 2) the knowledge and critical evaluation of the different programs adopted in different areas could be of the utmost importance in continuously improving our results, always keeping in mind that the main objective is to ensure the best quality of care for every patient affected with thalassemia.

ACKNOWLEDGMENT

The author thanks M.G. Zurlo, MD, Cattedra di Puericultura Milano, for her helpful advice and criticism in the organization of this paper.

REFERENCES

1. Modell B: Total management of thalassaemia major. Arch Dis Child 52:489, 1977.
2. Cao A, Gabutti W, Masera G, Vullo C: Protocollo per la terapia della β-thalassemia. Consiglio Nazionale delle Ricerche and Associazione Italiana di Ematologia ed Immunoematologia Pediatrica. Genova 1981.
3. Sirchia G, Parravicini A, Rebulla P, Fattori L, Milani S: Evaluation of three procedures for the preparation of leukocyte-poor and leukocyte-free red blood cells for transfusion. Vox Sang 38:197, 1980.

The Management of the Improved Prognosis in Thalassemia Major

Bernadette Modell, MB, PhD

DESFERRIOXAMINE AND SURVIVAL

Regular iron chelation with desferrioxamine given intramuscularly, or more recently subcutaneously, has been shown to produce various beneficial effects, such as negative iron balance [1, 2], arrest of hepatic damage [3], and reversal of biochemical signs of liver injury [4]. Figure 1, based on data from Modell et al [6, 7], shows that it has also improved the survival of thalassemic patients in Britain. The study includes only patients over 16 years of age who have received im Desferal, as well as those (the same and others) who more recently have been receiving larger doses subcutaneously by "the pump." Though there is now good evidence for the extension of life by desferrioxamine, the final evaluation of its beneficial effects in terms of longevity could take up to 60 years.

Deaths can still occur in the older group of well-chelated patients. However, in general, these have not been primarily due to iron overload, but to rejection of treatment, or from infection or complications of infections, in splenectomized patients. It may be that the scene has changed, and the two main threats to life in thalassemic patients may now be noncompliance with treatment and overwhelming infection. This gives splenectomy a new importance, since there can be no doubt that splenectomy leaves a lifelong susceptibility to infection in at least some patients, though it is possible that patients whose spleens were removed in early life are most susceptible.

OPTIMUM TREATMENT FOR LONG-TERM SURVIVAL

For young and newly presenting patients we now need to stand back and reevaluate the design of treatment, with the aim of avoiding hypersplenism and preventing splenectomy, in order to provide the best long-term prognosis. Hy-

Birth Defects: Original Article Series, Volume 18, Number 7, pages 329–337
© 1982 March of Dimes Birth Defects Foundation

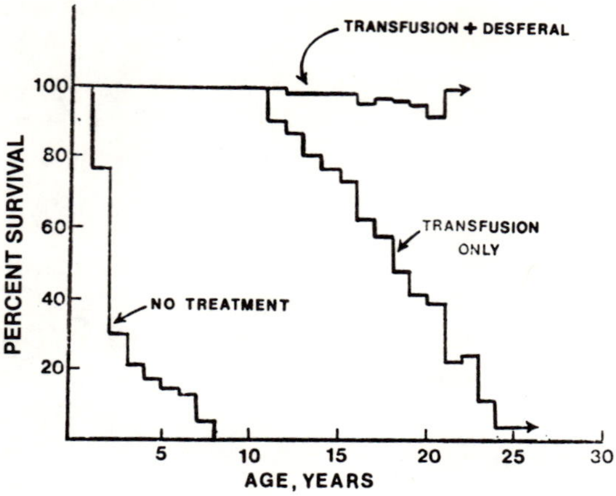

Fig. 1. Summary of data from a retrospective study of all British thalassemic patients who would have been 16 years old or more in 1980, including Dr. E. Letsky's and Dr. D. Flynn's patients from the Great Ormond Street Hospital controlled trial of desferrioxamine [3, 5]. The statistical analysis is reported elsewhere [6, 7]. The patients were divided into 2 groups — those who had received desferrioxamine 500 mg or more 5 days a week or more for 2 years or more (the "chelated" group) and those who had received less than this or none (the "unchelated" group). The lines show the percent survival of the patients who should have reached a certain age. For instance, of "chelated" patients who should have passed through the age of 20 before 1980, 5% did not because they had died. However, 100% of the small group of patients who should have passed through the age of 21 by 1980 were still alive, whereas only 22% of "unchelated" patients who should have reached 21 did so. The numbers of older patients who have been chelated in the long term are still quite small, which makes accurate statistical analysis difficult. A more sophisticated form of analysis has been used by Modell et al [6] with essentially similar results.

persplenism seems to be more common among some types of patients than among others. For instance, about 90% of London Cypriot patients, who generally have homozygous β^{+}-thalassemia, have developed severe hypersplenism and required splenectomy [7], but hypersplenism has been much less common among patients in Ferrara with homozygous β^{o}-thalassemia (G. Vullo and M. Lucci, personal communication). It has also been shown that high transfusion can reduce or retard the development of hypersplenism in Cypriot patients with thalassemia [8]. Finally, in many cases, especially in β^{o}-thalassemia, the "supertransfusion" scheme favored by Propper et al [9] (ie transfusing from 11 to 15 Hb gm/dl, mean about 13 gm/dl) does not ultimately increase the amount of blood required.

Putting all these observations together, it therefore seems that new patients presenting with severe transfusion-dependent thalassemia major (not thalassemia intermedia) should be started on a regular "supertransfusion" regimen with the objective of clearing thalassemic cells from the peripheral blood, and so removing the stimulus to hypersplenism. The hope that this approach would achieve the best possible long-term prognosis by preserving the spleen.

In general, in the past, we have hesitated to remove the spleen unless the blood requirement was increased to twice the expected level or more [8], and this policy should still be followed. In some cases, hypersplenism can be reduced by a short course of steroids, and it may be that a trial of intensive high transfusion plus prednisolone should be tried in young hypersplenic patients in an effort to get hypersplenism under control, rather than proceeding straight to splenectomy. However, if a patient's blood requirement remains at more than twice basal, and especially if there is thrombocytopenia, there is no resort other than splenectomy. This should be preceded, or followed, by immunization with polyvalent pneumococcal vaccine, and with prophylactic penicillin V 125 mg bd, *provided that the patient takes it regularly.* If the patient proves unreliable, as most do in their teens or as young adults, it is best not to give prophylactic penicillin, or to give regular injections of long-acting penicillin at transfusion, so as to be clear where you stand should the patient present with an infection.

PSYCHOLOGIC ASPECTS OF IMPROVED SURVIVAL

Because of improved treatment, there is now an increasing group of patients of adolescent and adult age who are facing a set of difficult physical and emotional problems that we have not encountered before. As the birthrate of new patients with thalassemia major is falling drastically, it seems that we have a limited cohort of patients who have difficult problems now, and will continue to have them all their lives. I would like to discuss the management of this group of patients.

The simple knowledge that a disease is fatal is in itself responsible for a great deal of suffering, because it leads to despair. The fact that thalassemia can no longer be confidently described as a fatal disease has brought about an enormous amelioration of the effect of the illness on the family, but now the anxieties of the older patients, the doctors, and all the other patients are focused on the well-being of the oldest age group. Their confidence and everyone else's rises steadily as they continue to lead rewarding lives, but their position is particularly stressful. This is a strong reason why special efforts should be made for them.

Table 1 shows the timing of the main advances in the treatment of thalassemia. High transfusion was introduced by Wolman [10], and the intramuscular use of desferrioxamine by Sephton-Smith in 1964 [1]. Propper introduced the improved method of administering desferrioxamine by subcutaneous infusion of larger doses in 1975, and "supertransfusion" in 1977. Consequently the prognosis has improved progressively, from about 10 years in 1960, to around 16 years by 1970 (when patients still used to die of tranfusional iron overload before desferrioxamine treatment was widely adopted), to an open-ended prognosis by 1980. The older patients have survived all these phases. Their perception of their disease has undergone a constant evolution, and many of them now have complicated physical problems (Table 2) due to the late point in their lives at which control of iron overload was achieved. It is to be hoped that similar problems will be avoided by younger patients who are treated by high transfusion and adequate chelation therapy from the start.

Thalassemic patients usually start attending the clinic by themselves at about 12 years of age, and it is at this time that they begin to encounter more complicated physical and emotional problems. Many of the physical difficulties summarized in Table 1 have important emotional consequences, and the depression they cause is possibly the greatest danger now to the lives of the older patients, because they have available a passive means of committing suicide by failing to take their Desferal.

There is often a tendency among adolescents with chronic disease, such as diabetes, to reject treatment because of a combination of depression with the adolescent need to be "normal." Rejection of treatment can occur in thalassemia, especially if the patient has no long-standing stable relationship with a particular doctor or nurse who can encourage and support him. The danger of denying the disease is greatest among the few whose physical development through puberty has been normal; unfortunately they often reject the idea that there is anything seriously wrong with them, together with the treatment that would preserve their normality. They may have sexual relations, marry and reproduce, and come for their transfusions regularly, but they may refuse regular desferrioxamine treatment, especially if they have not had it from childhood. They may also try to avoid contact with other patients with thalassemia, especially those who are physically less "normal" than they, because this undermines their psychologic defenses; provision may have to be made for this, for instance by transferring them to an adult clinic or arranging a special time for their visits.

Patients who have obvious problems with puberty have no opportunity to pretend they are normal, especially if everyone treats them as children when they are 20, which is a very painful experience. These patients often achieve an impressive psychologic balance and both give and receive a great deal of mutual support in a peer group of thalassemic patients. Unfortunately, some patients in this age group still die; this of course presents a serious emotional problem every time it happens. Under these circumstances frank discussion and reliable support are required.

The main emotional problems of young adults with thalassemia are summarized in Table 3, which is intended to show that adaptation to death can all too easily lead to death. Some of the simple physical steps that can be taken to counteract the problems and help the patients value their lives are discussed below and summarized in Table 3.

TABLE 1. Timing of Developments in the Control of Thalassemia

Treatment	Decade 1960	1970	1980
1. Blood	.... Wolman [10] ↓	High transfusion →	→
2. Iron chelation im	Sephton-Smith [1] ↓	20 mg/kg/day →	....
sc		Propper [9] 25–45 mg/kg/day ↓ →	→
3. Splenectomy when indicated	.. →	→	→
Prognosis	7–10 years	16–20 years	open-ended
Antenatal diagnosis		→	→

im = intramuscular
sc = subcutaneous

TABLE 2. Physical Problems of Thalassemic Patients More Than 12 Years Old

Failure of { growth - dwarfism*; puberty - hypogonadism* }

Endocrinopathy - { hypoparathyroidism; diabetes*; hypothyroidism; GH deficiency }

Cardiac disease
Hepatic disease
Risk of postsplenectomy infection
Danger of death*

*Major causes of emotional stress

ADAPTATION TO DEATH

Most patients have spent a lifetime coming to terms with death, but now they are faced with the new task of coming to terms with life and hope, and this is not easy. In coming to terms with death, some were bitter and despairing, though some managed to adjust, and all had an undercurrent of depression which combined with failure of puberty to produce passive behavior. This made them compliant patients, but the contrast with the usual storms of adolescence was striking

TABLE 3. Problems of Adolescents With Thalassemia Major

Feature	Associated with:	Result	Counteraction
1. Adaptation to death	depression; living for the moment; caring for others; religion	Depression leading to death	Adaptation to life (← Adult commitment)
2. Rejection of treatment	despair; "testing"; need to be normal		Responsibility for treatment (→ Adult commitment)
3. Failure of puberty, infertility	feelings of inadequacy		Replacement therapy (→ Adult commitment)
4. Difficulty in employment	feelings of inadequacy		Strong support (→ Adult commitment)
5. Isolation	major problem		Peer group
6. Transfer to adult physician	the wrong moment		day care; adolescent unit; careful overlapping/graded transfer

and distressing to those who understood its meaning. The introduction of hope (and replacement therapy) has produced a more aggressive approach to the problems of their lives, and the combination of a continuing need to live every day to the fullest (because their prognosis is uncertain) with the challenge to work at creating a life for themselves (because of new realistic hope) sometimes leads to excessively lively or assertive behavior. This should be accepted, and explained to medical and nursing staff, as a highly desirable alternative to the previous passivity and depression, even when it causes mild disturbances of medical routine. (For instance, our older patients who have cars often discharge themselves from hospital at 3:00 am when a transfusion has finished.)

REJECTION OF TREATMENT

This is the greatest danger to the life of adolescents at present, and is partly a rejection of dependence. It can be counteracted by giving the patients as much responsibility as possible for their own treatment, eg in the selection of veins for blood-taking or transfusion, allowing those who so wish to set up their own transfusions, discussing transfusion and chelation treatment with them as partners and collaborators, and arranging the management routine as conveniently as possible for each patient. They need (and want) *continual* pressure and encouragement to continue their chelation therapy, and this takes time. It is worth noting that children who have started receiving regular injections early, so that they can barely remember a time when they did not have them, do not seem to have as much difficulty continuing them through puberty, so we hope this problem will decrease with time.

IMPAIRED SEXUAL DEVELOPMENT

People in general are held to life by their responsibilities to others, as expressed in their family life and at work. Thalassemics should be encouraged to aspire to adult sexual relationships, to work, and to marriage, because they will best look after themselves if they feel something important depends on their continuing health. Therefore, replacement therapy is of the greatest importance. Even those patients who have passed through a normal puberty should be continuously monitored, since secondary impotence or amenorrhea is common, may not be mentioned spontaneously and can be extremely demoralizing if not treated. The doctor can conscientiously support patients in aiming for normal adult goals *providing they are taking their desferrioxamine regularly.* Steps that increase their commitment to life improve their treatment and in a self-confirming way prolong life, as indicated in Table 2.

DIFFICULTY IN OBTAINING EMPLOYMENT

This differs according to the country in which the patients live, and their doctors' ability to support them. In Britain, thalassemic patients have not had major difficulties, though most are employed below their potential. One student (our first) has just obtained an honors degree in Biochemistry. In the long term, the thalassemic patients' lives may depend on their ability to gain employment, and they should receive the fullest encouragement in their efforts. Most find it difficult or embarassing to attend a clinic or come for transfusion during the day, as they do not want to take time off from work or from studying for exams, so evening or weekend treatment should be provided.

ISOLATION

This can be effectively countered by putting older patients in touch with each other so that those who wish can form a peer group. The most lively section of the British Parents' and Patients' Association, the UK Thalassaemia Society,* is the 40–50-strong older patients' group, which meets weekly for social activities.

CONCLUSIONS

1) Thalassemic children should be under the long-term care of a single individual, so that the strong relationship they establish with their doctor in childhood can be used to their advantage when they most need it, during adolescence and early adult life. At this time, when they must achieve independence of their parents, and yet are dependent, they need the doctor to fulfill a parent-like supporting role. Because of the many physical complications of the disease, this role cannot be fulfilled adequately by the paramedical staff.

2) If the patients must be transferred from pediatric to adult care at 14–16 years of age, the changeover should be done gradually, and when the patients themselves feel ready for it.

3) Day-transfusion using washed or frozen red cells is the optimal system, since it allows children, adolescents, and adults to be treated by the same team and avoids the traumas of transfer.

4) Many adolescents and young adults are working for exams, or find it difficult or embarrassing to take time off from work. An evening clinic is a necessity for them, and evening transfusion would be ideal.

5) Measures which increase adult commitment are crucially important in helping the patients to survive mentally and physically. Therefore, replacement ther-

*Address: UK Thalassaemia Society, 107 Nightingale Lane, London, N8 England.

apy with sex hormones should be given adequately and early, and all possible support should be provided to help these patients obtain and retain jobs.

6) The acceptance that doctor and patient are partners in the struggle against thalassemia, and *full* information about the disease and treatment, is necessary to preserve the patients' autonomy and self-respect.

REFERENCES

1. Sephton-Smith RS: Chelating agents in the diagnosis and treatment of iron overload in thalassaemia. Ann NY Acad Sci 119:776–788, 1964.
2. Propper RD, Shurin SB, Nathan DG: Reassessment of the use of desferrioxamine B in iron overload. N Engl J Med 294:1421–1423, 1976.
3. Barry M, Flynn DM, Letsky EA, Risdon RA: Long-term chelation therapy in thalassaemia major: Effect on liver iron concentration, liver histology, and clinical progress. Br Med J 2:16–20, 1974.
4. Hoffbrand AV, Gorman A, Laulicht M et al: Improvement in iron status and liver function in patients with transfusional iron overload with long-term subcutaneous desferrioxamine. Lancet 1:947–949, 1979.
5. Letsky EA: A controlled trial of long-term chelation therapy in homozygous β-thalassemia. In Bergsma D, Cerami A, Peterson CM, Graziano JH (eds): "Iron Metabolism and Thalassemia." New York: Alan R Liss for The National Foundation-March of Dimes, BD:OAS XII(8)31–41, 1976.
6. Modell B, Letsky EA, Flynn DM, Peto R, Weatherall DJ: Survival and desferrioxamine in thalassaemia major. Br Med J 284:1081–1084, 1982.
7. Modell B, Berdoukas V: "The Clinical Approach to Thalassaemia." (In preparation)
8. Modell B: Total management of thalassaemia major. Arch Dis Child 52:489–500, 1977.
9. Propper RD, Button LN, Nathan DG: New approaches to the transfusion management of thalassaemia. Blood 55:55–60, 1980.
10. Wolman IJ: Transfusion therapy in Cooley's anaemia: Growth and health as related to long-range hemoglobin levels. A progress report. Ann NY Acad Sci 119:736–747, 1964.

Reduction of Iron Overload in Thalassemia

Sergio Piomelli, MD, and Joseph Graziano, PhD

Repeated blood transfusions, the basis of therapy for the thalassemia syndromes, have invariably led to the development of secondary iron overload associated with multiple organ dysfunctions [1,2]. Three approaches to the reduction of iron overload have been evaluated in our laboratory: splenectomy, transfusion with young red blood cells, and chelation therapy with deferoxamine. While the first two approaches are aimed at reducing iron input, the studies of chelation therapy have been designed to increase iron output such that iron balance may be achieved in patients of various ages. We will take this opportunity to review our recent work in this field, emphasizing that iron overload can be effectively dealt with *only* through a program which minimizes blood intake *and* achieves good compliance with chelation therapy, while maintaining the hemoglobin concentration in the normal range.

SPLENECTOMY

Prior to the development of current hypertransfusion regimens which are designed to maintain the hemoglobin concentration and prevent the numerous consequences of erythroid expansion, the decision to remove the spleen was invariably based on the development of overt hypersplenism, with splenic engorgement, anemia, thrombocytopenia, and leukopenia [3]. Because there is an increased risk of fatal infections after splenectomy [4,5], and because the presence of the spleen probably prevents early iron-induced damage to the liver, the decision to remove the spleen has rarely been an easy one. The usefulness and timing of splenectomy have been even less clear-cut since the advent of hypertransfusion therapy, which prevents overt hypersplenism in early childhood [4,6,7].

We therefore assessed the role and optimal age for splenectomy [8] in a large group of hypertransfused patients followed at 3 institutions in New York City (Columbia Presbyterian-Babies' Hospital, Cornell-New York Hospital, and New

Birth Defects: Original Article Series, Volume 18, Number 7, pages 339–346
© 1982 March of Dimes Birth Defects Foundation

York University-Bellevue Hospital). Transfusion records for the year 1978 were comprehensively reviewed, and only patients whose mean pretransfusion hemoglobin concentrations were 10 gm/dl or greater, ie only those who were truly hypertransfused, were included in the data analysis. Prior to 1978, most patients had been maintained at a lower hemoglobin concentration for some period in their lives, while a subgroup of 8 patients had been hypertransfused since the time of diagnosis. Frozen red blood cells had been used almost exclusively to minimize leukoagglutinin reactions.

When the blood requirements were calculated and analyzed as a function of age, there were striking differences between the splenectomized and nonsplenectomized groups (Table 1), despite the fact that the mean pretransfusion hemoglobin concentrations of both groups were identical (10.9 gm/dl). Before the age of 6 years, the blood requirement of 11 nonsplenectomized cases was 211 ml/kg/yr, which is comparable to that seen in older splenectomized patients. However, after the age of 6 years, the presence of the spleen resulted in a substantial increase in blood requirement and iron load (Table 1). The difference between the 2 groups of patients is graphically shown in Figure 1, which illustrates that in nonsplenectomized patients, the transfusion requirement increased steadily with age ($p < 0.03$), while in splenectomized patients the transfusion requirement remained relatively constant with age.

We interpret these data to indicate that splenectomy reduces the rate of iron loading, even in hypertransfused patients with Cooley anemia. The blood requirements of 8 patients, who were hypertransfused since the time of diagnosis, were not different from those of other nonsplenectomized patients who had begun hypertransfusion only recently. Thus, while the initiation of hypertransfusion early in life prevents overt hypersplenism and has numerous other beneficial effects [6,7,9], it does not eliminate the ultimate need for splenectomy. Since the completion of this analysis, we have adapted the practice of removing the spleen when the annual blood requirement exceeds 250 ml/kg/yr. Following splenectomy, the requirement invariably falls to approximately 200 ml/kg/yr; in 10 patients who have reached one year postsplenectomy, the mean transfusion requirement fell from 327 ml/kg/yr to 198 ml/kg/yr, a 39% reduction in the annual iron load.

TABLE 1. Mean Transfusion Requirement (ml/kg/yr)

Patient Group	0-5 yrs	6-10 yrs	11-15 yrs	16-20 yrs	21-25 yrs	26-30 yrs
Nonsplenectomized	211 (11)*	262 (20)	295 (11)	277 (4)	— (0)	— (0)
Splenectomized	— (0)	223 (1)	224 (7)	187 (12)	199 (8)	195 (5)

*Number of patients

YOUNG RED CELL TRANSFUSIONS

In 1973 [10], based on in vitro experiments utilizing an arabinogalactane (stractan) density gradient technique [11] capable of separating red cells according to age, our laboratory proposed that it might be possible someday to isolate young red cells for transfusion into patients with thalassemia major. Subsequent studies in rabbits demonstrated prolonged survival in vivo of the less dense fractions of red cells as compared to unfractionated blood [12]. In 1980, Propper and co-workers [13] reported that continuous flow blood cell separators, which also utilize differences in cell densities to achieve cell fractionation, could be adapted to isolate very young red blood cells with improved survival for transfusion into patients with Cooley anemia. However, the pheresis approach to young cell separation is extremely expensive, requires highly motivated blood donors, and is associated with some risk to the donors [14]. To our knowledge, the use of continuous flow blood cell separators for the collection of young red cells has been abandoned by all major centers as a practical approach to the treatment of thalassemia major.

During the past 2 years, we have been successful in developing simple and relatively inexpensive methods for isolating young red cells from ordinary units of fresh or frozen blood [15,16]. These methods utilize the IBM-2991 Blood Cell

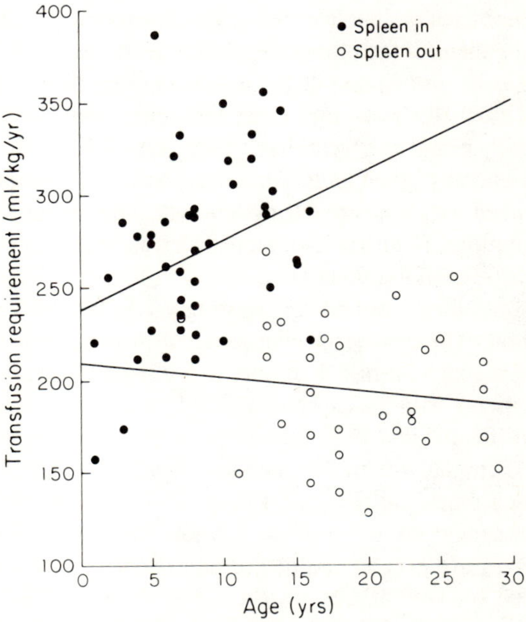

Fig. 1.

Figs. 1–3 from Graziano J et al: Chelation therapy in B-Thalassemia major. III. The role of splenectomy in achieving iron balance. J Pediatr 99:695, 1981, with permission.

Processor, an instrument which was originally designed to deglycerolize frozen blood, or wash a unit of fresh blood. The key to the method, whose important details have been described elsewhere [16], is a centrifugation step initiated when the red cell boundary reaches the centerport of the instrument. During that centrifugation, the most dense cells migrate to the outside of the centrifuge head, while the lighter cells distribute toward the center. When red cells subsequently are slowly expressed through the centerport, they can be collected in an age-dependent sequence, youngest cells first [16]. Based on in vitro measurements of pyruvate kinase, an age-dependent red cell enzyme, we have determined that the resolution of the IBM-2991 technique in fractionating fresh blood units is excellent, comparable to that which can be achieved with the arabinogalactane (stractan) density gradient method in the laboratory. We estimate that given this resolution of cell separation, chronic transfusion with the lightest (''youngest'') 50% of blood units would result in a 30% reduction in the annual transfusion requirement and iron load.

In the United States, most chronically transfused patients are transfused with frozen-deglycerolized red cells in order to minimize the incidence of leukocyte reactions. When one isolates the lightest 50% of the red cells from a blood unit by the IBM-2991 technique, virtually all of the white cells are found with the young red cells. Since the chronically transfused patient would receive a proportionally larger ratio of white cells/red cells, blood freezing becomes even more important. We have therefore explored the ability of the IBM-2991 technique to isolate young red cells from previously frozen units of blood. We have been completely unsuccessful in isolating young red cells from units frozen by the low-glycerol technique and deglycerolized manually [17]. However, we have devised a method whereby blood units frozen by the high-glycerol technique [18] can be deglycerolized and fractionated by age with one operation of the IBM-2991, with a resolution of cell fractionation which is only slightly poorer than that achieved with fresh blood units [16].

The ultimate proof of any method for isolating young red cells for transfusion is the demonstration of improved in vivo survival in patients with thalassemia major. We have completed a limited number of 51Cr red cell survival studies in splenectomized patients with thalassemia major. In one patient, packed red cells which were sham-fractionated but remixed prior to 51Cr labeling yielded the typical radiochromium half-life of 29 days. In two patients who received the top 50% of whole blood units, half-lives of 40 and 42 days were obtained, while in one patient who received the top 30% of a whole blood unit, a half-life of 56 days was obtained. Furthermore, radiochromium survivals of 41 and 43 days have been obtained in two patients who received the top 50% of blood units which were previously frozen by the low-glycerol technique [16]. These preliminary studies confirm our in vitro pyruvate kinase data which indicate that the IBM-2991 is capable of isolating a relatively young population of red cells for transfusion.

The effect and the cost of chronic young red cell transfusions remain to be established. It is quite possible that the size of the reduction in transfusion requirement may not warrant the additional effort and expense of young cell preparation. In particular, in geographic areas where the supply of blood is inadequate, this technique is probably of no use since it will undoubtedly waste some blood; the development of an adequate blood donor program should be given a higher priority. The clinical usefulness of the "oldest" portion of blood units must be evaluated in order to minimize the potential waste of blood. Nevertheless, we are hopeful that this new approach to transfusion therapy will significantly reduce the rate of iron loading in chronically transfused patients.

Our laboratory has embarked upon a long-term clinical evaluation of young red cell transfusions in a large group of splenectomized patients whose previous transfusion requirements have been carefully established. During the coming year, we will measure the reduction in the annual transfusion requirement and iron load, and determine the actual financial costs of young red cell transfusion therapy. Until the actual benefits and costs of such therapy are established, we feel that it would be premature for this technique to enter widespread use.

CHELATION THERAPY

During the past 5 years, it has been well established that slow subcutaneous infusions of deferoxamine are capable of achieving iron balance in most chronically transfused patients [7,8,18-20]. Although repeated subcutaneous drug infusions are obviously not the ideal mode of therapy, and in some cases result in serious compliance problems, for now we must face the fact that the development of an effective oral chelating agent does not appear likely in the immediate future [21]. Since all drugs are potentially toxic, particularly if used daily for extremely prolonged periods of time, we have approached deferoxamine therapy in very young thalassemics with the aim of finding the minimal effective dose required to achieve iron balance. While one could successfully argue that in older patients, who are at greater risk to potentially fatal iron-induced organ dysfunction, higher doses of drug are justifiable, the use of unnecessarily high drug doses in young children seems unwarranted. While there is no question that persistent use of subcutaneous (sc) deferoxamine appears safe, one still must proceed with caution; we know of no other situation where a child is constantly exposed to a drug for life.

We have measured the mean daily urinary iron excretion in response to 8-hour sc deferoxamine infusions of 20 mg/kg in a large series of splenectomized and nonsplenectomized patients. In most patients, there is a substantial day-to-day variability for reasons which remain unclear. (By measuring white cell ascorbic acid concentrations on days when urinary iron excretion was determined, we have eliminated daily variations in ascorbic acid status as a possible explanation for daily urinary iron variability; within a given patient, white cell ascorbate remains relatively constant from day to day.) The mean daily urinary excretion of iron increased as a function of age, with no significant difference between splenectomized and nonsplenectomized patients (Fig. 2). Thus, removal of the spleen does not reduce the response to sc infusions of 20 mg/kg deferoxamine.

For each patient, we have computed the annual iron load for the year 1978, and have projected the annual iron balance according to the formula below:

$$\text{Iron Balance (\%)} = \frac{\text{mean urinary iron (mg/day)} \times 365 \text{ days/yr}}{\text{1978 iron load (mg/yr)}} \times 100$$

It is intuitively obvious that the achievement of iron balance must become more difficult, ie require a higher drug dose, as the annual blood requirement and iron load increase. It is therefore not surprising that we have been able to demonstrate a significant negative correlation ($p < 0.001$) between the projected iron balance (at 20 mg/kg) and the transfusion requirement (Fig. 3). Among patients between 10 and 17 years of age, 8 of 11 splenectomized patients were in negative iron balance, whereas only 2 of 11 patients with intact spleens were in balance. These findings support the concept that, if one is to minimize drug dose and drug

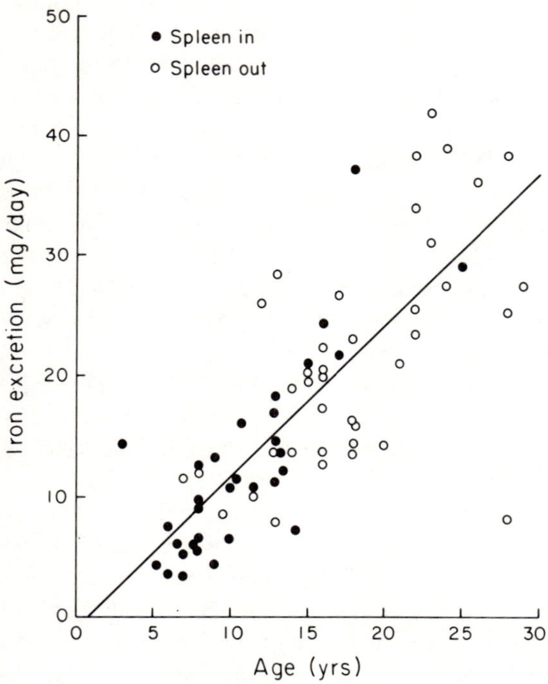

Fig. 2.

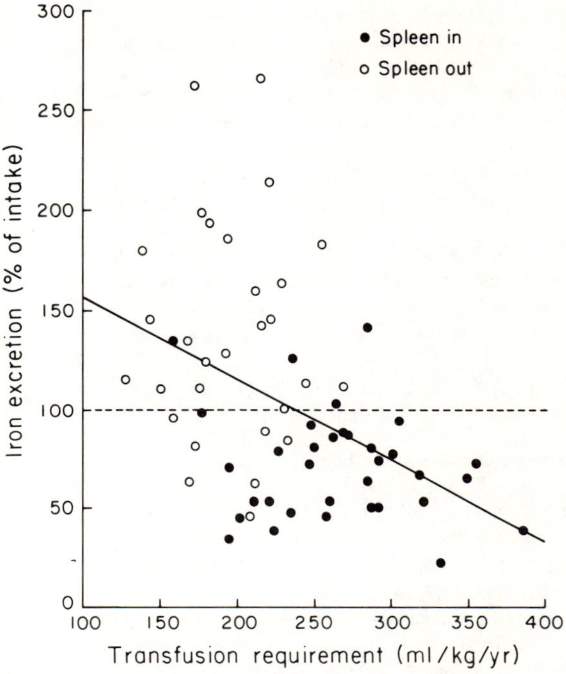

Fig. 3.

costs, the spleen should be removed when the transfusion requirement exceeds 250 ml/kg/yr, which almost always occurs between 6 and 8 years of age (Fig. 1).

In conclusion, through a combination of therapeutic approaches, it is now possible to minimize the accumulation of iron in chronically transfused patients. As a result, we believe that the prognosis for young children with thalassemia major, in whom it should be possible to prevent the sequelae of iron overload, has changed dramatically. We should not be discouraged if chronic deferoxamine therapy does not completely reverse the consequences of extensive fibrotic organ damage which has developed over a period of many years in the older patient population. It is in the younger population where persistent use of chelation therapy will probably have its most pronounced effect.

REFERENCES

1. Ellis JT, Schulman I, Smith CH: Generalized siderosis with fibrosis of liver and pancreas in Cooley's (Mediterranean) anemia. Am J Pathol 30:287, 1954.
2. Engle MA: Cardiac involvement in Cooley's anemia. Ann NY Acad Sci 119:694, 1964.
3. Bouroncle BA, Doan CA: Cooley's anemia: Indications for splenectomy. Ann NY Acad Sci 119:709, 1964.

4. Modell B: Total management of thalassemia major. Arch Dis Child 52:489, 1977.
5. Smith CH, Erlandson ME, Stern G, Hilgartner MW: Postsplenectomy infection in Cooley's anemia. Ann NY Acad Sci 119:748, 1964.
6. Piomelli S, Karpatkin MH, Arzanian M, Zamani M, Becker MH, Geneiser N, Danoff SJ, Kuhns WJ: Hypertransfusion regimen in patients with Cooley's anemia. Ann NY Acad Sci 232:186, 1974.
7. Weiner M, Karpatkin MH, Hart D, Seaman C, Vora SK, Henry WL, Piomelli S: Cooley anemia: High transfusion regimen and chelation therapy. Results and perspective. J Pediatr 92:653, 1978.
8. Graziano JH, Piomelli S, Hilgartner M, Giardina P, Karpatkin M, Andrew M, LoIacono N, Seaman C: Chelation therapy in β-thalassemia major. III. The role of splenectomy in achieving iron balance. J Pediatr 99:695, 1981.
9. Wolman IJ: Transfusion therapy in Cooley's anemia: Growth and health as related to long range hemoglobin levels. A progress report. Ann NY Acad Sci 119:736, 1964.
10. Corash L, Piomelli S, Seaman C, Camisa C: High resolution separation of blood cell types by density gradient centrifugation. Sixteenth meeting of the Amer Soc Hematol: Abstract No. 88, 1973.
11. Piomelli S, Lurinsky G, Wasserman LR: The mechanism of red cell aging. I. Relationship between cell age and specific gravity evaluated by ultracentrifugation in a discontinuous density gradient. J Lab Clin Med 69:659, 1967.
12. Piomelli S, Seaman C, Reibman J, Tytun A, Graziano J, Tabachnik N, Corash L: Separation of younger red cells with improved survival in vivo: An approach to chronic transfusion therapy. Proc Natl Acad Sci USA 75:3474, 1978.
13. Propper RD, Button LN, Nathan DG: New approaches to the transfusion management of thalassemia. Blood 55:55, 1980.
14. Corash L, Klein H, Deisseroth A, Shafer B, Rosen S, Beman J, Griffith P, Nienhuis A: Selective isolation of young erythrocytes for transfusion support of thalassemia major patients. Blood 57:599, 1981.
15. Graziano JH, Seaman C, Leong J, Ingalls L, Piomelli S: A comparison of three methods for separating young red cells for transfusion into patients with thalassemia major. (Abstract) Pediatr Res 14:534, 1980.
16. Graziano JH, Piomelli S, Seaman C, Cohen AR, Kelleher JF Jr, Schwartz E, Wang T: A simple technique for preparation of young red cells for transfusion from ordinary units. Blood 59:865–868, 1982.
17. Rowe AW: Preservation of blood by the low glycerol-rapid freeze process. In Valeri CR et al (eds): "Red Cell Freezing: A Technical Workshop." Washington DC: American Association of Blood Banks, 1973, pp 55–72.
18. Propper RD, Cooper B, Rufo RR, Nienhuis AW, Anderson WF, Bunn HF, Rosenthal A, Nathan DG: Continuous subcutaneous administration of deferoxamine in patients with iron overload. N Engl J Med 297:418, 1977.
19. Graziano JH, Markenson A, Miller DR, Chang H, Bestak M, Meyers P, Pisciotto P, Rifkind A: Chelation therapy in β-thalassemia major. I. Intravenous and subcutaneous deferoxamine. J Pediatr 92:648, 1978.
20. Piomelli S, Graziano JH, Karpatkin M, Dudell GG, Hart D, Hilgartner MW, Khanna K, Valdes-Cruz LM, Vora S: Chelation therapy, transfusion requirement and iron balance in young thalassemic patients. Ann NY Acad Sci 344:409, 1980.
21. Cerami A: The future of new iron chelating drugs. In Martell AE, Anderson WF, Badman DG (eds): "Development of Iron Chelators for Clinical Use." Amsterdam: Elsevier-North Holland, 1981, pp 197–200.

Subcutaneous Desferrioxamine: The Effect of Three Years' Treatment on Liver, Iron, Serum Ferritin, and Comments on Echocardiography

D.M. Flynn, MD, FRCP, DCH, **A.V. Hoffbrand,** DM, FRCP, FRCPath,
and Dina Politis, MD

Subcutaneous desferrioxamine (scDF) is now widely used in the treatment of patients with thalassemia major who require regular blood transfusions. This expensive and difficult treatment is given in the hope of reversing or preventing potentially lethal cardiac or other organ damage caused by iron overload. As yet, there is no definite evidence that scDF can achieve this aim, although regular intramuscular DF has some proven benefits on growth and liver fibrosis [1,2], and may well improve the life expectancy of children with thalassemia major.

As previously described [3], we have used scDF for up to 5 years in a group of patients in London and Athens with thalassemia major who were receiving regular transfusions. The results have shown an initial fall in iron stores in all patients, which has been sustained in those keeping to intensive chelation therapy. Figure 1 shows the results of serial liver iron concentrations in 19 patients during treatment with scDF; a definite and striking fall is observed. This was associated with a reduction in liver size assessed clinically in these patients, and a fall in total liver iron, despite the continuing blood transfusions, was clearly shown.

Figure 2 shows serial serum ferritin levels in patients, and again a fall is observed. The fall in serum ferritin within the first year is greatest with patients whose ferritin levels were highest at the start of therapy. The mean fall was less in the second year than the first, and again, less in the third than the second year of therapy. Only 4 or 5 of our patients have serum ferritin levels $< 1{,}000$ μg/liter despite the use of scDF in doses of about 80 mg/kg infused over 12 hours. With the fall in iron stores, the amount of urine iron in response to scDF also falls. The implication is that it may be difficult to remove the "last" part of the iron stores.

The serum ferritin, however, has been criticized as a measure of iron overload especially when serum ferritin is over 3,500 μg/liter [4] and the transfused load is $>$ 100 units. However, recent work by Chapman et al [5] has shown that the

Birth Defects: Original Article Series, Volume 18, Number 7, pages 347–353
© 1982 March of Dimes Birth Defects Foundation

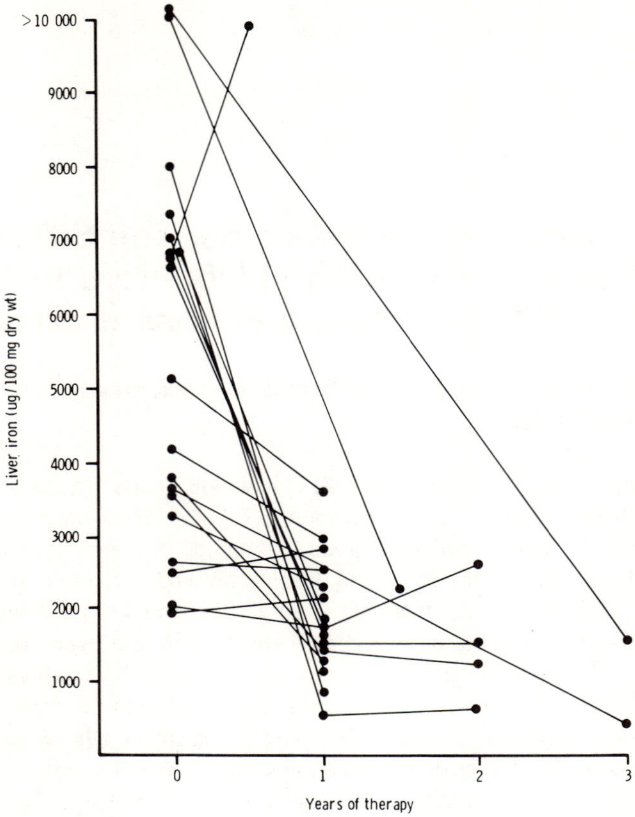

Fig. 1. Iron content of serial liver biopsies in patients on scDF therapy, for up to 3 years.

well-known ascorbic acid deficiency in patients with the highest iron overload disturbs the normal close relation between serum ferritin and transfusional iron load. Ascorbic acid deficiency appears to cause serum ferritin to underestimate the iron load. This was dramatically shown in the interesting patient reported by Cohen et al [6].

In a previous paper, serum ferritin concentrations were plotted against units transfused in unchelated patients whose ascorbic acid status was unknown [7]. The two variables are fitted better by a log curve than by a straight line. However, it is likely that those patients, with more than 100-200 units transfused had ascorbic acid deficiency which caused the serum ferritin to underestimate the transfused load, and this may have contributed to the flattening of serum ferritin

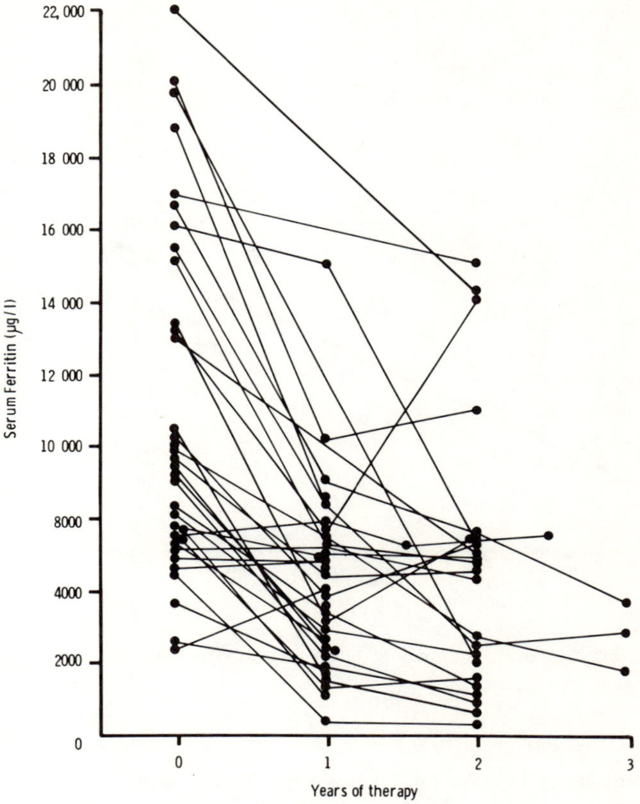

Fig. 2. Serial serum ferritin levels in patients on scDF therapy.

concentration in relation to units transfused. When the relation between serum ferritin and units transfused was examined in ascorbic acid replete patients [5], the points were well fitted by a straight line (Fig. 3, $r = 0.82$, $p < 0.0005$).

The fall in iron stores in these patients has been associated with an improvement in organ function. Serial liver function tests in 35 thalassemic patients treated with scDF for a period of 3 years or more showed a striking fall in serum aspartate transaminase concentrations in the majority of cases, demonstrating an actual reversal in pathology despite continuing blood transfusions (Fig. 4).

Substantial endocrine damage occurs in patients with thalassemia major who have received multiple blood transfusions. As yet, there is no definite evidence that this endocrine damage can be reversed by removing iron. However, an increase in the serum thyroxine level has occurred during scDF therapy in 8 of our patients. Further follow-up of this and other endocrine functions is important.

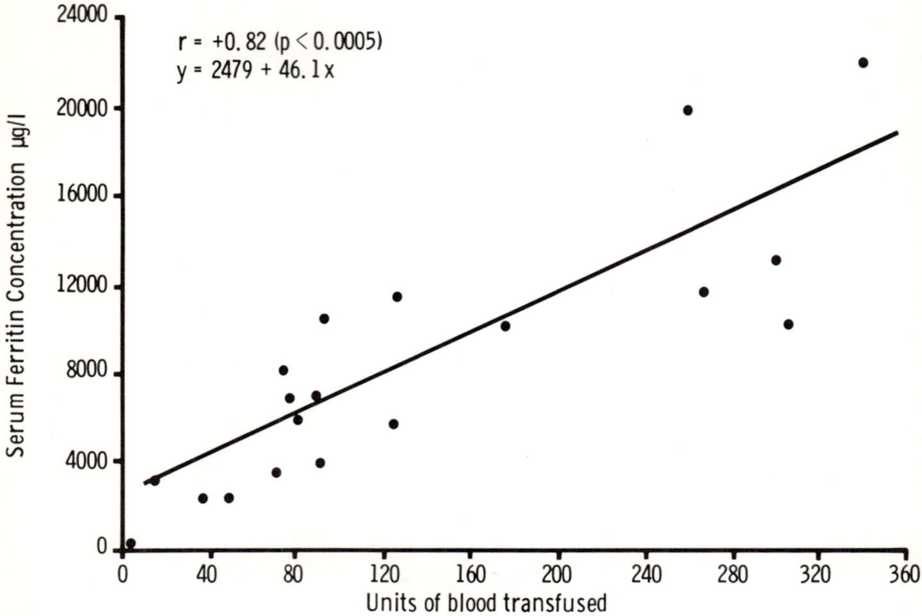

Fig. 3. Serum ferritin levels and units of blood transfused in patients who were ascorbic acid replete, and before chelation.

In a recent study [8], we have shown that serum immunoreactive trypsin is often abnormal in thalassemic patients. Both high and low values were seen in patients less than 12 years of age, whereas, in patients over 12 years the results were low, in general, suggesting a more severe degree of pancreatic exocrine damage. Serial observations of serum trypsin will be used.

Thus, it is clear that scDF used regularly may lessen iron load and improve liver function despite the continued need for transfusion. Far more important is the question of what effect on life expectancy this has. Before the introduction of iron chelation therapy, patients nearly always died of cardiac failure with arrhythmias rather than of liver failure. It may be that sufficient iron will remain, despite intense chelation, to cause enough cardiac damage to prevent worthwhile improvement in life expectancy even though function in other organs has improved. It is clear that the amount of functional damage in different organs is not proportional to their iron concentrations. On one hand, the heart contains relatively little iron—even in heavily iron overloaded subjects—and, at postmortem, has a lower iron concentration than many other organs of the body. On the other hand, the liver may contain 5% or more of its dry weight as iron, but fatal liver failure is very rare, although liver function tests are abnormal at an early stage.

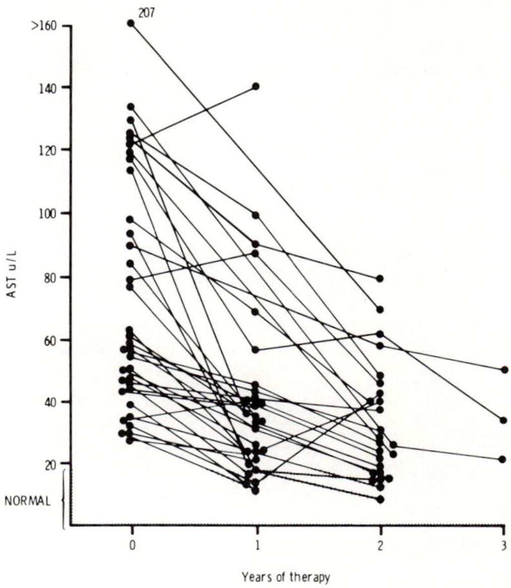

Fig. 4. Serial aspartate transaminase levels in thalassemic patients on scDF therapy.

Deaths from cardiac failure in unchelated patients occur after 200-400 units of blood have been transfused. In order to determine whether chelation is preventing serious cardiac damage it is worth having accurate estimates of early cardiac damage in these patients. Only two published studies have addressed the problem of early cardiac dysfunction in these patients. Kaye and Owen [9] studied cardiac arrhythmias with 24-hour ECG monitoring and showed a greater incidence of arrhythmias in heavily transfused patients. A more recent publication [10] showed that the systolic ejection fraction during exercise was an earlier sign of cardiac damage than x ray or conventional ECG. Neither study showed a linear relationship between units of blood transfused and the degree of cardiac damage. Therefore, so far there is no accurate index of the likely rate of cardiac deterioration with increasing iron load so that the results of chelation therapy on heart function can be monitored in the individual patient.

We have used echocardiography to measure left ventricular internal dimension in diastole (LVIDd) and have found a linear relationship between heart size and blood transfused. Using the normal values for LVIDd, based on examining 105 children and young people [11], we have calculated the mean and SD expected in patients of any given size. The SD score

$$(\text{SD score} = \frac{(\text{observed value})-(\text{expected value})}{\text{SD}})$$

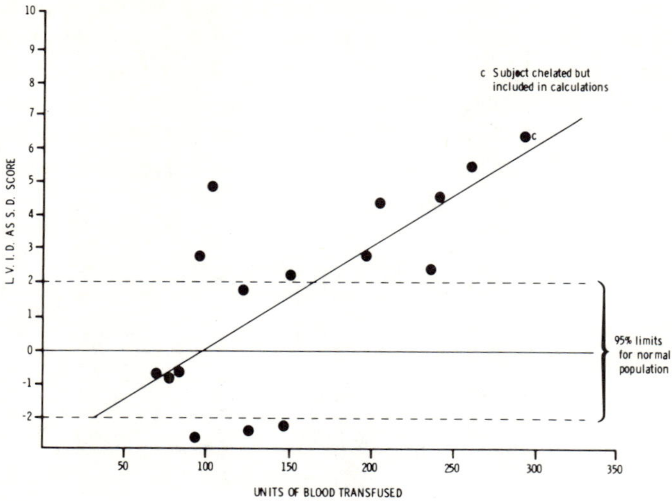

Fig. 5. LVID diastole as SD score and units of blood transfused in thalassemic patients before chelation.

of any particular patient among our group has been calculated and, in serial repeated measurements on a normal growing child, this should nearly always lie between ± 2 SD.

We have plotted the relation between LVIDd expressed as a SD score against units of blood transfused before our patients had received scDF. There is a correlation ($p < 0.01$) which is stronger at > 150 units of blood transfused (Fig. 5). For younger (and less transfused) patients the correlation is less strong. One patient (indicated by C on the graph) had received intramuscular DF for 12 years before the present study. Although his serum ferritin was only 1,000 μg/liter at the time, the heart size was as large as expected from the number of units transfused rather than from the serum ferritin, and the correlation coefficients were not influenced by his insertion or removal from the sample. Long-term intramuscular DF therefore does not appear to have prevented an increase in his heart size.

The advantage of this technique is that it is noninvasive, but it is not as reproducible as one would wish. LVIDd measurements before and after transfusion (the patients were transfused from approximately 9—13 gm/dl) were different, although no net change was seen. The largest difference in successive measurements was 2.7 SDs.

Ideally, one would like to have long-term serial observations in a number of patients over a period of time before they have been chelated (ie longitudinal rather than cross-sectional data). However, it now seems unethical to withhold scDF from patients with thalassemia major. We have used the regression line to predict what change in heart size is to be expected in patients who are not chelated, but are continuing to receive blood transfusions. Although we have now obtained serial measurements of LVIDd in a number of patients during scDF chelation, the SD scores have not yet consistently fallen more than 2.7 SDs below the regression line in Figure 5. In one patient who was followed serially, however, there was a fall of more than 2.7 SDs below the prechelation LVIDd (rather than the regression line) while on continued chelation, suggesting a definite improvement in heart function.

A few of our patients are failing to use scDF as intensively in subsequent years as in the first few months or year of therapy, partly because of the failure of the patients themselves to observe symptomatic improvement other than in skin pigmentation. Improvement in heart function would be a strong incentive for them to remain on intensive scDF therapy.

CONCLUSION

Subcutaneous desferrioxamine, if used intensively, will lower liver iron concentrations, reduce serum ferritin to near normal levels, and reverse liver dysfunction. Although evidence in one of our patients suggests that scDF may reverse cardiac pathology, further studies are needed on this point as well as to see whether endocrine function can be improved with this intensive chelation.

REFERENCES

1. Barry M, Flynn DM, Letsky EA, Risdon RA: Long-term chelation therapy in thalassemia major: Effect on liver iron concentration, liver histology, and clinical progress. Br Med J 2:16, 1974.
2. Risdon RA, Barry M, Flynn DM: Transfusional iron overload: The relation between tissue iron concentration and hepatic fibrosis in thalassaemia. J Pathol 83:116, 1975.
3. Hoffbrand AV, Gorman A, Laulicht M, Garidi M, Economidou J, Georgipoulou P, Hussain MAM, Flynn DM: Improvement in iron status and liver function in patients with transfusional iron overload with long-term subcutaneous desferrioxamine. Lancet 1:947, 1979.
4. Worwood M: Serum ferritin. CRC critical reviews. Clin Lab Sc 10:171, 1979.
5. Chapman RWG, Hussain MAM, Gorman A, Laulicht M, Politis D, Flynn DM, Sherlock S, Hoffbrand AV: Effect of ascorbic acid deficiency on serum ferritin concentration in patients with β-thalassemia major and iron overload. J Clin Pathol 35 (5):487–490, 1982.
6. Cohen A, Cohen IJ, Schwartz E: Scurvy and altered iron stores in thalassaemia major. N Engl J Med 304:158, 1981.
7. Letsky EA, Miller F, Worwood M, Flynn DM: Serum ferritin in children with thalassaemia regularly transfused. J Clin Pathol 27:652, 1974.
8. Hussain MAM, Dandona P, Fedail SS, Ramdial L, Flynn DM, Hoffbrand AV: Serum immunoreactive trypsin in β-thalassaemia major. J Clin Pathol 45:970, 1981.
9. Kaye SB, Owen M: Cardiac arrhythmias in thalassaemia major: Evaluation of chelation treatment using ambulatory monitoring. Br Med J 1:342, 1978.
10. Leon MB, Booer JS, Bacharach SL, Green MV, Benz EJ, Griffith P, Nienhuis AW: Detection of early cardiac dysfunction in patients with severe beta thalassaemia and chronic iron overload. N Engl J Med 301:1143, 1979.
11. Henry WL, Ware J, Gardin JM, Hepner SI, McKay J, Weiner M: Echocardiographic measurements in normal subjects. Circulation 57:278, 1978.

Therapy of HBsAg-Negative Chronic Active Hepatitis in Transfusion-Dependent Thalassemia Major

Stefano De Virgiliis, MD, F. Argiolu, MD, M. Rais, MD, P. Cossu, MD, C. Toccafondi, MD, G. Sanna, PhD, G. Cornacchia, PhD, A. Nucaro, PhD, A. Ferreli, MD, and Antonio Cao, MD

Transfusional chronic active hepatitis (CAH), due to non-A, non-B, or to B-virus infection, is a frequent complication of thalassemia major [1-3]. While there is universal agreement concerning the use of intensive iron chelation by subcutaneous desferrioxamine in the treatment of this complication [3-5], the use of steroids is not universally accepted.

In CAH occurring in nonthalassemic patients, steroid treatment was seen to be ineffective or even detrimental in HBsAg-positive cases [6], while histologic improvement has been found in the HBsAg-negatives [7-9]. Recently, a restricted cortisone trial, carried out in prevalently HBsAg-negative CAH complicating thalassemia major, showed reduction of inflammatory activity with disappearance of piecemeal necrosis and with no effect on the evolution to cirrhosis [4]. Herein, we review the results of a prospective nonrandomized methylprednisolone trial associated with intensive iron chelation, carried out on a group of transfusion-dependent thalassemia major patients with HBsAg-negative CAH, probably due to non-A non-B-virus.

PATIENTS

Thirty-four thalassemia major patients ($\beta°$-thalassemia homozygotes), with biopsy features of CAH and no HBsAg in the serum by solid phase radioimmunoassay (RIA), were included in this study. For 4 years they followed a transfusion regimen designed to maintain a minimum hemoglobin level of 9 gm/dl. Chelation therapy was carried out from 3–8 years with intramuscular desferrioxamine (750 mg/day for ages 3–9, and 1 gm/day over 9 years of age, 6 days a week), and subsequently 6 days a week with 12 hour/day subcutaneous infusion by means of a portable pump (HP4 HH model, Carandina Lab., Bondeno-

Birth Defects: Original Article Series, Volume 18, Number 7, pages 355–360
© 1982 March of Dimes Birth Defects Foundation

Ferrara, Italy). The desferrioxamine subcutaneous dose was established on an individual basis as the lowest dose inducing maximal excretion, after evaluation of desferrioxamine-induced iron elimination obtained with 1 gm, 1.5 gm, and 2 gm, administered for 3 consecutive days. During the trial, the patients were taking 100 mg ascorbic acid/day.

After a detailed presentation of the pros and cons of prednisolone treatment, the parents of 18 of 34 patients gave informed consent. These 18 patients were treated with 6 methylprednisolone at a dose of 50 mg/M^2/day for 7 days; then the dose was reduced by 8 mg/M^2/week, until a maintenance dose of 8-16 mg/day was reached.

The remaining 16 patients, who were comparable to the treated group in age, clinical features (including transfusional iron load), laboratory findings, and chelation therapy, were considered as controls (Table 1).

All patients had monthly serum GPT determination, 3-month liver function tests, 6-month serum ferritin assessments and desferrioxamine-induced iron elimination, and liver biopsy at 1 year.

Treatment was continued until liver biopsy showed disappearance of piecemeal or bridging necrosis associated with restriction of inflammatory infiltrate to the portal tracts. The patients were considered to have attained biochemical remission when serum GPT returned to normal levels. Relapse was considered to have occurred when normal GPT levels increased to more than twice the value observed in remission.

METHODS

HBsAg, anti-HBs, anti-HBc, and anti-HAV were determined by solid phase RIA (Ausria II-125 Ausab, Corab™ and Havab™, Abbott).

Twenty-four hour urinary iron excretion was evaluated by atomic absorption spectrophotometry (spectrophotometer IL model 551).

Serum ferritin was assayed by means of a kit (Ramco Lab., Houston, Texas) at a serum dilution of 1:1000.

Liver function tests were carried out by means of standard methods.

Statistical evaluation was carried out by means of one-tailed and double-tailed Student's *t*-test and χ^2-test. The cumulative incidence of biochemical remission in each group of patients was calculated according to the distribution-free two-sample test proposed by Gehan [10].

RESULTS

Clinical Observations

Pertinent clinical and laboratory data are summarized in Table 1. All patients were anti-HBs and/or anti-HBc-positive and HBsAg-negative. Anti-HAV was detected in 25 patients.

At the beginning of the trial, both treated and nontreated patients had increased γ-globulins and γ-GT and reduced albumin levels with no statistically significant difference. Eleven patients in the treated and 10 in the nontreated group had been splenectomized.

Iron Chelation

The 24-hour urinary iron excretion after increasing doses of desferrioxamine are shown in Table 2. There is a statistically significant ($p < 0.05$) higher excretion with 60 than 40 mg/kg, while no significant difference can be seen between eliminations found with 60 and 80 mg/kg. Since individual dose-response curves were found highly variable, the dose for the trial was selected on an individual basis (40 to 80 mg/kg).

TABLE 1. Baseline Clinical and Biochemical Features of 34 Thalassemia Major Patients With HBsAg-Negative Chronic Active Hepatitis Who Were Treated (or Not) With Prednisolone.

	Prednisolone Group	Control Group
Cases	18	16
Age (years)	8 ± 2.4	8.6 ± 3.8
Transfusional iron load (g)	13.4 ± 2.6	13.2 ± 5.5
Liver iron (mg/gm dry weight)	24 ± 13	22 ± 6
Serum ferritin (ng/ml)	3444 ± 1790	3100 ± 1370
Serum GPT (mU/ml)	84 ± 26	72 ± 29
Serum γGT (mU/ml)	38 ± 27	28 ± 24
Serum ChE (mU/ml)	3125 ± 935	4115 ± 1481
Serum bilirubin (mg/100 ml)	1.89 ± 1.48	1.45 ± 0.65
Serum proteins (gm/100 ml)	7.20 ± 0.75	7.60 ± 0.92
Serum albumins (%)	45 ± 4.6	43 ± 8
Serum γ-globulin (%)	30 ± 4.8	32.7 ± 6.4
Prothrombin ratio	1.12 ± 0.09	1.10 ± 0.009
Anti-HBs	14/18	14/16
Anti-HBc	6/18	7/16

TABLE 2. Twenty-Four Hour Urinary Iron Excretion After Increasing Doses of Desferrioxamine and Iron Balance in 34 Thalassemia Major Patients With HBsAg-Negative Chronic Active Hepatitis Who Were Treated or Not With Prednisolone.

Urinary iron (mg/24 hr) after different doses of desferrioxamine (12hr subcutaneous infusion)			Iron Balance (% of intake eliminated)
40 mg/kg	60 mg/kg	80 mg/kg	
14.33±7.61	18.30±9.82	19.79±7.96	252.88±88.14

The estimation of the percentage of transfusional iron that can be eliminated showed that all chronic hepatitis patients may be put into near iron balance, and most of them have a substantial net iron excretion (Table 2).

Ferritin levels, after the one-year trial, were unmodified or slightly reduced in both groups of patients with no significant differences.

Serum GPT

Prednisolone-treated patients consistently showed lower mean GPT levels than controls; the difference between means being significant ($p<0.05$) at 4, 8, 12, 15, 18, and 24 months (Fig. 1).

At the end of the trial, GPT levels were significantly reduced ($p<0.05$) in the prednisolone-treated group, while no significant difference was seen in the controls (Fig. 1).

Remission

At follow-up, 15 of 18 patients taking prednisolone, and 6 of 16 controls went into remission. As can be seen from the actuarial curves, the percentage of remission was significantly higher in the prednisolone group (T 8 months: $Z= 1.98437$, $p<0.025$; T 24 months: $Z= -2.45293$, $p<0.01$) (Fig. 2).

Relapse

In patients taking prednisolone, relapse occurred both in the 1st year and in the 2nd year in 1 case. The respective figures in controls were 3 and 1.

Histology

Follow-up liver histology revealed much less portal inflammation and piecemeal necrosis in the prednisolone group, the difference between the 2 groups being statistically significant (χ^2-test, $p<0.01$).

Mortality and Complications

During the period of study there were no deaths and no complications related to treatment in either group of subjects.

CONCLUSION

This prednisolone trial in thalassemia major patients with HBsAg-negative chronic active hepatitis had a favorable effect on the biochemical remission and liver histology, the active process reverting to chronic persistent hepatitis. From these results it seems that prednisolone treatment is indicated in thalassemia major patients with HBsAg-negative CAH. However, prednisolone must be used in conjunction with intensive iron chelation by subcutaneous desferrioxamine on a

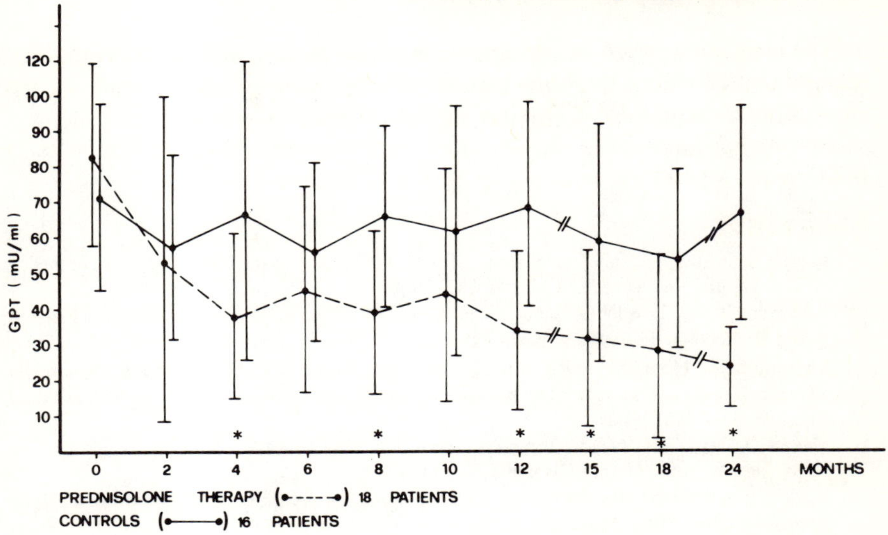

Fig. 1. Serial determinations of serum alanine aminotransferase in thalassemia major patients with HBsAg-negative chronic active hepatitis who were receiving (dotted line) or not (solid line) prednisolone treatment. Values represent geometric means ± SD expressed in mU/ml. An asterisk indicates $p<0.05$ at the time marked. Horizontal lines represent the upper limit of normal values.

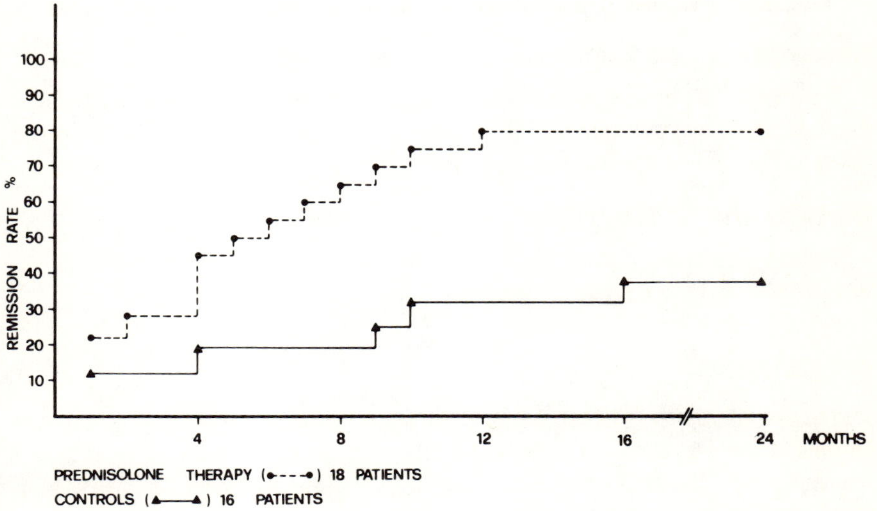

Fig. 2. Cumulative rate of biochemical remission in thalassemia major patients with HBsAg-negative chronic active hepatitis receiving (dotted line) or not (solid line) prednisolone treatment (T 8 months: $Z= 1.98437$, $p<0.025$; T 24 months: $Z= -2.45293$, $p<0.01$).

schedule individually selected from dose-response curves, in order to obtain iron balance and reduce the liver iron burden. Whether this approach can prevent or impede the progression to cirrhosis can be assessed only after a much longer period of observation.

REFERENCES

1. Masera G, Jean G, Gazzola G, Novakova M: Role of chronic hepatitis in development of thalassemic liver disease. Arch Dis Child 51:680, 1976.
2. Papaevangelau G, Frosner G, Economidau J, Parcha S, Roumeliotou A: Prevalence of hepatitis A and B infections in multiply transfused thalassemic patients. Br Med J 1:689, 1978.
3. De Virgiliis S, Fiorelli G, Fargion S, Cornacchia G, Sanna G, Cossu P, Murgia V, Cao A: Chronic liver disease in transfusion-dependent thalassemia: Hepatitis B virus marker studies. J Clin Pathol 33:949, 1980.
4. Masera G, Jean G, Conter V, Terzoli S, Mauri RA, Cazzaniga M: Sequential study of liver biopsy on thalassemia. Arch Dis Child 55:800, 1980.
5. Modell B: Advances in the use of iron-chelating agents for the treatment of iron overload. Prog Hematol 11:267–312, 1979.
6. Lam KC, Lai CL, Trepo BS, Wu BC: Deleterious effect of prednisolone in HBsAg positive chronic active hepatitis. N Engl J Med 304:380, 1981.
7. Cook GC, Mulligan R, Sherlock S: Controlled prospective trial of corticosteroid therapy in active chronic hepatitis. Q J Med 40:159, 1971.
8. Soloway RD, Summerskill WHJ, Baggenstass AH: Clinical, biochemical and histological remission of severe chronic acute liver disease. A controlled study of treatments and early prognosis. Gastroenterology 63:820, 1972.
9. Schalm SW, Summerskill WHJ, Gitmick GL, Elveback L: Contrasting features and responses to treatment of severe chronic active liver disease with and without hepatitis B antigen. Gut 17:781, 1976.
10. Gehan EA: A generalized Wilcoxon test for comparing arbitrarily singly-censored samples. Biometrika 52:203, 1965.

Allogeneic Bone Marrow Transplantation for Blood Cell Disorders

E. Donnall Thomas, MD

For some 25 years it has been recognized that transplantation of marrow from one individual to another might constitute effective therapy for the following conditions:

1. Failure of the myeloid marrow organ. Although much of the original research in marrow transplantation was directed toward reconstitution of the marrow after lethal irradiation damage, the most common, practical application is for the treatment of the patient with severe aplastic anemia.

2. Malignancies of the bone marrow. Most of the effort has been directed toward the patient with leukemia, with the intention of administering "supralethal" chemoradiotherapy in order to destroy the malignant cell population, and along with it the normal cell population, and to replace the normal myeloid marrow by transplantation.

3. Hereditary diseases of the marrow. The aim of this approach is to destroy the genetically abnormal marrow and replace it with normal marrow from another individual. Very little work has been done in this area because of the risks of marrow transplantation on the one hand, and because most of these patients can live for a period measured in years on conventional treatment.

A brief summary of what has been accomplished under the first 2 headings above follows.

SEVERE APLASTIC ANEMIA

This summary refers to patients prepared for engraftment with cyclophosphamide, 50 mg/kg on each of 4 days, followed by marrow from an HLA-

Birth Defects: Original Article Series, Volume 18, Number 7, pages 361–369
© 1982 March of Dimes Birth Defects Foundation

identical sib. Initially, patients with severe aplastic anemia were transplanted only after failure of conventional treatment [1]. Most of these patients had been treated with steroids and androgens, and all had received multiple blood transfusions. Many were infected or refractory to platelet transfusions at the time of transplantation. For these end-stage patients, most transplant centers have reported long-term survival and apparent cure in 40-50% of the patients. The early Seattle experience is shown in Figure 1 [2]. Deaths were due to marrow graft rejection in approximately one-third of the patients, and the other deaths were due to graft-versus-host disease (GVHD), opportunistic infections, and occasionally to cardiac failure or bleeding problems.

In the canine model, it was demonstrated that minor transplantation antigens contained in blood products could sensitize the recipient and result in subsequent rejection of the marrow graft [3]. Accordingly, an effort was made to identify patients with severe aplastic anemia and to bring them to transplantation before transfusions had to be given. Figure 1 shows the survival curve of the first 39 such patients transplanted in Seattle [4]. It appears that approximately 80% of

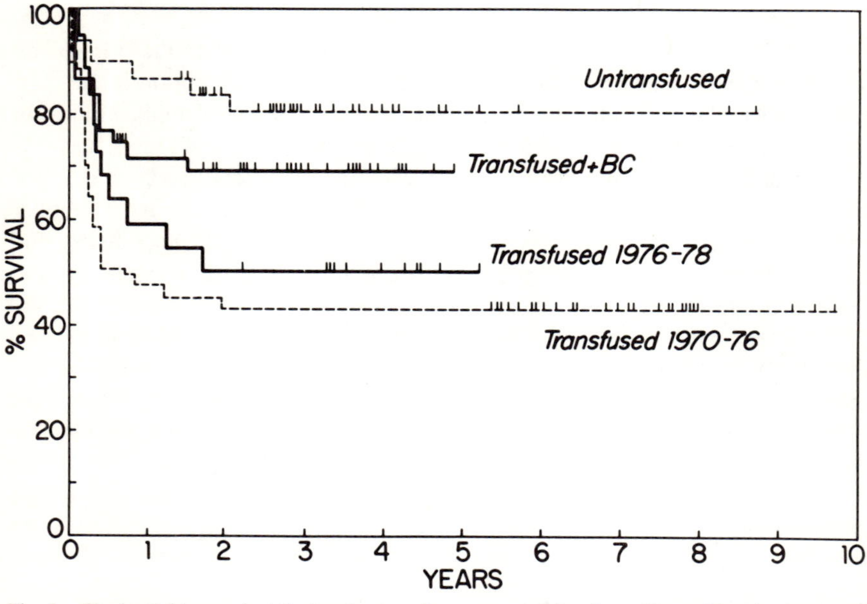

Fig. 1. Kaplan-Meier product limit estimates of percent surviving for patients with aplastic anemia treated by cyclophosphamide and a marrow graft from an HLA-identical family member. Shown are the survival curves of 60 transfused patients grafted between 1970 and 1976 and 22 patients grafted between 1976 and 1978 and given marrow only. Forty-three transfused patients were given marrow and buffy coat cells (BC). Also shown is the survival curve of 39 untransfused patients. Tick marks indicate surviving patients.

these patients will be cured, while 20% die of problems largely related to GVHD and opportunistic infections.

At the time of diagnosis, many patients with severe aplastic anemia require transfusions as a matter of urgent medical necessity. These patients, therefore, will have had multiple transfusions even if they come to transplantation early in the course of the disease. In the canine model it had been demonstrated that leukocytes from the peripheral blood (buffy coat cells) could serve as a source of donor cells for transplantation [5]. A proportional hazard regression analysis of the human cases in Seattle showed that the likelihood of marrow graft rejection decreased with an increasing number of donor marrow cells infused [6]. Accordingly, in transfused patients it was decided to supplement the marrow graft with donor buffy coat cells (4 units obtained on each of 5 days). Figure 1 shows the Kaplan-Meier survival curve for 43 transfused patients given marrow and buffy coat and demonstrates that approximately 70% of these patients are apparently cured of the disease (unpublished data).

ACUTE LEUKEMIA

Between 1970 and 1976, 110 patients with acute leukemia in end-stage relapse were transplanted from HLA-identical sibs. Ten of these patients were prepared with 1,000 rad total body irradiation and the next 100 were given cyclophosphamide at 60 mg/kg on each of 2 days followed by the total body irradiation [7]. Thirteen of these patients are living in remission 6–11 years later; they have received no further antileukemic therapy, and they appear to be cured of the disease. The overall survival for this group of patients was, of course, poor, but the important point is that some of these end-stage patients actually can be cured of the disease.

Since it appeared possible to cure some patients, it was logical to carry out marrow transplants earlier in the course of the disease in patients known to have a poor prognosis [8, 9]. Of particular interest are those patients with acute nonlymphoblastic leukemia transplanted in first remission [9]. The first 19 of these patients were reported in 1979 and Figure 2 shows the Kaplan-Meier survival curve for these patients updated to February 1, 1981. Only 2 patients have had a recurrence of leukemia. The principal causes of death are GVHD, interstitial pneumonia, and opportunistic infections. As of December 1980, this series has now been extended to 82 patients and the Kaplan-Meier survival curve continues to show a long plateau at approximately 55%.

THE EFFECT OF AGE

The above summaries describe patients ranging in age from 1 to 50 years. All marrow transplant studies have shown a worse survival for each decade of increasing age due apparently to an increasing incidence and severity of GVHD.

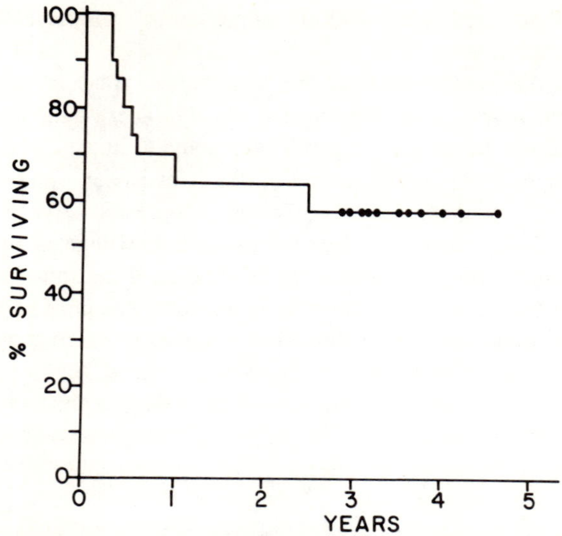

Fig. 2. Kaplan-Meier product limit estimates of percent surviving for 19 patients with acute nonlymphoblastic leukemia transplanted in remission. The dots indicate surviving patients.

APPLICATION OF MARROW TRANSPLANTATION TO INHERITED BLOOD DISORDERS

Animal Studies

In 1967, Steinmuller and Motulsky [10] described studies of the treatment of hereditary spherocytosis in peromyscus (deer mice) by radiation and allogeneic bone marrow transplantation. In 1976, Weiden et al [11] described the treatment of severe hereditary hemolytic anemia related to pyruvate kinase deficiency in Basenji dogs by total body irradiation and marrow transplantation from nonanemic histocompatible littermates. In both of these animal models, marrow transplantation successfully corrected the hereditary blood dyscrasia. Of interest, and relevant to marrow grafting for thalassemia, the iron overload of the transplanted Basenji dogs was reversed with the passage of years [12]. Marrow transplantation has also been successful in overcoming the cyclic neutropenia of the grey Collie dog [13, 14].

Studies in Humans

A few efforts have been made to transplant marrow in patients with thalassemia. These efforts were made before the "current state-of-the-art" for marrow transplantation and details have not been reported. Lucarelli et al ([15] and unpublished data) have recently carried out pilot experiments utilizing fetal hematopoietic tissue transplantation in patients with thalassemia, but these studies, as yet, are only of a preliminary nature.

THE POTENTIAL OF MARROW TRANSPLANTATION FOR THE TREATMENT OF THALASSEMIA

In considering marrow transplantation for a patient with thalassemia, it will be essential to select a patient who is known to have a severe form of the disease, who has had a minimum number of transfusions, and who has an HLA-identical sib (either normal or heterozygous). The patient should not have significant iron toxicity and, for best results, should not be over 5 years of age. In this setting, based on the results for aplastic anemia and acute leukemia described above, it may be anticipated that approximately one-third of the patients will die in the first 2 or 3 months after marrow transplantation from graft rejection, acute GVHD, or opportunistic infections.

Additionally, there may be a risk of partially disabling chronic GVHD which is rare in children (< 10%). The major questions, then, are: 1) Is the risk of early death offset by the reasonable expectation that more than one-half of the patients will be cured and able to lead normal lives? 2) Is the current conventional treatment of thalassemia sufficient to assure a normal life for most patients? 3) What is the relative cost effectiveness of the 2 approaches? Marrow transplantation is an expensive procedure but, if successful, no further expense is involved. Current conventional treatment is certainly less expensive initially but may be more costly over time periods measured in years.

Preparation of the Recipient for Marrow Transplantation

If a decision is made to transplant a patient with thalassemia, a major unresolved question is that of how to prepare the recipient for the transplant. The routine regimen for preparation of patients with severe aplastic anemia has been cyclophosphamide, 50 mg/kg on each of 4 days. It may well be that the cyclophosphamide regimen alone will suffice for preparation of patients with thalassemia, as it has been quite effective in permitting engraftment in normal rodents, dogs, and monkeys (with a presumably normal marrow) that have not been sensitized by blood transfusions. Preparation with cyclophosphamide alone has been successful in the majority of transfused patients with severe aplastic anemia, and in a series of end-stage transfused patients with leukemia (there was a high incidence of recurrence of leukemia in the latter patients). Our follow-up of patients with aplastic anemia prepared with cyclophosphamide alone now extends beyond 9 years without recognized late untoward sequelae.

It must be kept in mind that patients with aplastic anemia represent a special case, since the disease has produced nearly complete marrow aplasia. Thus, the preparative regimen does not have to create "space" for the transplant to grow but need only immunosuppress the recipient so that the graft will be accepted. When the myeloid marrow space is already occupied by a hypercellular marrow, as would be the case with thalassemia, the usual regimen of cyclophosphamide may not be sufficient for eradication of the genetically abnormal marrow. For example, Camitta et al prepared an infant with neutrophil dysfunction and a hyperplastic marrow with antithymocyte serum, procarbazine, and cyclophosphamide (50 mg/kg × 4) followed by marrow from an HLA-identical sib [16]. The graft did not "take" and there was rapid regeneration of the patient's own marrow. It is unsafe to give total doses of cyclophosphamide of more than 200 mg/kg because of the risk of cardiac toxicity.

Some studies have been done utilizing other agents in conjunction with cyclophosphamide. Kapoor et al [17] have recently reported 3 cases of Wiskott-Aldrich syndrome prepared with busulfan 2 mg/kg/d × 4 days and cyclophosphamide, 50 mg/kg/d × 4 days. Engraftment of HLA-identical sib marrow was successful and the recipients were alive 12, 8, and 6 months later. A Wiskott-Aldrich patient in Seattle was successfully transplanted 16 months ago with the same regimen except that a single dose of dimethyl busulfan (4 mg/kg) was used in place of busulfan (unpublished data).

Other studies have used cyclophosphamide with total body irradiation. For example, Parkman et al prepared a Wiskott-Aldrich patient for transplantation utilizing cytosine arabinoside, 150 mg/square meter/day, for 7 days, followed by cyclophosphamide [18]. The graft was only transiently successful. The patient was successfully regrafted and a second patient successfully grafted utilizing antithymocyte globulin and total body irradiation. Santos et al have utilized large doses of busulfan in conjunction with cyclophosphamide and have successfully grafted patients with acute leukemia in remission [19]. In patients with aplastic anemia, Gale et al [20] have followed the usual cyclophosphamide regimen with 300 rad total body irradiation with a decrease in the incidence of graft rejection but, unfortunately, no improvement in overall survival. The leukemic patients and the animal studies described above have involved total body irradiation. Because of the potential late damaging effects of irradiation, including carcinogenesis, it would seem unwise to employ total body irradiation for young patients with thalassemia.

In summary, the standard cyclophosphamide (CY) regimen might be adequate for preparation for engraftment of the patient with thalassemia. However, several marrow transplant centers have used busulfan or dimethyl busulfan in addition to CY without a recognized increase in toxicity. Therefore, combined drugs appear to be preferable.

FUTURE PLANS

Over the past decade there has been a steady improvement in the long-term survival of patients undergoing marrow transplantation. Further improvement can be expected to result from current studies of new immunosuppressive agents, such as cyclosporin A and monoclonal antibodies that react with T cells or T-cell subsets, for the prevention and treatment of GVHD. In Seattle, a randomized trial is underway to determine the role of interferon in the prevention of viral interstitial pneumonia following marrow transplantation. Other areas of intensive research involve nutritional support, the treatment of herpes infections with Acyclovir, and the use of newer antifungal agents for prevention and treatment of opportunistic fungal infections. A successful conclusion to any of these research endeavors should result in a further improvement in the safety of and long-term survival after marrow transplantation. Similarly, it is to be hoped that there will be corresponding improvement in other methods of treating the patient with thalassemia as discussed at this conference.

LATE COMPLICATIONS

Not only with irradiation but also with other conditioning regimens, late genetic effects are of concern (2 women with aplastic anemia prepared with CY have subsequently given birth to normal children). As stated in an earlier editorial [21], "The eventual cure of patients with a homozygous genetic disorder not only will free them of the disease but also may enable them to procreate, resulting in new problems for the genetic counselor." This statement, of course, will apply to any form of successful treatment.

CONCLUSION

At present, marrow transplantation is the only procedure that offers the promise of being able to cure the patient with homozygous thalassemia. The safety of marrow transplantation is now such that it should be possible to cure well over one-half of the patients. Marrow transplantation should be cost effective when compared to prolonged conventional therapy. It is time to offer transplantation to carefully selected patients in a setting of fully informed consent.

ACKNOWLEDGMENT

I thank my colleagues Drs. Dean Buckner and Rainer Storb for advice and criticism in the preparation of this manuscript.

REFERENCES

1. Thomas ED, Buckner CD, Storb R, Neiman PE, Fefer A, Clift RA, Slichter SJ, Funk DD, Bryant JI, Lerner KG: Aplastic anaemia treated by marrow transplantation. Lancet 1:284–289, 1972.
2. Storb R, Thomas ED, Weiden PL, Buckner CD, Clift RA, Fefer A, Fernando LP, Giblett ER, Goodell BW, Johnson FL, Lerner KG, Neiman PE, Sanders JE: Aplastic anemia treated by allogeneic bone marrow transplantation: A report on 49 new cases from Seattle. Blood 48:817–841, 1976.
3. Storb R, Kolb HJ, Graham TC, Kane PJ, Thomas ED: The effect of prior blood transfusions on hemopoietic grafts from histoincompatible canine littermates. Transplantation 14:248–252, 1972.
4. Storb R, Thomas ED, Buckner CD, Clift RA, Deeg HJ, Fefer A, Goodell BW, Sale GE, Sanders JE, Singer J, Stewart P, Weiden PL: Marrow transplantation in thirty "untransfused" patients with severe aplastic anemia. Ann Intern Med 92:30–36, 1980.
5. Storb R, Kolb HJ, Graham TC, Erickson V, Thomas ED: The effect of buffy coat-poor blood transfusion on subsequent hemopoietic grafts. Transplantation 15:129–136, 1973.
6. Storb R, Prentice RL, Thomas ED: Marrow transplantation for treatment of aplastic anemia. An analysis of factors associated with graft rejection. N Engl J Med 296:61–66, 1977.
7. Thomas ED, Buckner CD, Banaji M, Clift RA, Fefer A, Flournoy N, Goodell BW, Hickman RO, Lerner KG, Neiman PE, Sale GE, Sanders JE, Singer J, Stevens M, Storb R, Weiden PL: One hundred patients with acute leukemia treated by chemotherapy, total body irradiation, and allogeneic marrow transplantation. Blood 49:511–533, 1977.
8. Thomas ED, Sanders JE, Flournoy N, Johnson FL, Buckner CD, Clift RA, Fefer A, Goodell BW, Storb R, Weiden PL: Marrow transplantation for patients with acute lymphoblastic leukemia in remission. Blood 54:468–476, 1979.
9. Thomas ED, Buckner CD, Clift RA, Fefer A, Johnson FL, Neiman PE, Sale GE, Sanders JE, Singer JW, Shulman H, Storb R, Weiden PL: Marrow transplantation for acute nonlymphoblastic leukemia in first remission. N Engl J Med 301:597–599, 1979.
10. Steinmuller D, Motulsky AG: Treatment of hereditary spherocytosis in peromyscus by radiation and allogeneic bone marrow transplantation. Blood 29:320–330, 1967.
11. Weiden PL, Storb R, Graham TC, Schroeder ML: Severe hereditary haemolytic anaemia in dogs treated by marrow transplantation. Br J Haematol 33:357–362, 1976.
12. Weiden PL, Hackman RC, Deeg HJ, Graham TC, Thomas ED, Storb R: Long-term survival and reversal of iron overload after marrow transplantation in dogs with congenital hemolytic anemia. Blood 57:66–70, 1981.
13. Weiden PL, Robinett B, Graham TC, Adamson J, Storb R: Canine cyclic neutropenia. A stem cell defect. J Clin Invest 53:950–953, 1974.
14. Dale DC, Graw RG Jr: Transplantation of allogeneic bone marrow in canine cyclic neutropenia. Science 183:83–84, 1974.
15. Lucarelli G, Izzi T, Porcellini A, Delfini C, Polchi P, Moretti L, Manna A, Grilli G: Fetal liver transplantation in aplastic anemia and acute leukemia. In Lucarelli G, Fliedner TM, Gale RP (eds): "Fetal Liver Transplantation. Current Concepts and Future Directions." Amsterdam: Excerpta Medica, 1980, pp 284–299.
16. Camitta BM, Quesenberry PJ, Parkman R, Boxer LA, Stossel TP, Cassady JR, Rappeport JM, Nathan DG: Bone marrow transplantation for an infant with neutrophil dysfunction. Exp Hematol 5:109–116, 1977.
17. Kapoor N, Kirkpatrick D, Blaese RM, Oleske J, Hilgartner MH, Chaganti RSK, Good RA, O'Reilly RJ: Reconstitution of normal megakaryocytopoiesis and immunologic functions in Wiskott-Aldrich syndrome by marrow transplantation following myeloablation and immunosup-

pression with busulfan and cyclophosphamide. Blood 57:692–696, 1981.
18. Parkman R, Rappeport J, Geha R, Belli J, Cassady R, Levey R, Nathan DG, Rosen FS: Complete correction of the Wiskott-Aldrich syndrome by allogeneic bone-marrow transplantation. N Engl J Med 298:921–927, 1978.
19. Santos GW, Elfenbein GJ, Tutschka PJ: Bone marrow transplantation—Present status. Transplant Proc 11:182–188, 1979.
20. Gale RP, Ho W, Feig S, Champlin R, Tesler A, Arenson E, Ladish S, Young L, Winston D, Sparkes R, Fitchen J, Territo M, Sarna G, Wong L, Paik Y, Bryson Y, Golde D, Fahey J, Cline M: Prevention of graft rejection following bone marrow transplantation. Blood 57:9–12, 1981.
21. Thomas ED: Marrow transplantation for nonmalignant disorders. (Editorial) N Engl J Med 298:963–964, 1978.

Index

[redacted]